Orthopedic Emergencies

Melvin C. Makhni • Eric C. Makhni
Eric F. Swart • Charles S. Day
Editors

Orthopedic Emergencies

Springer

Editors
Melvin C. Makhni, MD, MBA
Department of Orthopedic Surgery
Columbia Presbyterian Medical Center
New York, NY, USA
orthopedicemergencies@gmail.com

Eric C. Makhni, MD, MBA
Sports Medicine
Department of Orthopedic Surgery
Henry Ford Hospital
Wayne State University
Detroit, MI, USA

Eric F. Swart, MD
Orthopedic Trauma
Department of Orthopedics and Physical Rehabilitation
University of Massachusetts Medical Center
Worcester, MA, USA

Charles S. Day, MD, MBA
Orthopedic Surgery
Harvard Medical School
Boston, MA, USA

ISBN 978-3-319-31522-5 ISBN 978-3-319-31524-9 (eBook)
DOI 10.1007/978-3-319-31524-9

Library of Congress Control Number: 2016935868

Design and Illustrations by Svetlana N. Makhni

Printed on acid-free paper

This Springer imprint is published by Springer Nature
The registered company is Springer International Publishing AG Switzerland

To our Team: the most innovative, driven mentors, colleagues, and friends—a constant source of inspiration and motivation. Thank you for all the hard work and for making these years of work so exciting.

To our Teachers—at Columbia, Shock Trauma, and Harvard, thank you for an outstanding decade of training in the fundamentals of orthopedic surgery, trauma, and medicine. It is an honor to share your insights and teachings with the world.

To our Families—for sharing in this experience, and every experience, and for being the most loving, supportive parents, siblings, and better halves we could imagine. Nothing in our lives would be possible without your love and support.

Contents

Part I Emergency Orthopedic Evaluation
Alex Ha, Navid Behrooz, and Chris Rafie

Initial Trauma Assessment 3

Initial Cervical Spine Management 7

Damage Control Orthopedics 11

Part II True Orthopedic Emergencies
Jamal Shillingford

Compartment Syndrome 15

Open Fracture 17

Septic Joint 21

Traumatic Arthrotomy 23

Necrotizing Fasciitis 25

High-Pressure Injection Injury 27

"Open Book" Pelvis/Hemodynamically Unstable Pelvis Fracture 31

Gunshot Wound 33

Part III Spine
Melvin C. Makhni, Neil Sardesai, Comron Saifi,
K. Daniel Riew, and Steven C. Ludwig

Incomplete Spinal Cord Injury (SCI) 37

Cauda Equina Syndrome 41

Fracture in DISH/AS 45

Atlanto-axial Fractures and Instability 49

Dens Fracture 53

Subaxial (C3-C7) Cervical Spine Fractures 57

Central Cord Syndrome 61

Thoracolumbar Fractures 65

Compression Fracture 71

Spinous Process and Transverse Process Fractures 75

Burst Fracture 79

Chance Fracture 83

Thoracolumbar Fracture-Dislocation 87

Sacral Fracture 91

Vertebral Osteomyelitis 95

Part IV Shoulder and Upper Arm
Manish Noticewala, David Trofa, Robert L. Parisien,
Luke Nicholson, and Eric C. Makhni

Glenohumeral Dislocation 101

Proximal Humerus Fracture 111

Clavicle Fracture 117

Acromioclavicular (AC) Joint Injury 123

Sternoclavicular (SC) Joint Injury 127

Septic Arthritis of the Shoulder 131

Glenoid and Scapula Fracture 133

Humerus Shaft Fracture 137

Distal Humerus Fractures 145

Olecranon Fracture 151

Radial Head Fracture 157

Elbow Dislocation 163

Coronoid Fracture 169

Elbow Capitellar Fracture 173

Radius and Ulna Shaft Fractures 177

Part V Wrist and Hand

Stephanie Gancarzyk, Robert L. Parisien, and Joseph Lombardi

Distal Radius Fracture 183

DRUJ Injury 189

Carpal Fracture (Excluding Scaphoid) 193

Scaphoid Fracture 201

Scapholunate Instability 205

Perilunate Dislocation 209

Tendon Lacerations 215

Finger Fractures and Dislocations 221

Digit Amputations 231

Foreign Bodies in the Hand and Wrist 237

Hand Infections 239

Part VI Pelvis and Lower Extremity

Eric F. Swart and Joseph Laratta

Acetabular Fractures 245

ACL Rupture 251

Distal Femur Fracture 253

Femoral Head Fracture 257

Femoral Shaft Fracture 259

Hip Dislocation (Native) 265

Hip Dislocation (Total Hip Arthroplasty) 269

Impending Fractures 273

Intertrochanteric/Subtrochanteric Fracture 277

Femoral Neck Fracture 283

Knee Dislocation 289

Meniscus Tear 293

Quadriceps or Patellar Tendon Rupture 295

Patella Fractures 299

Patella Dislocation 303

Pelvic Ring Injuries ... 307

Periprosthetic Hip Fracture ... 311

Periprosthetic Knee Femur Fracture ... 315

Tibia-Fibula Shaft Fracture ... 319

Tibial Plateau Fracture ... 325

Part VII Foot and Ankle
Thomas Hickernell and Jon-Michael Caldwell

Achilles Tendon Rupture ... 331

Ankle Fracture ... 335

Calcaneus Fracture ... 347

Proximal Fifth Metatarsal Fracture ... 351

Lisfranc Injury ... 355

Metatarsal Fractures ... 359

Tarsal Navicular Fracture ... 361

Tibial Plafond (Pilon) Fracture ... 365

Talar Neck Fracture ... 371

Lateral Process of Talus Fracture ... 375

Phalanx Fractures of the Foot ... 379

Part VIII Pediatrics
Daniel Miller, Katie Rosenwasser, Anny Hsu, and Jeanne Franzone

Sedation for the Pediatric Patient ... 385

Casting and Immobilization in the Pediatric Patient ... 389

Child Abuse-Non-accidental Trauma (NAT) ... 393

Salter–Harris Classification ... 397

Clavicle Fracture ... 401

Proximal Humerus Fracture ... 405

Humeral Shaft Fracture ... 409

Supracondylar Humerus Fracture (SCHFx) ... 413

Lateral Condyle Fracture 419

Medial Epicondyle Fracture 423

Distal Humerus Physeal Separation 427

Radial Head Subluxation (Nursemaid's Elbow) 431

Radial Neck Fracture 433

Both-Bone Forearm Fracture 437

Distal Radius Fracture 443

Monteggia Fracture 447

Galeazzi Fracture 451

Pelvic Fracture 453

Avulsion Fractures of the Pelvis 457

Hip Pain: Septic Hip vs. Transient Synovitis 461

Hip Dislocation 465

Slipped Capital Femoral Epiphysis 469

Hip Fracture 473

Femur Fracture 477

Distal Femur Physeal Fracture 481

Tibial Eminence Fracture 485

Tibial Tubercle Fracture 489

Toddler's Fracture 493

Ankle Fractures 497

Part IX Emergency Sideline Management of Athletic Conditions
Jeremy Alland and Sonya Makhni

Concussion 505

Heat Illness 507

Exercise-Associated Hyponatremia (EAH) 509

Sudden Cardiac Arrest (SCA) 511

Asthma 513

Frostbite 515

Appendix A: Physical Exams Overview ... 517
Danica Vance and Maggie Wright

Distal Extremity Exam ... 518

Spine Exam ... 519

Shoulder Exam ... 526

Elbow Exam ... 528

Wrist Exam ... 531

Hand Exam ... 536

Hip Exam ... 542

Knee Exam ... 544

Foot and Ankle Exam ... 549

References ... 554

Appendix B: Procedure Guides ... 555
William Giles Stuart Mackenzie

General Principles of Casting and Splinting ... 556

Upper Extremity Immobilization ... 557

Lower Extremity Immobilization ... 572

Reduction Techniques ... 579

Local Anesthesia and Blocks ... 586

Intraarticular Injections and Aspirations ... 589

Saline Load Testing ... 594

Skeletal Traction ... 596

Nailbed Laceration Repair ... 597

Compartment Check with "Stryker Needle" ... 600

Gardner Wells Tongs Traction ... 601

References ... 602

Index ... 605

Contributors

Jeremy Alland Rush Medical College, Chicago, IL, USA

Navid Behrooz Department of Emergency Medicine, New York-Presbyterian, The University Hospital of Columbia, New York, NY, USA

Jon-Michael Caldwell Department of Orthopaedic Surgery, Columbia Presbyterian Medical Center, New York, NY, USA

Jeanne Franzone Department of Orthopaedic Surgery, Columbia Presbyterian Medical Center, New York, NY, USA

Stephanie Gancarzyk Department of Orthopaedic Surgery, Columbia Presbyterian Medical Center, New York, NY, USA

Alex Ha Department of Orthopaedic Surgery, Columbia Presbyterian Medical Center, New York, NY, USA

Thomas Hickernell Department of Orthopaedic Surgery, Columbia Presbyterian Medical Center, New York, NY, USA

Anny Hsu Department of Orthopaedic Surgery, Columbia Presbyterian Medical Center, New York, NY, USA

Joseph Laratta Department of Orthopaedic Surgery, Columbia Presbyterian Medical Center, New York, NY, USA

Joseph Lombardi Department of Orthopaedic Surgery, Columbia Presbyterian Medical Center, New York, NY, USA

William Stuart Mackenzie Department of Orthopaedic Surgery, Columbia Presbyterian Medical Center, New York, NY, USA

Melvin C. Makhni Department of Orthopaedic Surgery, Columbia Presbyterian Medical Center, New York, NY, USA

Eric C. Makhni Department of Orthopaedic Surgery, Henry Ford Hospital, Wayne State University, Detroit, MI, USA

Sonya Makhni Icahn School of Medicine at Mount Sinai, New York, NY, USA

Daniel Miller Department of Orthopaedic Surgery, Columbia Presbyterian Medical Center, New York, NY, USA

Luke Nicholson Tufts University School of Medicine, Boston, MA, USA

Manish Noticewala Department of Orthopaedic Surgery, Columbia Presbyterian Medical Center, New York, NY, USA

Robert L. Parisien Orthopaedic Surgery Resident, Boston University Medical Center, Boston, MA, USA

Christopher Rafie Department of Orthopaedic Surgery, Columbia Presbyterian Medical Center, New York, NY, USA

Katie Rosenwasser Department of Orthopaedic Surgery, Columbia Presbyterian Medical Center, New York, NY, USA

Comron Saifi Department of Orthopedic Surgery, Rush University Medical Center, Chicago, IL, USA

Neil Sardesai Department of Orthopedics, University of Maryland Medical Center, Baltimore, MD, USA

Jamal Shillingford Department of Orthopaedic Surgery, Columbia Presbyterian Medical Center, New York, NY, USA

Eric F. Swart Department of Orthopedics and Physical Rehabilitation, University of Massachusetts Medical Center, Worcester, MA, USA

David Trofa Department of Orthopaedic Surgery, Columbia Presbyterian Medical Center, New York, NY, USA

Danica Vance Department of Orthopaedic Surgery, Columbia Presbyterian Medical Center, New York, NY, USA

Maggie Wright Department of Orthopaedic Surgery, Columbia Presbyterian Medical Center, New York, NY, USA

Introduction

The goal of this book is to be a practical reference for any and all who manage orthopedic conditions in the emergency setting. It is the culmination of years of experience by several orthopedic practitioners in varying stages of their careers. We have purposely tried to make the book a quick, handy reference rather than a comprehensive text or manual on orthopedic trauma. Therefore, we included the most pertinent and important factors to consider when evaluating and managing these patients.

We understand that many of you all may have your own tips, tricks, and insights into managing orthopedic emergencies, and we always welcome your thoughts, comments, criticisms, or suggestions. Therefore, if you have any additional thoughts or images that you would like to share with us for consideration for inclusion in future editions, please email us at orthopedicemergencies@gmail.com.

Thank you again for your support and all the best.

Melvin C. Makhni
Eric C. Makhni
Eric F. Swart
Charles S. Day

Part I
Emergency Orthopedic Evaluation

Alex Ha, Navid Behrooz, and Chris Rafie

Initial Trauma Assessment 3

Initial Cervical Spine Management 7

Damage Control Orthopedics 11

Initial Trauma Assessment

Initial management of trauma begins with the primary survey before orthopedic intervention is performed.

Primary Survey

A. Airway maintenance with C-spine stabilization
B. Breathing and ventilation, listening for breath sounds bilaterally
C. Circulation, and hemorrhage control
D. Disability, with assessment of neurological status (Glasgow Coma Scale, and motor and sensory function)
E. Exposure/environment—undress patient to further evaluate trauma, but avoid hypothermia

Secondary Survey

History
   Complete Physical Exam

Positioning/Log Rolling

- Pregnant women into left lateral decubitus to prevent blockage of inflow to heart and subsequent hypotension
- Spinal immobilization after trauma requires log rolling onto a rigid long board

M.C. Makhni et al. (eds.), *Orthopedic Emergencies*,
DOI 10.1007/978-3-319-31524-9_1

- Prevents secondary injury, alleviate possible cord compression, and establish spinal stability
- Do not manipulate any patients with kyphosis or scoliosis while on a backboard
- Paralyzed patient on the rigid board for more than a few hours can be at risk for developing pressure ulcers

Minimum of four people is required for log rolling

Member A—At the patient's head; responsible for maintaining manual inline stabilization of the head and cervical spine; orchestrates the other three members

Members B and C—Adjacent to each other along the same side of the patient to maintain a neutral anatomic alignment of the entire vertebral column while log rolling

Member D—Responsible for positioning the spine board; also palpates the spinous processes and paraspinal muscles throughout the vertebral column to assess for step-offs and points of tenderness

Initial Imaging

XR: AP chest, AP pelvis, and lateral cervical spine
CT: c-spine/chest/abdomen/pelvis is part of the initial protocol at some institutions

Intubation

- Airway managed with intubation for obtunded patients or those in severe pain
- Neck manipulation may potentially displace unstable cervical spine
- If there is high suspicion for cervical spine trauma, consider cricothyroidotomy

FAST Exam

- Focused assessment of abdomen with sonography for trauma
- Allows detection of free fluid at the perihepatic space, perisplenic space, pericardium, and the pelvis

Pelvic Sheet/Binder

- Place sheet underneath patient at level of greater trochanter
- For a sheet, tightening requires three people: one on each side to pull, and one person to clamp at top and bottom levels of sheet. Sheet should be folded so it's no more than about 20 cm wide
- Once tightened/clamped, the abdomen should still be exposed (to allow general surgery access for possible laparotomy if needed). Holes can be cut as needed for windows if needed by vascular surgery for access

Pelvic binders are applied in a similar manner with the same principles, but the exact steps are specific to the binder type.

Initial Cervical Spine Management

All trauma patients are assumed to have cervical spine injury until proven otherwise. Have a high index of suspicion for c-spine pathology especially in obtunded and polytrauma patients

Imaging

Immediate lateral c-spine XR
Complete XR series of c-spine (as well as other affected regions)
C-spine CT commonly obtained immediately for diagnosis and surgical planning
C-spine MRI indicated for suspected spinal cord injury or to further evaluate cervical spine ligamentous integrity

C-Spine Clearance

Asymptomatic

Clearance possible by physical exam alone if:

- Alert with no evidence of intoxication or distracting injuries
- Negative physical exam
  - Complete neurological exam (see Appendix A)
  - Palpation for midline spinal tenderness
  - ROM 45° rotation

M.C. Makhni et al. (eds.), *Orthopedic Emergencies*,
DOI 10.1007/978-3-319-31524-9_2

Symptomatic

XR c-spine: AP, lateral, odontoid

If need of swimmer's/oblique views, obtain CT instead
Flexion-extension views not usually performed acutely in ED

Low threshold to obtain CT c-spine (especially if need additional CT imaging)
MRI if neurologic deficit or concern for spinal cord or ligamentous injury

Not examinable (intoxicated, concurrent distracting injuries, or obtunded)

Cervical immobilization until able to clear c-spine clinically (if temporarily non-examinable) or radiographically (if obtunded)
Serial re-evaluations
CT (especially if urgency or if not expected to be imminently examinable)
Consider MRI in addition to CT

Types of Cervical Collars (Fig. 1)

Miami-J Collar—Rigid collar w/greatest cervical ROM restriction in all planes
Aspen Collar—Rigid collar with similar ROM as Philadelphia Collar
Philadelphia Collar—Rigid collar w/similar cervical ROM as Aspen Collar
Soft Collar—Flexible, but higher risk of further cervical spine damage

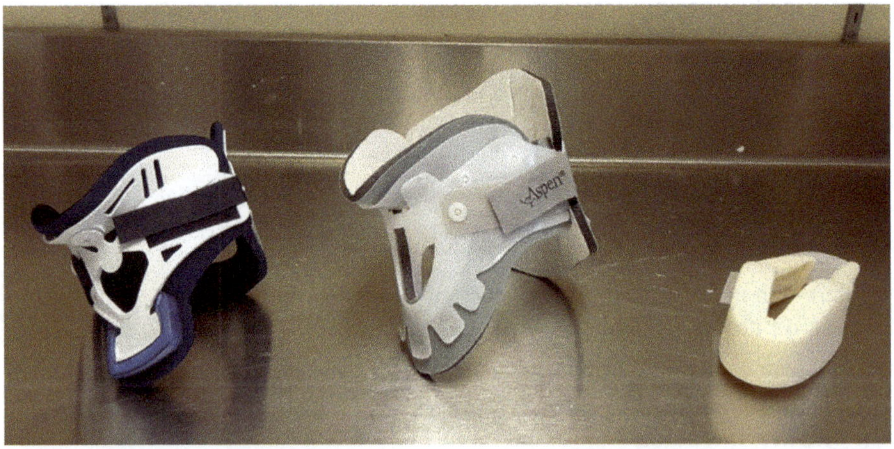

Fig. 1 Cervical collars (from *left* to *right*, Miami-J, Aspen, Soft Collar)

References

Anderson PA, Lindsey RW, Schoenfeld AJ, Harris MB, Guagala Z. Clearing the Cervical Spine in the Blunt Trauma Patient. J Am Acad Orthop Surg. 2010;18(3):149–59.

Bransford RJ, Alton TB, Patel AR, Bellabarba C. Upper cervical spine trauma. J Am Acad Orthop Surg. 2014 Nov;22(11):718–29. doi:10.5435/JAAOS-22-11-718.

Mosenkis, Robert. CITECH Test Report,Citech #: 490–421, February 28, 2001.

Tescher, AN, Rindflesch AB, Youdas JW, Jacobson TM, Downer LL, Miers AG et al. Range-of-motion restriction and craniofacial tissue-interface pressure from four cervical collars. J Trauma 2007;63(5):1120–26.

Damage Control Orthopedics

The initial treatment decisions for borderline or unstable polytrauma patients hinges on their physiologic state. The benefits and risks of early vs. delayed surgical intervention are weighed when deciding initial treatment strategy in these patients.

- Timing for definitive fracture fixation especially in polytrauma patients controversial
- Delayed definitive fixation in borderline or unstable polytrauma patients
  - Can avoid “second-hit” to body and decrease chance of developing acute respiratory distress syndrome, multisystem failure, or death
  - However, delay in definitive treatment associated with inferior outcomes in otherwise stable patients
- DCO involves temporary stabilization with plan for delayed definitive treatment
  - Physiologic and metabolic management
  - Pelvic binder/sheet
  - Skeletal traction
  - External fixation
- End-organ hypoperfusion is assessed with multiple markers
  - Lactate level >2.5 mmol/L (best marker for end-organ hypoperfusion)
  - Urine output less than 30 cc/h
  - MAP >60
  - HR <100
  - Base deficit outside the normal range of −2 to 2
- Careful monitoring of patients with multiple of the following parameters:
  - SBP <90 mmHg
  - Platelets <70,000
  - Temperature <35 °C
  - Significant soft tissue damage

M.C. Makhni et al. (eds.), *Orthopedic Emergencies*,
DOI 10.1007/978-3-319-31524-9_3

Other indications for DCO

Hemodynamic instability with associated trauma to pelvis/abdomen
Pulmonary contusions/respiratory distress
Bilateral femur fractures
Polytrauma with significant head injury
Increased injury severity score

References

Andersen LW, Mackenhauer J, Roberts JC, Berg KM, Cocchi MN, Donnino MW. Etiology and therapeutic approach to elevated lactate levels. Mayo Clinic Proc Mayo Clinic. 2013;88(10):1127–40.

Pape HC, Giannoudis PV, Krettek C, Trentz O. Timing of fixation of major fractures in blunt polytrauma: role of conventional indicators in clinical decision making. J Orthop Trauma. 2005;19(8):551–62.

Pape HC, Tornetta 3rd P, Tarkin I, Tzioupis C, Sabeson V, Olson SA. Timing of fracture fixation in multitrauma patients: the role of early total care and damage control surgery. J Am Acad Orthop Surg. 2009;17:541–9.

Part II
True Orthopedic Emergencies

Jamal Shillingford

Compartment Syndrome 15
Open Fracture 17
Septic Joint 21
Traumatic Arthrotomy 23
Necrotizing Fasciitis 25
High-Pressure Injection Injury 27
"Open Book" Pelvis/Hemodynamically Unstable Pelvis Fracture 31
Gunshot Wound 33

Compartment Syndrome

What It Is

- Elevated fascial compartment pressures leading to decreased blood flow within the compartment.

Why It's an Emergency

- Decreased blood flow can lead to irreversible ischemic injury with resultant nerve and muscle damage.

How "Emergent" Is It?

- **Truly emergent. Irreversible changes occur in muscles and nerves within 4–8 h.**

When to Be Suspicious

- The key to treatment is early recognition and compartment fasciotomies of the affected limb.
- Increasing pain requirements after an acute injury, usually in the 24–48-h window.
- Sensory changes (paresthesias) and vascular changes (decreased pulses) are usually late findings.

M.C. Makhni et al. (eds.), *Orthopedic Emergencies*,
DOI 10.1007/978-3-319-31524-9_4

How to Diagnose

- Compartment syndrome is primarily a clinical diagnosis
- Historical hallmarks: pain, pallor, paresthesias, pulselessness, paralysis
- Swelling with firmness
- Pain out of proportion to injury and exam *IMPORTANT*
  - Earliest and most sensitive finding
  - Difficult to assess in sedated, polytrauma, child patients, or patient with significant nerve damage
  - Pain with passive stretch of the muscles within the compartment
  - Increasing narcotic requirement
- Stryker needle pressure measurement when exam findings are equivocal or inconclusive or patient is obtunded (polytrauma or sedated)
  - Absolute pressure above 30 mmHg concerning
  - "Delta P" = difference between diastolic pressure and compartment pressure less than 30 mmHg also concerning

How to Treat

- Definitive treatment is emergent fasciotomy/compartment release

References

Hammerberg EM, Whitesides Jr TE, Seiler 3rd JG. The reliability of measurement of tissue pressure in compartment syndrome. J Orthop Trauma. 2012;26(1):24–31.

McQueen MM, Court-Brown CM. Compartment monitoring in tibial fractures. The pressure threshold for decompression. J Bone Joint Surg Br. 1996;78(1):99–104.

Olson SA, Glasgow RR. Acute compartment syndrome in lower extremity musculoskeletal trauma. J Am Acad Orthop Surg. 2005;13(7):436–44.

Open Fracture

What It Is

- A fracture where the bone has violated the soft-tissue envelope and broken through the skin
- Beware of threatened skin (e.g.: in tongue-type calcaneus fracture or ankle fracture dislocation), which could convert into open fracture

Why It's an Emergency

- Since the skin has been violated, there is a much higher risk for infection following fracture treatment.
- Additionally, it usually requires higher energy for the bone to break the skin (compared to a closed fracture of the same area), so there are often multiple other soft-tissue injuries involved.

How "Emergent" Is It?

- **Urgent.** Although historically the treatment goal has been operative I+D within 6 h, recent literature has questioned if this truly affects infection rates or outcomes.
- General consensus is currently:
  - **Immediate/emergent IV antibiotics** (as soon as possible)
  - Urgent operative debridement (but not necessarily emergently)
  - For underequipped/non-trauma centers, time to transfer to an appropriate level 1 facility has also been shown to correlate with outcomes

M.C. Makhni et al. (eds.), *Orthopedic Emergencies*,
DOI 10.1007/978-3-319-31524-9_5

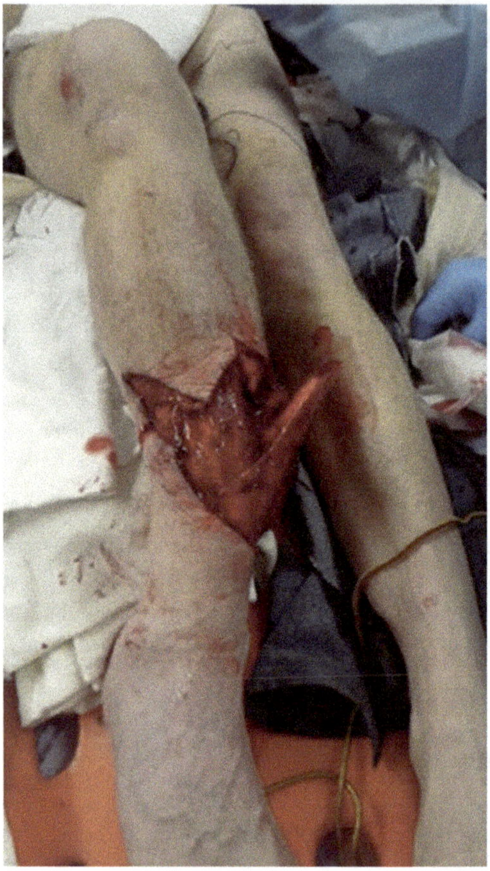

Open fracture of tibia and fibula

When to be Suspicious

- **Any violation of the skin within the zone of injury around the fracture should be considered an open fracture until proven otherwise.**
- Checking for "veinous oozing" out of laceration, or probing laceration, may provide information but these are not sensitive enough to be definitively diagnostic.

How to Diagnose

- Diagnosis is clinical—any break in skin around a fracture is presumed to be an open fracture. No gold standard for diagnosis other than exploration in OR accompanied by I+D.

How to Treat

- Immediate antibiotics:
  - First-generation cephalosporin for all open fractures
  - Consider adding aminoglycoside for Gustilo/Anderson grade 3
  - Consider adding penicillin for farm injuries or possible bowel contamination
- Tetanus prophylaxis
- Immediate removal of gross contamination in ED (although no formal ED I+D)
- Coverage of wound with saline or betadine gauze—minimize exposures of wound after initial evaluation
- Definitive treatment is thorough irrigation and debridement in OR

References

Hauser CJ, Adams Jr CA, Eachempati SR, Council of the Surgical Infection Society. Surgical Infection Society guideline: prophylactic antibiotic use in open fractures: an evidence-based guideline. Surg Infect (Larchmt). 2006;7(4):379–405.

Saveli CC, Belknap RW, Morgan SJ, Price CS. The role of prophylactic antibiotics in open fractures in an era of community-acquired methicillin-resistant Staphylococcus aureus. Orthopedics. 2011;34(8):611–6. doi:10.3928/01477447-20110627-25. quiz 617.

Zalavras CG, Patzakis MJ. Open fractures: evaluation and management. J Am Acad Orthop Surg. 2003;11(3):212–9.

Septic Joint

What It Is

- Bacterial infection of a synovial joint

Why It's an Emergency

- The combination of the bacteria and inflammatory response ("pus under pressure") can cause rapid erosion of the cartilage with irreversible joint destruction.
- Occasionally, an infected joint can be a bacterial source in a septic patient, and treatment of the sepsis requires timely source control.

How "Emergent" Is It?

- **Usually emergent**—The longer diagnosis and treatment are delayed, the more damage to the joint occurs, sometimes on the order of hours.

When to Be Suspicious

- Classic presentation is a painful effusion or a new effusion in a patient who has known bacteremia.

M.C. Makhni et al. (eds.), *Orthopedic Emergencies*,
DOI 10.1007/978-3-319-31524-9_6

How to Diagnose

- Initial diagnosis is from clinical exam, which usually includes an effusion and pain with joint passive micromotion, although these are not always present.
- Serum inflammatory markers (CBC with differential, ESR, CRP) should also be part of initial work-up - unreliable in immunosuppressed patients.
- In the pediatric population, the "Kocher Criteria" determine the risk of hip infection. If >3 of these are present, 90 % chance of septic joint.
    - Inability to bear weight
    - Temperature >101.3 °F
    - WBC >12 k
    - ESR >40 mm/h
    - CRP >2.0 mg/dL
- Definitive diagnosis is from arthrocentesis (see joint aspiration techniques in "Appendix B").
    - Stat WBC count + PMN % should be available within hours. Under 30 k makes septic joint very unlikely. Over 50 k makes it more likely
        - Fluid should also be sent for crystal examination to eval for crystalline arthropathy as well, although he presence of crystals doesn't definitively rule out infection
    - Culture from aspirate usually not back within 2 days, so less important for immediate emergent decision making

How to Treat

- Treatment of septic joint is surgical irrigation and debridement (either open or arthroscopic) + broad-spectrum IV antibiotics until cultures and sensitivities back.

References

Kocher MS, Mandiga R, Murphy JM, Goldmann D, Harper M, Sundel R, et al. A clinical practice guideline for treatment of septic arthritis in children: efficacy in improving process of care and effect on outcome of septic arthritis of the hip. J Bone Joint Surg Am. 2003;85-A(6):994–9.

Margaretten ME, Kohlwes J, Moore D, Bent S. Does this adult patient have septic arthritis? JAMA. 2007;297(13):1478–88.

Shah K, Spear J, Nathanson LA, McCauley J, Edlow JA. Does the presence of crystal arthritis rule out septic arthritis? J Emerg Med. 2007;32(1):23–6.

Traumatic Arthrotomy

What It Is

- A deep traumatic laceration that extends through the joint capsule

Why It's an Emergency

- A laceration into the joint exposes the normally sterile intra-articular contents to external contamination, and can imminently become a septic arthritis.

How "Emergent" Is It?

- **Urgent**. Diagnosis must be made in a timely manner and should be taken to the OR expeditiously, although not truly emergent if antibiotics have been started.

When to Be Suspicious

- Any penetrating trauma around a joint should be evaluated for potential traumatic arthrotomy.

M.C. Makhni et al. (eds.), *Orthopedic Emergencies*,
DOI 10.1007/978-3-319-31524-9_7

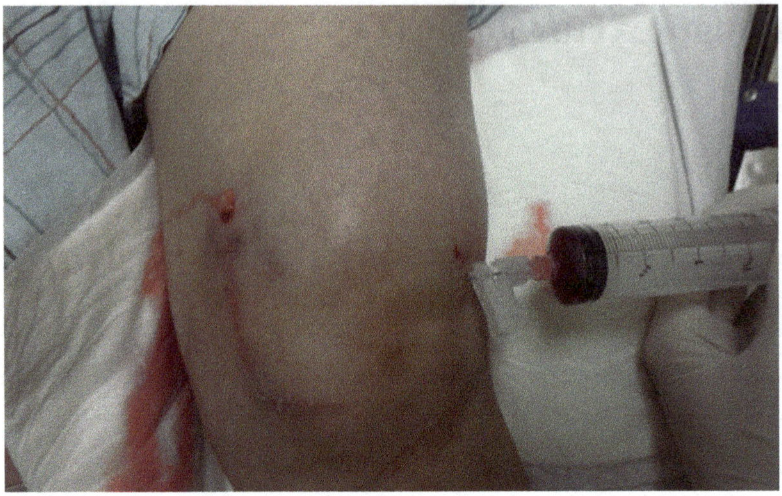

Fig. 1 Positive saline load test

How to Diagnose

- Physical exam of wound and probing may be enough to confirm intra-articular involvement. However, when unclear, the saline load test is considered the best diagnostic test (Appendix B: Saline load of knee technique). In this test, arthrocentesis of the joint in question is performed, preferably with a portal away from the area of injury, and with a large-bore needle (at least 18G) sterile saline is injected into the joint while the laceration site is watched for saline extravasation. Sometimes over 150ccs is required for larger joints with more distensible capsules (e.g., the knee) (Fig. 1).
- CT scan of knee can detect intra-articular air, indicating traumatic arthrotomy.

How to Treat

- Treatment is immediate IV antibiotics (typically a first-generation cephalosporin) and urgent operative irrigation and debridement of the laceration and arthrotomy with joint irrigation, and possible synovectomy.

References

Metzger P, Carney J, Kuhn K, Booher K, Mazurek M. Sensitivity of the saline load test with and without methylene blue dye in the diagnosis of artificial traumatic knee arthrotomies. J Orthop Trauma. 2012;26(6):347–9.

Konda SR, Davidovitch RI, Egol KA. Computed tomography scan to detect traumatic arthrotomies and identify periarticular wounds not requiring surgical intervention: an improvement over the saline load test. J Orthop Trauma. 2013;27(9):498–504.

Necrotizing Fasciitis

What It Is

- Polymicrobial soft-tissue infection that travels rapidly along fascial planes - can be both limb and life threatening.

Why It's an Emergency

- This is an extremely rapidly progressive infection that can spread on the order of hours.

How "Emergent" Is It?

- **Emergent**. Untreated it can progress to limb-threatening or life-threatening extent within hours.

When to Be Suspicious

- Rapidly progressive soft-tissue infection
  - Often minimal erythema (infection spreads faster than immune system can respond with inflammation)
  - "Dirty dishwater" drainage
  - Subcutaneous crepitus

M.C. Makhni et al. (eds.), *Orthopedic Emergencies*,
DOI 10.1007/978-3-319-31524-9_8

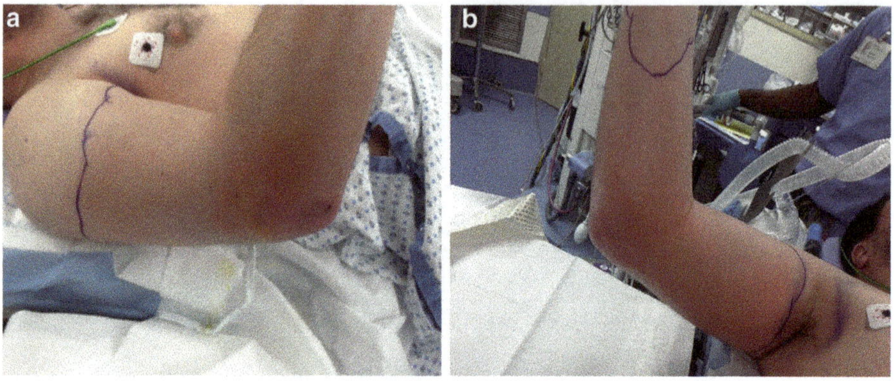

Fig. 1 Necrotizing fasciitis around the elbow

How to Diagnose

- Clinical diagnosis—no lab or imaging work-up definitive
- Emergent frozen section in OR can be confirm diagnosis, but shouldn't delay treatment (Fig. 1)

How to Treat

- Emergent fasciotomy/radical debridement and I+D, often requiring wide margins of soft-tissue excision
  - Broad-spectrum antibiotics after I+D
- Consider amputation when infection is life threatening

References

Bellapianta JM, Ljungquist K, Tobin E, Uhl R. Necrotizing fasciitis. J Am Acad Orthop Surg. 2009;17(3):174–82.

Ozalay M, Ozkoc G, Akpinar S, Hersekli MA, Tandogan RN. Necrotizing soft-tissue infection of a limb: clinical presentation and factors related to mortality. Foot Ankle Int. 2006;27(8):598–605.

High-Pressure Injection Injury

What It Is

- A soft-tissue injury (usually around the hands) caused by high-pressure injection devices

Why It's an Emergency

- Despite the often benign appearance of the injury (Fig. 1), the soft-tissue damage beneath the skin is often extensive (Fig. 2). Additionally, the material injected is often toxic/damaging to tissues as well, and can continue to cause damage after injection.

How "Emergent" Is It?

- **Emergent**—Time to operative debridement is one of the major determinants of outcome after these injuries, and should be done as quickly as possible.

When to Be Suspicious

- Any patient with a punctate wound from a possible pressure injection. History taking is critical in these patients, and a detailed report of exactly how the injury occurred and what device caused it is imperative.

M.C. Makhni et al. (eds.), *Orthopedic Emergencies*,
DOI 10.1007/978-3-319-31524-9_9

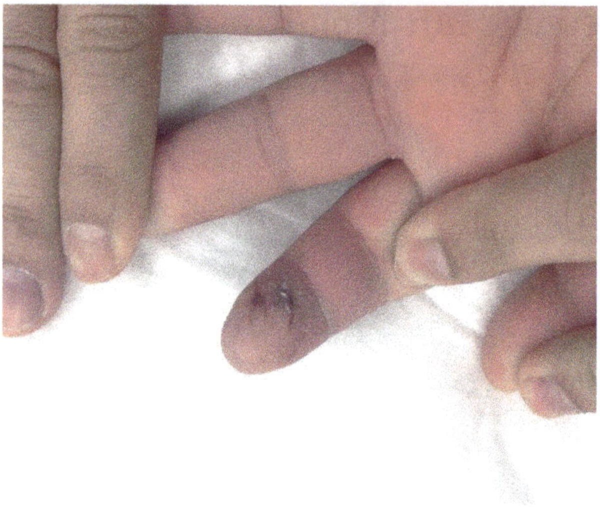

Fig. 1 Clinical appearance of injection injury

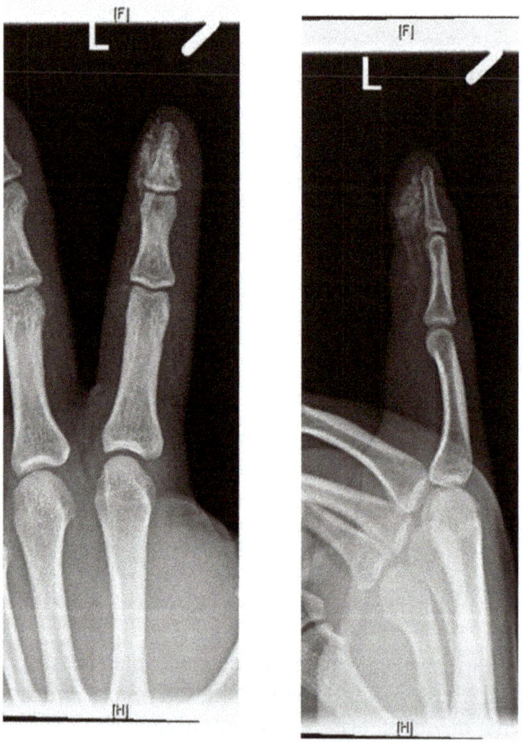

Fig. 2 Radiographic appearance of injection injury

How to Diagnose

- Diagnosis is exclusively off history, since physical exam is often initially benign.

How to Treat

- Treatment is emergent operative irrigation and debridement, removal of foreign material, and initiation of broad-spectrum antibiotics.

References

Amsdell SL, Hammert WC. High-pressure injection injuries in the hand: current treatment concepts. Plast Reconstr Surg. 2013;132(4):586e–91. doi:10.1097/PRS.0b013e31829f4bb4.

Bekler H, Gokce A, Beyzadeoglu T, Parmaksizoglu F. The surgical treatment and outcomes of high-pressure injection injuries of the hand. J Hand Surg Eur Vol. 2007;32(4):394–9. Epub 2007 Mar 30.

“Open Book” Pelvis/Hemodynamically Unstable Pelvis Fracture

What It Is

- “Open book” pelvis refers to a pelvic ring injury where the entire pelvis becomes unstable. Multiple arteries and veins course along the inside of the pelvis and can cause significant bleeding.

  (Open Book Pelvis)

Why It’s an Emergency

- Until the pelvis is stabilized, the intra-pelvic bleeding can continue, which makes this a life-threatening emergency.

How “Emergent” Is It?

- **Truly emergent.** This is life threatening and complications can occur on the order of minutes.

When to Be Suspicious

- High-energy trauma patients with persistent hemodynamic instability

M.C. Makhni et al. (eds.), *Orthopedic Emergencies*,
DOI 10.1007/978-3-319-31524-9_10

How to Diagnose

- Part of the secondary survey of ATLS protocol should involve checking pelvic stability on exam.
- Additionally, basic ATLS protocol should also include an AP pelvis X-ray.

How to Treat

- Initial treatment is immediate placement of pelvic binder or wrapping with pelvic sheet (see section "Pelvic Sheet/Binder application," in chapter "Initial Trauma Assessment"), which usually provisionally stabilizes the pelvis enough to initiate further work-up.
- Secondary treatment may involve some combination of angiography/embolization by interventional radiology, open pelvic packing by general surgery, and/or emergent operative pelvic stabilization (external fixation +/− posterior SI fixation).

References

Croce MA, Magnotti LJ, Savage SA, Wood 2nd GW, Fabian TC. Emergent pelvic fixation in patients with exsanguinating pelvic fractures. J Am Coll Surg. 2007;204(5):935–9.

Krieg JC, Mohr M, Ellis TJ, Simpson TS, Madey SM, Bottlang M. Emergent stabilization of pelvic ring injuries by controlled circumferential compression: a clinical trial. J Trauma. 2005;59(3):659–64.

Manson TT, Nascone JW, Sciadini MF, O'Toole RV. Does fracture pattern predict death with lateral compression type 1 pelvic fractures? J Trauma. 2010;69(4):876–9.

Gunshot Wound

What It Is

- Penetrating ballistic injuries that can cause fractures or soft-tissue damage (Fig. 1)

Why It's an Emergency

- The bullet/shot injury can cause damage to neurovascular structures or cause unstable fractures.

How "Emergent" Is It?

- **Mixed**. The urgency of treatment is a function of the underlying soft-tissue/bony injury, rather than the presence of a gunshot wound itself.

When to Be Suspicious

- Based on both history and physical exam. Gunshot wounds are usually clinically apparent, provided that a thorough secondary survey has been performed and all skin exposed.

M.C. Makhni et al. (eds.), *Orthopedic Emergencies*,
DOI 10.1007/978-3-319-31524-9_11

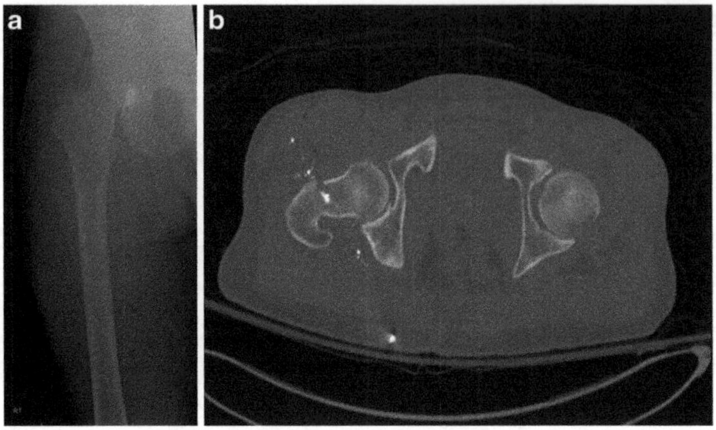

Fig. 1 Radiograph (**a**) and CT scan (**b**) of a gunshot wound involving the femoral neck

How to Diagnose

- Clinically diagnosed by thorough secondary survey.

How to Treat

- Low-velocity wounds are treated as if they were closed fractures despite the skin injuries:
  - Tetanus, oral antibiotics, local wound care
- High-velocity wounds may require I+D if soft-tissue envelope is severely damaged/compromised.

References

Bartlett CS, Helfet DL, Hausman MR, Strauss E. Ballistics and gunshot wounds: effects on musculoskeletal tissues. J Am Acad Orthop Surg. 2000;8(1):21–36.

Geissler WB, Teasedall RD, Tomasin JD, Hughes JL. Management of low velocity gunshot-induced fractures. J Orthop Trauma. 1990;4:39–41.

Part III
Spine

Melvin C. Makhni, Neil Sardesai, Comron Saifi, K. Daniel Riew, and Steven C. Ludwig

Incomplete Spinal Cord Injury (SCI) 37
Cauda Equina Syndrome 41
Fracture in DISH/AS 45
Atlanto-axial Fractures and Instability 49
Dens Fracture 53
Subaxial (C3-C7) Cervical Spine Fractures 57
Central Cord Syndrome 61
Thoracolumbar Fractures 65
Compression Fracture 71
Spinous Process and Transverse Process Fractures 75
Burst Fracture 79
Chance Fracture 83
Thoracolumbar Fracture-Dislocation 87
Sacral Fracture 91
Vertebral Osteomyelitis 95

Incomplete Spinal Cord Injury (SCI)

Spinal cord injury with sparing of sensorimotor function below the level of injury including perirectal sensation. The prognosis and functional outcomes are significantly better for incomplete vs. complete SCIs, and should be managed urgently for optimal chance of neurologic recovery.

History

Do you have any extremity weakness, loss of sensation, and/or paresthesias?
Are you having back pain?
Do you have a history of spinal disorders?

Physical Exam

- Maintain cervical spine in stable position
- Inspect and palpate posterior spine
- Assess for tenderness palpation or step-off deformity
- Trauma Evaluation (Appendix A)
- Complete Neurologic Evaluation (Appendix A)
  - Full neurological exam including cranial nerves, bulbocavernosus reflex, Babinski reflex, voluntary anal contraction, bladder sphincter, triceps/biceps/ankle/patellar reflexes, strength, and sensation (light touch and pinprick)
  - Bulbocavernosus reflex
    - Squeeze glans penis/pressure on clitoris/pull foley
    - Resultant anal sphincter contraction if reflex intact

M.C. Makhni et al. (eds.), *Orthopedic Emergencies*,
DOI 10.1007/978-3-319-31524-9_12

    - Must have bulbocavernosus reflex to indicate end of spinal shock
    - Cannot determine incomplete vs. complete SCI until this reflex returns
  - Sacral neural exam
    - Sacral sparing (sensory, or sensory/motor) signifies incomplete spinal cord injury *IMPORTANT*
      - perianal sensation
      - anal sphincter contraction
      - FHL motor function
  - Palpable/visible muscle contraction below injury level
  - Rectal exam—perianal sensation and sphincter tone

Diagnosis

Imaging

- XR in obtunded patient or patient w/pain, tenderness, and/or neurological symptoms
- MRI in obtunded or unreliable patient
- CT or MRI for patient with ankylosing spondylitis or diffuse idiopathic skeletal hyperostosis

Classification

Neurologic level: Lowest level with intact neurologic function

Clinical Classification

- 1: Central cord syndrome (most common) (see Chapter "Central Cord Syndrome")
- 2: Posterior cord syndrome (rare)
  - Loss of proprioception but preserved motor, light touch, and pain sensation
- 3: Brown-Sequard syndrome (best prognosis)
  - Secondary to complete cord hemi-transection from penetrating trauma
  - Ipsilateral motor, proprioception, and vibratory sensation deficits below the level of the injury. Contralateral pain and temperature deficit below the lesion

- 4: Anterior cord syndrome (worst prognosis)
  - Anterior spinal cord injury secondary to direct compression or injury to the anterior spinal artery that supplies the anterior 2/3 of the cord
  - Lower extremities affected more than upper extremities
  - Loss of motor, pain, and temperature sensation. Preserved proprioception/vibratory sensation

ASIA Impairment Scale

- A (Complete): No sensorimotor function in S4–S5
- B (**Incomplete**): Preserved sensation. No motor function below neurological level (sacral sensory sparing)
- C (**Incomplete**): Muscle function preserved but more than half of key muscles with strength ≤ 3 below the involved neurological level
- D (**Incomplete**): Muscle function preserved and more than half of key muscles with strength ≥ 3 below the involved neurological level
- E (Normal): Normal sensorimotor function

Treatment Plan

Initial Management

- ICU admission
- Immobilization
  - Externally immobilize (cervical orthosis, lateral support, tape across forehead, body straps, secure to backboard in adult) and protect spine especially during transport
  - Log rolling to prevent further injury
  - Use recessed head backboard for pediatric patient to avoid neck flexion in child
- Limit fluids in spinal shock
- Cardiac monitoring for bradycardia
- GI: NGT/bowel regimen for ileus ppx, H2 blocker for PUD ppx (especially if given steroids)
- Consider steroid protocol (within 8 h)
  - Methylprednisolone bolus of 30 mg/kg body weight
  - Infusion at 5.4 mg/kg/h for 23 h if ≤3 h, and 48 h if between 3 and 8 h
  - Do not give to patient >8 h from injury, GSW, pregnant, <13 years old, high risk for systemic infection, receiving steroids for other reasons, or for cauda equina syndrome

Surgery

- Emergent surgical decompression ± stabilization in patients with acute progressive neurological deficits the setting of cord compression may improve chance for recovery

References

Schouten R, Albert T, Kwon BK. The spine-injured patient: initial assessment and emergency treatment. J Am Acad Orthop Surg. 2012;20:336–46.

Gupta R, Bathen ME, Smith JS, Levi AD, Bhatia NN, Steward O. Advances in the management of spinal cord injury. J Am Acad Orthop Surg. 2010;18:210–22.

Cauda Equina Syndrome

Condition associated with compression of the nerve roots in the lumbosacral spine characterized by progressive low back pain, sciatica, lower extremity sensorimotor loss, and bowel and bladder dysfunction.

Overview

- Lesions involving the cauda equine are lower motor neuron lesions—patients may demonstrate varying degrees of lower extremity muscle weakness and sensory disturbance as well as decreased or absent reflexes.
- Can be caused by compression due to tumor, trauma, disc herniation, epidural hematoma or abscess, spinal surgical implants, etc.
- Neurogenic bladder dysfunction is an essential element of cauda equine syndrome. Dysfunction can be divided into two categories (retention and incontinence). The injury to lower motor neurons causes disruptions to reflex arcs that control bladder function. Loss of sensation of fullness and the inability to contract lead to retention and overflow incontinence.

History

- Do you have a history of cancer or risk factors for cancer?
- Did you have any trauma?
- Have you had fevers, chills, or recent weight loss?
- Do you have bowel/bladder dysfunction?
- Do you have saddle anesthesia or any other motor/sensory deficits?
- When did the symptoms begin?

M.C. Makhni et al. (eds.), *Orthopedic Emergencies*,
DOI 10.1007/978-3-319-31524-9_13

Physical Exam

- Trauma evaluation (Appendix A)
- Complete neurologic evaluation (Appendix A)
- Rectal examination for decreased tone, perianal sensation
- Neurogenic bladder dysfunction
- Post-void residual - can indicate urinary retention
- Bulbocavernosus reflex

Diagnosis

Imaging

Diagnostic imaging should be obtained in an expedient manner; however, when the diagnosis is strongly suspected and diagnostic tests are not available it may be appropriate to recommend transfer of patient to a facility that can obtain advanced imaging studies.

XR entire spine
MRI—allows for visualization of space-occupying lesions as well as other potential causes of compression of neural structures.
CT myelography—for patient unable to undergo MRI.

Treatment

Non-operative treatment reserved for medically unstable
Otherwise, surgical decompression of offending lesion (tumor, disc, abscess, etc.)
Timing of surgery

Once a diagnosis is made and advanced imaging studies performed and reviewed, should proceed to surgery
Discordance in literature for benefits of early versus delayed

Historical "48-h" window
RCT showing improved outcomes of surgery (<24 h) versus 48 h

References

Daniels EW, Gordon Z, French K, Ahn UM, Ahn NU. Review of medicolegal cases for cauda equina syndrome: what factors lead to an adverse outcome for the provider? Orthopedics. 2012;35(3):414–419.

Fehlings MG, Vaccaro A, Wilson JR, Singh A, W. Cadotte D, Harrop JS, et al. Early versus delayed decompression for traumatic cervical spinal cord injury: results of the Surgical Timing in Acute Spinal Cord Injury Study (STASCIS). PLoS One. 2012;7(2):1–8.

Spector LR, Madigan L, Rhyne A, Darden B 2nd, Kim D. Cauda equina syndrome. J Am Acad Orthop Surg. 2008;16:471–9.

Fracture in DISH/AS

A fracture in a patient with diffuse idiopathic skeletal hyperostosis (DISH) or ankylosing spondylitis (AS) must be monitored and managed aggressively. These fractures have high risk of immediate/delayed neurologic deterioration, as well as high mortality rate.

Overview

- AS: bamboo spine with diffuse ankylosis and ossification of ligaments, joints, and discs (Fig. 1)
- DISH: anterolateral ossification between 4+ successive vertebrae (Fig. 2)
- Most often in cervical spine and due to hyperextension
- 20 % 3-month mortality after trauma
- ⅔ fractures from low-energy trauma
- >50 % present with neurologic compromise (especially AS)
- 14 % have delayed neurologic deterioration
- 17 % diagnosed >24 h after injury
    - Half due to delay in seeking care, half from delay in MD diagnosis
    - 81 % who had diagnostic delay experienced neurologic compromise
- Usually fracture through vertebral body (especially with DISH), although can fracture through disc
- Fractures often unstable since surrounding ligaments and tissues fracture as well (Figs. 1 and 2)

M.C. Makhni et al. (eds.), *Orthopedic Emergencies*,
DOI 10.1007/978-3-319-31524-9_14

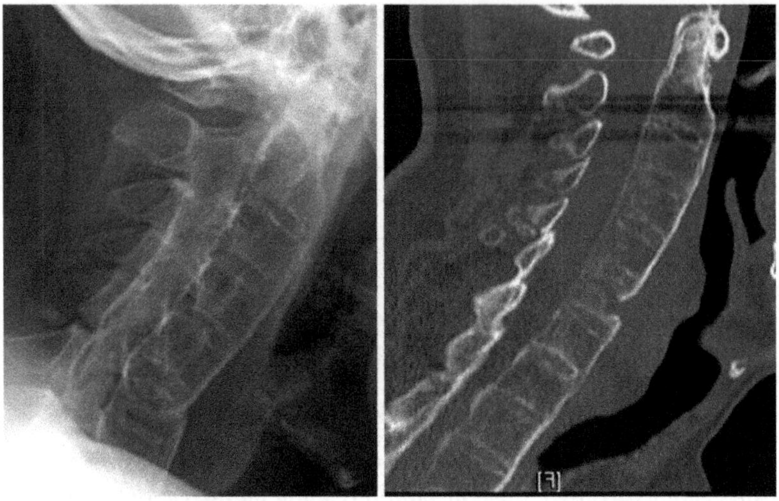

Fig. 1 AS—fracture through C6 body into C5–6 posterior elements

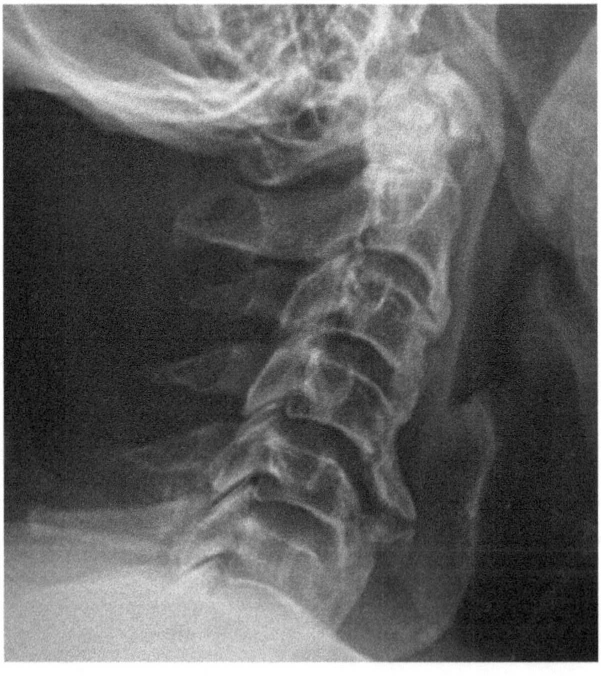

Fig. 2 DISH

History

- Do you have any weakness, numbness, or tingling?

Physical Exam

- Trauma evaluation (Appendix A)
- Serial complete neurologic exams (Appendix A)

Imaging

- C-spine XRs—AP, lateral
- C-spine CT—obtain for all to detect occult fractures *IMPORTANT*
- C-spine MRI—consider for neurologic deficit—assess hematoma
- Consider imaging of entire spine

Treatment Plan

Non-operative

- Indicated for stable fracture without neurologic compromise
- Immobilization with c-collar or halo
- Consider low-weight traction if displaced
- Must do serial neurologic exams to assess for progressive deficit *IMPORTANT*

Surgery

- Up to 83 % of patients may undergo operative fixation (especially with AS)
- More likely to lead to improved complication, mortality, and neurologic recovery rates but must give patients option of nonsurgical treatment due to high risks of surgery
- Indications
  - Neurologic compromise
  - Unstable fracture
  - Epidural hematoma

- Anterior versus posterior approach based on osteoporosis, location of hematoma, location of fracture
- High risk of nonunion, hardware failure, progressive deformity

References

Caron T, Bransford R, Nguyen Q, Agel J, Chapman J, Bellabarba C. Spine fractures in patients with ankylosing spinal disorders. Spine (Phila Pa 1976). 2010 May 15;35(11):E458–64.

Westerveld LA, Verlaan JJ, Oner FC.Spinal fractures in patients with ankylosing spinal disorders: a systematic review of the literature on treatment, neurological status and complications. Eur Spine J. 2009 Feb;18(2):145–56.

Whang PG, Goldberg G, Lawrence JP, Hong J, Harrop JS, Anderson DG, Albert TJ, Vaccaro AR. The management of spinal injuries in patients with ankylosing spondylitis or diffuse idiopathic skeletal hyperostosis: a comparison of treatment methods and clinical outcomes. J Spinal Disord Tech. 2009 Apr;22(2):77–85.

Atlanto-Axial Fractures and Instability

Loss of stability between C1 (atlas) and C2 (axis) may be caused by chronic degeneration (e.g., Down's syndrome, rheumatoid arthritis (RA), juvenile RA) or acute bony or ligamentous injury. Treatment depends on presence and etiology of instability.

Overview

Most commonly anterior displacement of C1 on C2 (can be posterior or lateral)
Present in up to ¾ of patients with RA due to transverse ligament (TAL) destruction
Atlanto-axial stability primarily due to transverse ligament, which maintains the odontoid to the anterior arch of C1

History

Have you had recent trauma?
Do you have other sites of pain along the spine?
Do you have any neurologic deficits? (e.g. weakness, numbness)

Physical Exam

Complete trauma evaluation (Appendix A)
Complete neurologic evaluation including tests for myelopathy (Appendix A)

M.C. Makhni et al. (eds.), *Orthopedic Emergencies*,
DOI 10.1007/978-3-319-31524-9_15

Imaging

C-spine XRs—AP, lateral, open mouth (odontoid) views

Flexion/extension films
Atlanto-dens interval (ADI)—posterior aspect of anterior ring of atlas to anterior dens
Posterior atlanto-dens interval (PADI)—posterior dens to anterior aspect of posterior ring of atlas (= SAC = space available for the cord)
Sum of lateral mass displacement

C-spine CT—can help to demonstrate rotational instability (Fig. 1)
C-spine MRI—obtain if neurologic deficit, or to visualize transverse ligament (TAL)

Classification

Instability determined by integrity of transverse ligament

Transverse Ligament Injuries

Type 1: midsubstance
Type 2: avulsion from C1 lateral mass

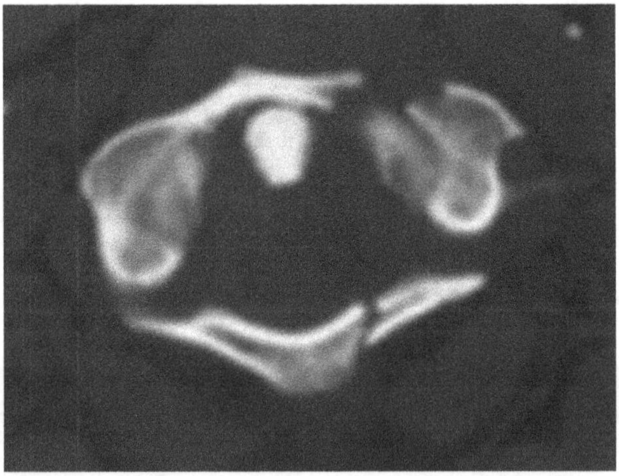

Fig. 1 Atlas fracture

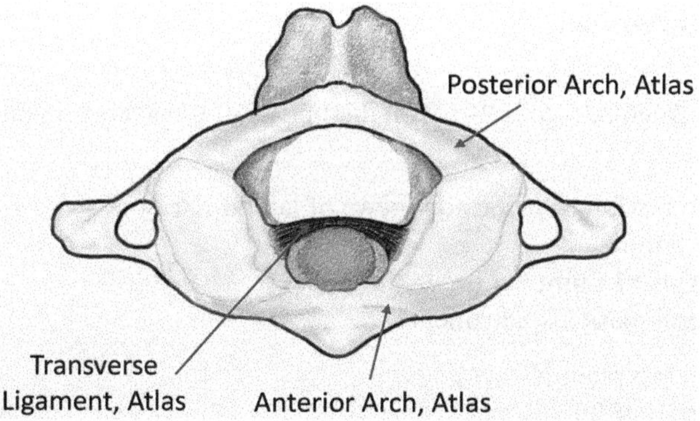

Fig. 2 Atlas fracture diagram

Atlas Fractures *(Descriptive of Fracture Location) (Fig. 2)*

Type 1: unilateral fracture of anterior or posterior arch
Type 2: bilateral fractures of anterior or posterior arch (Jefferson fracture)
Type 3: unilateral fracture of lateral mass

Dens Fractures (See Chapter "Dens Fractures")

Treatment Plan

Non-operative Treatment

Rigid cervical immobilization: any non-displaced fx without TAL rupture

- Type 1 atlas fracture
- Stable type 2–3 atlas fracture
- Consider type 2 transverse ligament ruptures (74 % heal non-operatively)

Surgical Indications

Unstable atlas fracture (types 2–3 with disruption of transverse ligament)
Instability

- >3.5 mm on flexion or extension views of lateral X-ray
- For child, >5 mm
- For RA, PADI <14 mm
- Sum of lateral mass displacement:
  - >8.1 mm (on plain X-rays)
  - >6.9 mm (on CT)
  - Will miss 60 % of TAL injuries seen on MRI, so order MRI if suspect

Progressive instability
Myelopathy
Neurologic deficits

Surgical Options

C1 fixation
C1–C2 fixation (trans-articular screw or temporary stabilization w/removal of rods when healed)
C1–C2 posterior arthrodesis

- Lateral mass screws less risk of complications
- Pedicle screws more rigid fixation

References

Boden SD, Dodge LD, Bohlman HH, Rechtine GR. Rheumatoid arthritis of the cervical spine. A long-term analysis with predictors of paralysis and recovery. J Bone Joint Surg Am. 1993;75(9):1282–97.

Dickman CA, Greene KA, Sonntag VK. Injuries involving the transverse atlantal ligament: classification and treatment guidelines based upon experience with 39 injuries. Neurosurgery. 1996;38:44–50.

Jackson RS, Banit DM, Rhyne 3rd AL, Darden 2nd BV. Upper cervical spine injuries. J Am Acad Orthop Surg. 2002;10(4):271–80. PMID:15089076.

Miller MD, Thompson SR, Hart JA. Review of orthopaedics. 6th ed. Elsevier; 2012. p. 595. Philadelphia, PA.

Dens Fracture

A fracture of the dens (otherwise known as the odontoid), which is the proximal process arising from C2 (the axis). Based on their location as well as patient characteristics, these can be treated non-operatively or surgically.

History

- Do you have other sites of pain along your spine?
- Do you have any weakness, numbness, or tingling?

Physical Exam

- Trauma evaluation (Appendix A)
- Complete neurologic exam (Appendix A)

Diagnosis

Imaging

- C-spine XRs—AP, lateral, open mouth (odontoid) views
- C-spine CT—consider for all dens fractures due to higher inter-rater reliability than XRs
- C-spine MRI—obtain if neurologic deficit, or suspected ligamentous instability

M.C. Makhni et al. (eds.), *Orthopedic Emergencies*,
DOI 10.1007/978-3-319-31524-9_16

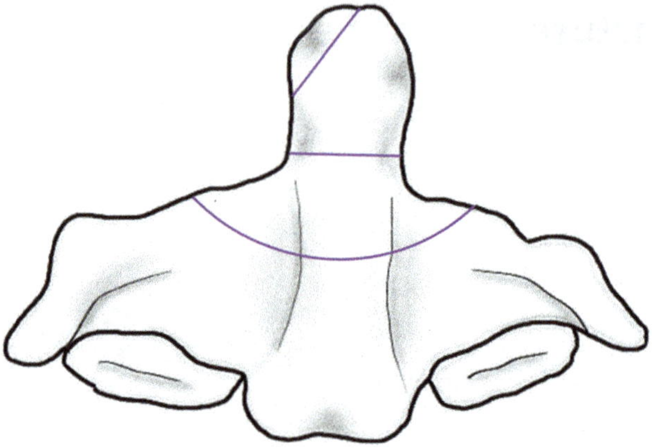

Fig. 1 Dens fracture diagram

- Sagittal fracture displacement: distance between anterior borders of proximal and distal fragments
- Fracture angulation: angle between posterior aspects of proximal and distal fragments

Classification

Anderson and D'Alonzo (Fig. 1)

- Type 1: tip of dens
  - Avulsion
  - Be suspicious for occipito-cervical dissociation
- Type 2: base of dens (Fig. 2)
  - High nonunion risk due to limited trabecular bony surface; distractive forces from apical ligament
- Type 3: body of axis (Fig. 3)
  - High healing rate due to large cancellous surface

Grauer classification

- Detailed classification of type 2 and type 3 fractures that helps predict management options (see References below)

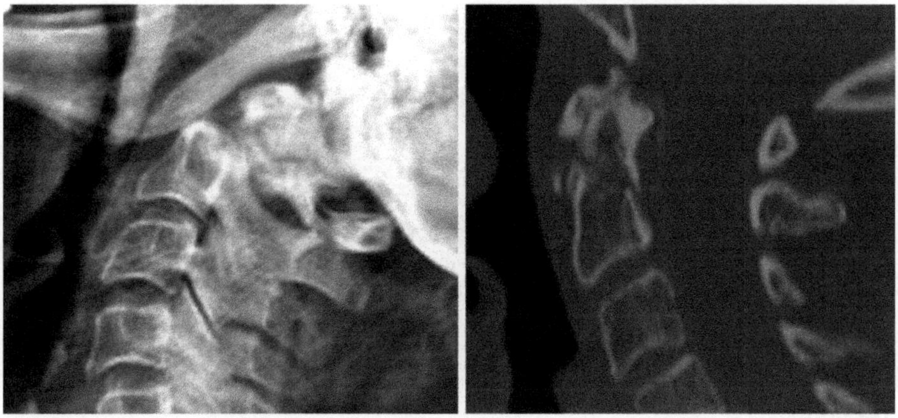

Fig. 2 Type 2 dens fracture

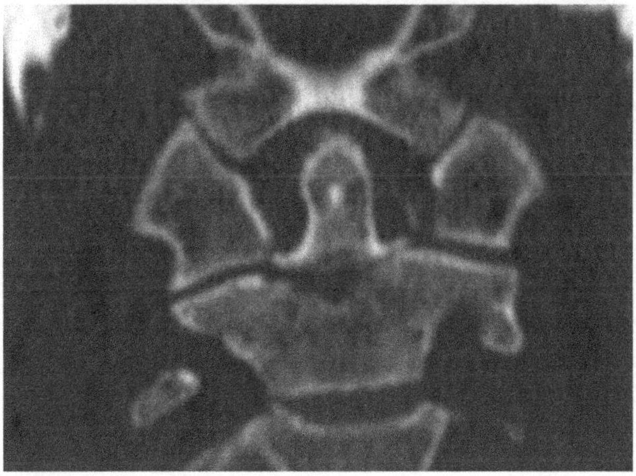

Fig. 3 Type 3 dens fracture

Treatment Plan

Non-operative

- C-collar, halo vest, cervico-thoracic orthosis
- Nearly all type 1 fractures heal with non-operative management
- Higher healing rates for type 3 compared to type 2
  - Type 2: C-collar 51 %, halo vest 65 % healing
  - Type 3: 90 + % healing with immobilization

- High morbidity/mortality of halo vests, especially in patients >70 years old (2× mortality than c-collar)
  - Aspiration, cardiac arrest, pin site infection, pin loosening
- Closed reduction with axial traction
  - If posterior displacement, cord impingement and neurologic symptoms
  - Secure airway prior to reduction to prevent respiratory compromise
  - Stabilize neck during intubation to avoid fracture displacement
  - Beware of over-distraction! *IMPORTANT*

Surgical

- Fixation (odontoid screw, trans-articular screw) vs. atlanto-axial arthrodesis
- 90 + % healing
- Indications:
  - Cord compression
  - Neurologic deficit
  - Instability
  - >2 mm secondary displacement compared to initial
  - High nonunion risk (relative)—if stable, can operate initially, or attempt non-operative management first. This will decrease chance of success of primary fixation, but still allow option for fusion if fails to improve. Risk factors:
    - ≥5 mm posterior displacement
    - Comminution
    - Fracture gap >1 mm
    - Fracture angulation >11 °
    - 4+ day delay in initiating treatment
    - Age >40 years old

References

Grauer JN, Shafi B, Hilibrand AS, Harrop JS, Kwon BK, Beiner JM, et al. Proposal of a modified, treatment-oriented classification of odontoid fractures. Spine J. 2005;5(2):123–9.

Hsu WK, Anderson PA. Odontoid fractures: update on management. J Am Acad Orthop Surg. 2010;18:383–94.

Subaxial (C3–C7) Cervical Spine Fractures

Subaxial fractures are evaluated primarily based on injury morphology and neurologic status, both of which are included in the SLIC classification system. Stability in this region is largely determined by the integrity of the posterior ligamentous complex.

History

- How much energy was involved in the trauma?
- Was there head strike?
- Do you have other sites of pain along your spine?
- Do you have any weakness, numbness, or tingling?

Physical Exam

- Absence of posterior c-spine midline ttp in cooperative patient strongly suggests lack of substantial c-spine injury
- Malrotation of head suggesting facet dislocations
- Inspect for signs of head trauma
- Trauma evaluation (Appendix A)
- Complete neurologic exam (Appendix A)

M.C. Makhni et al. (eds.), *Orthopedic Emergencies*,
DOI 10.1007/978-3-319-31524-9_17

Diagnosis

Imaging

- C-spine XRs—AP, lateral, flexion/extension views
  - Evaluate instability in cooperative patients
  - Must have normal mental status and a normal neurologic exam
  - Must visualize cervicothoracic junction to T1 *IMPORTANT*
- C-spine CT—required to evaluate fracture pattern and facet alignment
- C-spine MRI—necessary to evaluate for acute disc herniation or disrupted disco-ligamentous complex

Classification

<u>Sub-axial Cervical Spine Injury Classification System (SLIC)</u>

Morphology type

Normal (0)
Compression (1)
Burst (2)
Distraction (3)
Translational/rotational (4)

Neurologic Involvement

Intact (0)
Nerve root (1)
Complete cord (2)
Incomplete cord (3)
Continuous cord compression with deficit (+1)

Discoligamentous Complex

Intact (0)
Injury suspected/indeterminate (1)
Injury (2)

Treatment Plan

Non-operative Conditions

- SLIC score of 0–3 points
- Unilateral lateral pillar fracture
- Posterior column fracture

Non-operative vs. Operative Management

- SLIC score of 4 points
- Bilateral lateral pillar fractures

Operative Management

- SLIC score of 5–10 points
- Locked dislocated facets (unilateral or bilateral)
- Instability, demonstrated by spondylolisthesis
- Neurologic compromise due to vertebral body retropulsion

Non-operative

- For patients with SCI, consider IV methylprednisone based on the NASCIS II/III studies (see chapter "Incomplete Spinal Cord Injury")
- C-collar, halo vest, cervico-thoracic orthosis
- High morbidity/mortality of halo vests, especially in patients >70 years old (2x mortality than c-collar)
  - Aspiration, cardiac arrest, pin-site infection, pin loosening
- Closed reduction with axial traction and serial neurologic exams and imaging
  - Unilateral or bilateral facet dislocations
  - In alert patient
  - MRI to detect disc herniations prior to reduction in non-communicative patient

Surgical

- Anterior decompression, corpectomy, and fusion with instrumentation
  - Unstable burst, tear drop, or quadrangular fractures with cord compression
  - Primary anterior column pathology
- Posterior decompression and fusion with instrumentation
  - Indicated with posterior ligamentous complex disruption
  - Primary posterior column pathology

References

Helgeson MD, Gendelberg D, Sidhu GS, Anderson DG, Vaccaro AR. Management of cervical spine trauma: can a prognostic classification of injury determine clinical outcomes? Orthop Clin N Am. 2012;43(1):89–96.

Kwon BK, Vaccaro AR, Grauer JN, Fisher CG, Dvorak MF. Subaxial cervical spine trauma. JAAOS. 2006;14(2):78–89.

Vaccaro AR, Hulbert RJ, Patel AA, Fisher C, Dvorak M, Lehman RA, et al. The subaxial cervical spine injury classification system: a novel approach to recognize the importance of morphology, neurology, and integrity of the disco-ligamentous complex. Spine. 2007;32(21):2365–74.

Central Cord Syndrome

A form of incomplete spinal cord injury due to hyperextension often presenting with upper extremity motor weakness in older individuals. Surgical treatment and early intervention are controversial.

Overview

- Presentation ranges from distal UE weakness to quadriparesis
- Most patients affected have compression of cord in addition to predisposing decreased canal volume from spondylosis and osteophytes, stenosis, or OPLL
- Sacral sparing, and therefore incomplete spinal cord injury
- If motor status resolves, UE function last to return and often only partial hand functional improvement

History

- Mechanism of injury?
- Prior neck pain or stiffness?
- Neurologic deficits? Location/levels of deficits?

Physical Exam

- Trauma evaluation (Appendix A)
- Complete neurologic evaluation (Appendix A)

M.C. Makhni et al. (eds.), *Orthopedic Emergencies*,
DOI 10.1007/978-3-319-31524-9_18

- Sacral sparing (signifies incomplete SCI—see chapter "Incomplete Spinal Cord Injury")
  - FHL motor function
  - Anal sphincter contraction
  - Peri-anal sensation

Imaging

- C-spine XRs—AP, lateral, open mouth (odontoid) views
  - Chronic cervical spondylosis
- CT—better assessment of bony injury or other concomitant spinal fractures
  - Visualize entire spine with XR and/or CT
- MRI cord signal change indicating edema without hemorrhage
  - r/o soft-tissue disruption

Management

Non-operative Treatment

- Rigid cervical immobilization
  - Prevent motion injury
  - 6 weeks or until resolution of pain and neurologic symptoms
- ICU monitoring with MAP >85 mmHg
  - Maximal cord perfusion to improve chance for neurologic recovery
- Consider IV steroids
- Early neurologic improvement and absence of MRI cord signal changes are positive prognostic factors

Operative Treatment

- Trend towards surgery for central cord syndrome *IMPORTANT*
- Extent of decompression and stabilization dependent on pathology

- Indications:
  - Progressive neurologic deficit
  - Cervical instability
  - Structural cord compression—address spondylosis or chronic stenosis
- Results:
  - Best results in younger patients and those with compressive lesions
  - Unclear whether differences in outcomes between early and delayed surgery
  - However, STASCIS trial showed benefit of surgery <24 h after cervical spinal cord injury—so consider early intervention

References

Fehlings MG, Vaccaro A, Wilson JR, Singh A, W. Cadotte D, Harrop JS, et al. Early versus delayed decompression for traumatic cervical spinal cord injury: results of the Surgical Timing in Acute Spinal Cord Injury Study (STASCIS). PLoS One. 2012;7(2):1–8.

Nowak DD, Lee JK, Gelb DE, Poelstra KA, Ludwig SC. Central cord syndrome. J Am Acad Orthop Surg. 2009;17:756–65. PMID: 19948700.

Park MS, Moon S, Lee H, Kim T, Oh JK, Suh B, et al. Delayed surgical intervention in central cord syndrome with cervical stenosis. Global Spine J. 2015;5:69–72.

Riew KD, Kang DG. Central cord syndrome: is operative treatment the standard of care? Spine J. 2015;15(3):443–5.

Thoracolumbar Fractures

Thoracolumbar fractures are evaluated primarily based on injury morphology, neurologic status, and integrity of the posterior ligamentous complex. These are included in the TLICS classification system, which can help guide surgical decision making.

History

- Do you have other sites of pain along your spine?
- Do you have any weakness, numbness, or tingling?

Physical Exam

- Trauma evaluation (Appendix A)
- Complete neurologic exam (Appendix A)

Diagnosis

Imaging

- T/L XRs—AP, lateral
- T/L CT—required to evaluate fracture pattern (Fig. 1)
- T/L MRI—necessary to evaluate for acute disc herniation or disrupted disco-ligamentous complex

M.C. Makhni et al. (eds.), *Orthopedic Emergencies*,
DOI 10.1007/978-3-319-31524-9_19

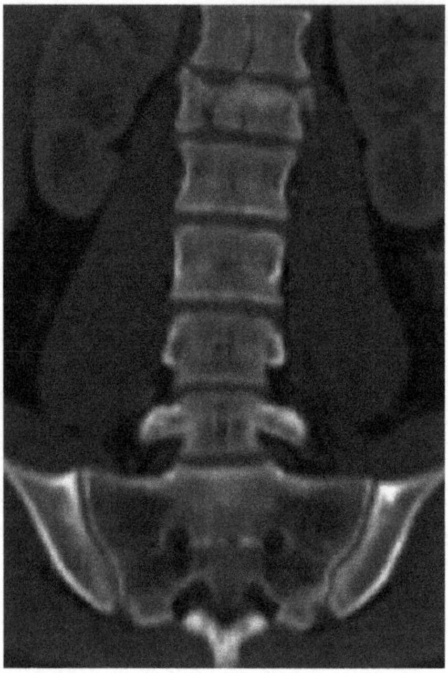

Fig. 1 Coronal CT

Classification

Denis 3—column model (Fig. 2)

Anterior column

- Anterior longitudinal ligament
- Anterior 2/3 of vertebral body and intervertebral disc

Middle column

- Posterior longitudinal ligament
- Posterior 1/3 of vertebral body and intervertebral disc
- Intervertebral foramina

Posterior column

- Posterior ligamentous complex (PLC)
  - Ligamentum flavum
  - Interspinous ligament

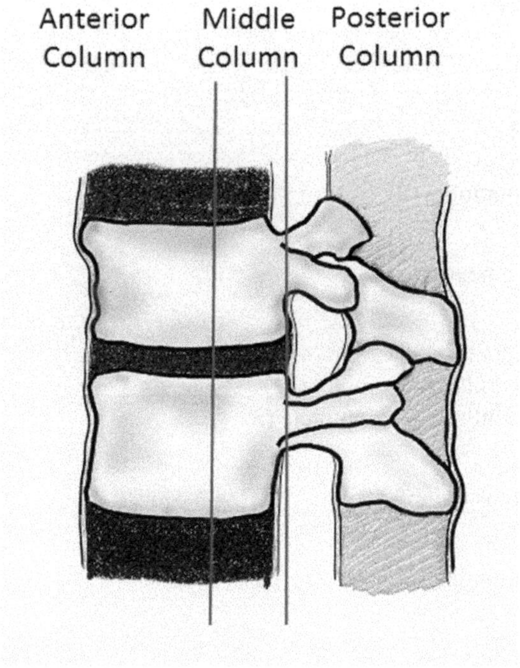

Fig. 2 Denis 3—column spine model

Supraspinous ligament
Facet capsules

Posterior elements

Pedicles
Facet joints
Transverse processes
Spinous process
Lamina

Spinal cord

TLICS: thoracolumbar injury classification and severity score

Descriptive of thoracolumbar trauma
Predicts need for surgical management

Description (Score)

Morphology type

Compression (1)
Burst (2)
Translational/rotational (3)
Distraction (4)

Neurologic involvement

Intact (0)
Nerve root (2)
Cord, conus medullaris—complete (2)
Cord, conus medullaris—incomplete (3)
Cauda equina (3)

Posterior ligamentous complex

Intact (0)
Injury suspected/indeterminate (2)
Injury (3)

Management

Non-operative Management (e.g., TLSO, LSO, Corset for Pain, No Intervention)

- TLICS 0–3
- Often indicated for spinous process fx, transverse process fx, and compression fx

Non-operative vs. Operative Management (Consider Percutaneous Stabilization)

- TLICS 4

Operative Management

- TLICS 5–10
- Indicated for instability, neurologic compromise with vertebral body retropulsion (Fig. 3)

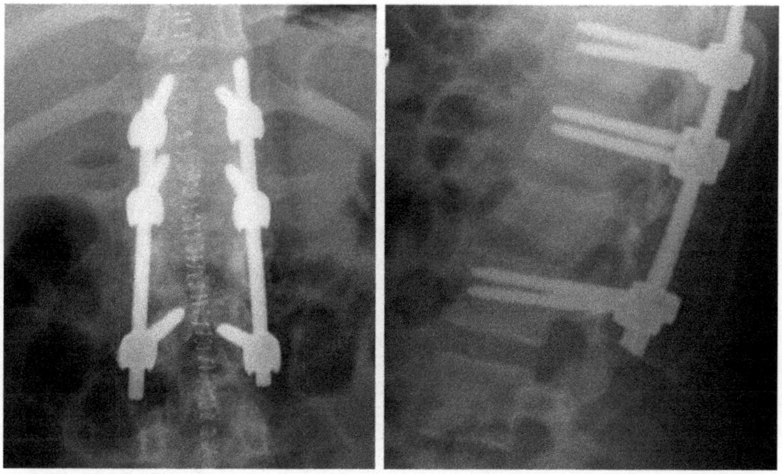

Fig. 3 Percutaneous stabilization

Treatment Plan

Non-operative

- For patients with SCI, consider IV methylprednisone (see chapter "Spinal Cord Injury")
- Soft corset, TLSO (thoraco-lumbo-sacral orthosis)

Surgical

- Posterior decompression and fusion with instrumentation
- Can consider percutaneous stabilization for indirect decompression (Figure 3)

References

Gelb D, Ludwig S, Karp J, Chung E, Werner C, Kim T, et al. Successful treatment of thoracolumbar fractures with short-segment pedicle instrumentation. J Spinal Disord Tech. 2010;23(5):293–301.

Vaccaro AR1, Lehman RA Jr, Hurlbert RJ, Anderson PA, Harris M, Hedlund R, Harrop J, Dvorak M, Wood K, Fehlings MG, Fisher C, Zeiller SC, Anderson DG, Bono CM, Stock GH, Brown AK, Kuklo T, Oner FC. A new classification of thoracolumbar injuries: the importance of injury morphology, the integrity of the posterior ligamentous complex, and neurologic status. Spine. 2005 Oct 15;30(20):2325–33.

Wood KB, Li W, Lebl DS, Ploumis A. Management of thoracolumbar spine fractures. Spine J. 2014;14(1):145–64.

Compression Fracture

Fragility fracture of the spine which rarely causes neurologic deficits and can often be treated nonoperatively, although cement augmentation may potentially improve pain relief and functional improvement.

Overview

- Most common fragility fracture
- Failure of anterior column from anterior (most common) or lateral flexion
- Associated with significant 2-year mortality
  - Rule out underlying metastatic etiology
  - Medical management to optimize bone quality
- Expected full resolution of pain and return to previous function
- Increased kyphosis from multiple adjacent fractures can compromise pulmonary function

History

- Did you have any preceding trauma?
- Have you ever had this type of pain before in your spine?
- Have you ever been diagnosed with osteoporosis?
- Do you have history or family history of cancer, or recent fevers, chills, or weight loss?
- Do you have any weakness, numbness, or tingling?

M.C. Makhni et al. (eds.), *Orthopedic Emergencies*,
DOI 10.1007/978-3-319-31524-9_20

Physical Exam

- Assess for focal sites of tenderness along entire spine
- Complete Neurologic Exam (Appendix A)

Imaging

- XRs entire spine (Fig. 1)
  - Loss of anterior column vertebral height and maintained posterior column
  - Assess for other sites of compression fractures *IMPORTANT*
  - Evaluate if local kyphosis (especially if multiple compression fractures)
  - Examine for possible lesions
- CT/MRI indicated if: neurologic deficit, lesions detected, insufficient plain films to rule out middle or posterior column compromise, to assess acuity of fractures, to diagnose occult fractures

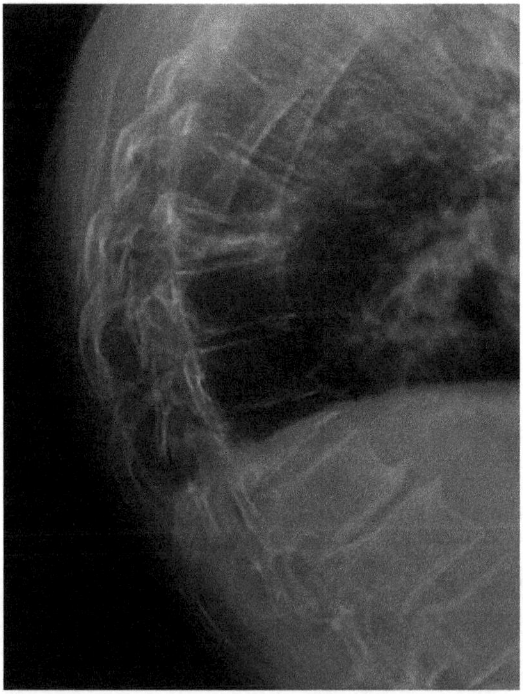

Fig. 1 Compression fractures

Classification

Stable—most common
Unstable—>50 % loss of vertebral height

>20° angulation
Multiple adjacent fractures
Disruption of middle/posterior columns (burst, chance fracture)

Treatment Plan

Nonoperative

- Early ambulation with pain control
- Extension orthosis—unclear benefit, no Level 1 or 2 evidence to support
- Serial imaging for 3 months to confirm no progression of fracture
- Medical management of osteoporosis
  - Consider bisphosphonates
  - Consider calcitonin for 1 month after injury

Surgery

- Kyphoplasty (expansion of vertebral body followed by cement augmentation)
- Vertebroplasty (injection of cement into vertebral body in situ)
- 2010 AAOS Guideline against vertebroplasty-unclear benefit of kyphoplasty
- Several prospective randomized trials since then
  - Most suggest improved pain relief and functional improvement with cement augmentation
  - Potential benefits up to 2 years
- Relative Indications
  - Pathologic fractures
  - Persistent pain >3–6 weeks
  - Patients hospitalized due to pain

References

Esses SI, McGuire R, Jenkins J, Finkelstein J, Woodard E, Watters WC, et al. The treatment of symptomatic osteoporotic spinal compression fractures. J Am Acad Orthop Surg. 2011;19(3):176–82.

Hazel WA, Jones RA, Morrey BF, Stauffer RN. Vertebral fractures without neurologic deficit. A long-term follow-up study. Bone Joint Surg Am. 1988;70(9):1319–21.

Savage JW, Schroeder GD, Anderson PA. Vertebroplasty and kyphoplasty for the treatment of osteoporotic vertebral compression fractures. J Am Acad Orthop Surg. 2014;22(10):653–64.

The Treatment of Symptomatic Osteoporotic Spinal Compression Fractures Guideline and Evidence Report. AAOS. 2010.

Spinous Process and Transverse Process Fractures

Fractures in the thoracic and lumbar spine that are nearly always stable and can be managed without intervention, although associated abdominal injuries must be sought. Rigid cervical immobilization may benefit patients with fractures in the cervical spine.

Overview

- Spinous process avulsion fracture as a result of hyperflexion
- Transverse process fracture due to pull from attached ligaments or paraspinal muscles
    - Thoracic and lumbar
        - 30 % associated with abdominal injuries
    - Cervical
        - 10 % with brachial plexus injury
        - 88 % with vertebral artery injury
- L5 TP fracture in patient with pelvic fracture represents avulsion of the iliolumbar ligament, and may indicate vertical pelvic instability * IMPORTANT *

History

- Do you have other pains along your neck and back?
- Do you have headache, nausea or vomiting, or neurologic symptoms?
    - r/o vertebral artery injury for cervical pathology

M.C. Makhni et al. (eds.), *Orthopedic Emergencies*,
DOI 10.1007/978-3-319-31524-9_21

Physical Exam

- Complete Trauma Exam (Appendix A)
- Complete Neurologic Exam (Appendix A)
- Abdominal exam

Imaging

- XRs: AP, lateral spine
- CT: as needed for further visualization (Figs. 1 and 2)
  - Can assess if fracture extends beyond fracture into lamina
  - Can rule out associated facet fracture or dislocation
- Vertebral Artery Angiograms
  - Can perform for all cervical transverse process fractures

Treatment Plan

Nonoperative

- Observation and analgesia
  - Nearly all isolated thoracic and lumbar spine process fractures

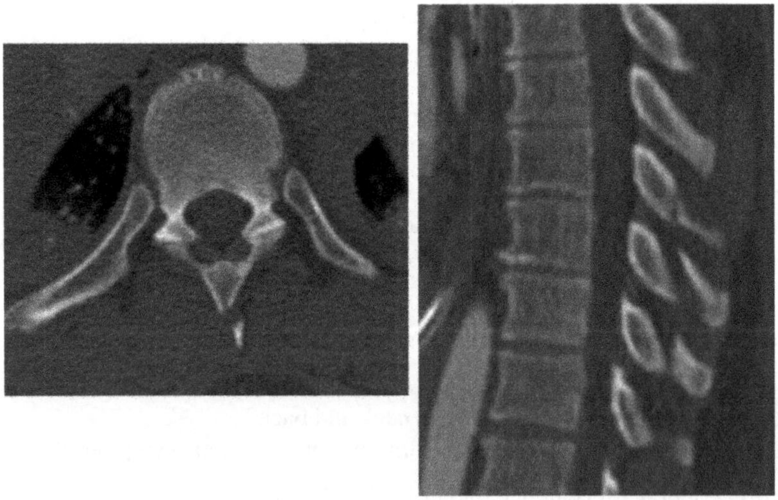

Fig. 1 Spinous process fracture

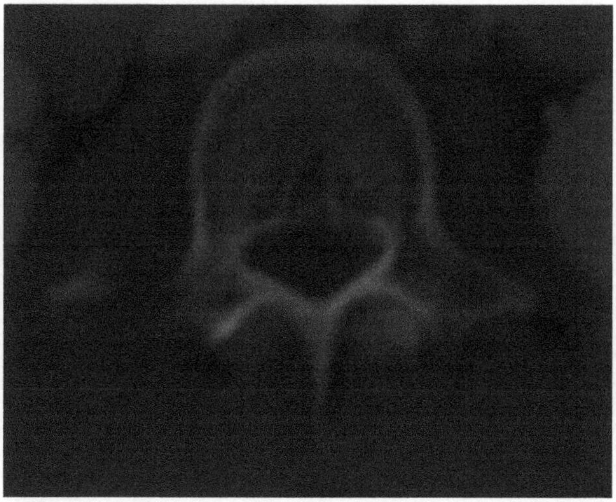

Fig. 2 Transverse process fracture

- Cervical collar
  - Consider for cervical fractures

Operative (Rare)

- If extension into lamina with spinal cord compromise, consider decompression ± fusion

Reference

Bradley LH, Paullus WC, Howe J, Litofsky NS. Isolated transverse process fractures: spine service management not needed. J Trauma. 2008;65(4):832–6.

Burst Fracture

A burst fracture is a fracture through the anterior and middle columns of the vertebra in the thoracolumbar region usually associated with significant trauma. Patients with stable fractures who are neurologically intact without posterior ligamentous complex disruption can usually be managed nonoperatively.

History

- Do you have other sites of pain along your spine?
- Do you have any weakness, numbness, or tingling?
- Are you able to urinate? Do you have bowel or bladder incontinence?
- Do you have pain along any of your extremities?

Physical Exam

- Trauma evaluation (Appendix A)
- Complete Neurologic Exam (Appendix A)

Diagnosis

Imaging

- Entire spine XRs—AP, lateral, oblique views
- T/L-spine CT—Evaluate extent of fracture, bony retropulsion (Fig. 1)

M.C. Makhni et al. (eds.), *Orthopedic Emergencies*,
DOI 10.1007/978-3-319-31524-9_22

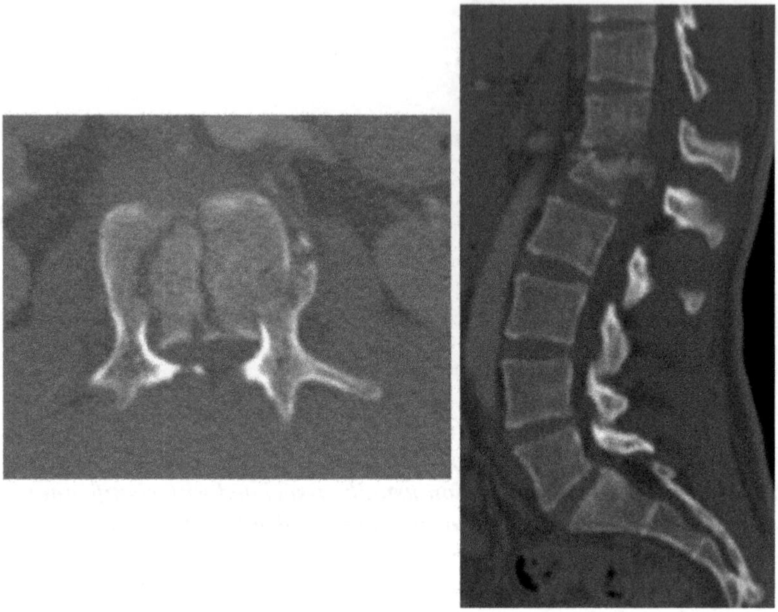

Fig. 1 L1 burst fracture

- T/L-spine MRI—Assess canal compromise, cord signal changes and compression of neural elements, edema, hemorrhage, and disruption in the posterior ligamentous complex (PLC)

Classification

- TLICS (see Chapter "Thoracolumbar Fractures")
- ASIA (see Chapter "Incomplete Spinal Cord Injury")

Treatment Plan

Nonoperative Treatment

- For stable burst fractures without neurologic compromise
  - Favorable results compared to surgical management
    - Short term: lower pain, less complications
    - Long term: lower pain, better function

- LSO (lumbar) vs. TLSO (thoracolumbar)
  - Pain control
  - Facilitates early function

Operative Indications

- Instability/disruption of PLC
- Neurologic deficit (attention also to bowel and bladder function)
  - Favorable results with early intervention <48 h
  - Incomplete SCI—to preserve function and prevent further deterioration
  - Complete SCI—to facilitate rehabilitation
- Progressive spinal deformity
- Progressive neurological deficit
- Inability to mobilize
- Polytrauma
- Inability to brace (e.g.: due to large habitus)

Surgical Options

- Posterior fusion
  - 1–2 levels above and below
  - ± Minimally invasive
- Decompression
  - Indications:
    - Incomplete neurological deficit
    - Severe radiculopathy secondary to posttraumatic canal stenosis
    - Bowel/bladder dysfunction
  - Direct: Remove retropulsed bone: laminectomy, extracavitary, transpedicular
    - Anterior corpectomy
    - Transpedicular approach
  - Indirect: Via ligamentotaxis, restoring height with posterior instrumentation

References

Spivak JM, Vaccaro AR, Cotler JM. Thoracolumbar spine trauma: II. Principles of management. J Am Acad Orthop Surg. 1995;3:353–60.

Wood KB, Buttermann GR, Phukan R, Harrod CC, Mehbod A, Shannon B, et al. Operative compared with nonoperative treatment of a thoracolumbar burst fracture without neurological deficit: a prospective randomized study with follow-up at sixteen to twenty-two years. J Bone Joint Surg Am. 2015;97(1):3–9.

Chance Fracture

A chance fracture is a flexion-distraction injury to the spine that involves all three columns. Bony chance fractures can often managed nonoperatively, while ligamentous disruption of the posterior column often necessitates operative stabilization.

Overview

- The posterior ligamentous complex (PLC) is comprised of:
  - Supraspinous ligament
  - Interspinous ligament
  - Ligamentum flavum
  - Facet joint capsules
- Bony chance fractures have potential to heal, while soft tissue 3 column injuries (e.g.: ligamentous, trans-discal) are unlikely to heal
- 10–15 % of chance fractures are associated with neurologic deficits

History

- Do you have other sites of pain along your spine?
- Do you have any weakness, numbness, or tingling?
- Do you have abdominal pain?
- Do you have any bowel or bladder difficulty or incontinence?

M.C. Makhni et al. (eds.), *Orthopedic Emergencies*,
DOI 10.1007/978-3-319-31524-9_23

Physical Exam

- Trauma evaluation (Appendix A)
- Complete Neurologic Exam (Appendix A)
- Seat belt sign

Diagnosis

Imaging

- Entire spine XRs—AP, lateral, oblique views
- T/L-spine CT—Evaluate extent of fracture, bony retropulsion (Fig. 1)
  - Assess for anterior compression, and fractures through spinous processes, lamina, pedicles, or vertebral body
  - >3.5 mm vertebral translation associated with PLC injury
- T/L-spine MRI—Assess canal compromise, cord signal changes and compression of neural elements, edema, hemorrhage
  - Also, assess signal intensity in posterior ligamentous complex (PLC)
  - Disruption of supraspinous AND interspinous ligaments on MRI associated with intra-op PLC disruption

Classification

- TLICS (see Chapter "Thoracolumbar Fractures")
- ASIA (see Chapter "Incomplete Spinal Cord Injury")

Treatment Plan

Nonoperative

- Treatment: TLSO to minimize resultant local posttraumatic kyphotic deformity
- Indications: Stable bony chance fracture

- Treatment: Hyperextension cast
- Indications: Stable bony chance fractures in children

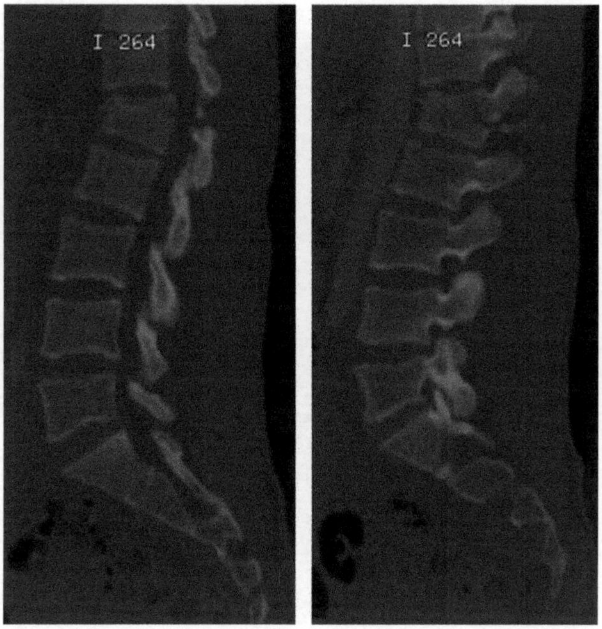

Fig. 1 L1 chance fracture

Operative

- Treatment:
  - Can not decompress without fusing, otherwise further destabilize
  - Posterior fusion: 1–2 levels above and below
- Indications:
  - Instability (soft-tissue chance injury, disruption of PLC)
  - Incomplete spinal cord injury—favorable results if surgery occurs within 24–48 h
  - Complete spinal cord injury (debatable)

References

Radcliff K, Su BW, Kepler CK, Rubin T, Shimer AL, Rihn JA, et al. Correlation of posterior ligamenous complex injury and neurological injury to loss of vertebral body height, kyphosis, and canal compromise. Spine. 2012;37(13):1142–50.

Vaccaro AR, Lee JY, Schweitzer KM, Lim MR, Baron EM, Oner FC, et al. Assessment of injury to the posterior ligamentous complex in thoracolumbar spine trauma. Spine J. 2006;6(5):524–8.

Thoracolumbar Fracture-Dislocation

A thoracolumbar fracture-dislocation is an inherently unstable injury pattern that involves disruption of all three spinal columns. These high-energy injuries are nearly always complete spinal cord injuries and are typically managed operatively for stabilization.

History (Most Likely Unable to Obtain)

- Do you have any strength or sensation distal to injury level?
- Do you have bowel or bladder function?

Physical Exam

- ATLS evaluation (Appendix A)
- Complete Neurologic Exam (Appendix A)
  - Bulbocavernosus reflex testing is necessary to differentiate spinal shock from SCI

Diagnosis

Imaging

- T/L XRs—AP, lateral
- T/L CT—Required to evaluate fracture pattern (Fig. 1)
- T/L MRI—Necessary for visualizing the spinal cord and posterior ligamentous complex

M.C. Makhni et al. (eds.), *Orthopedic Emergencies*,
DOI 10.1007/978-3-319-31524-9_24

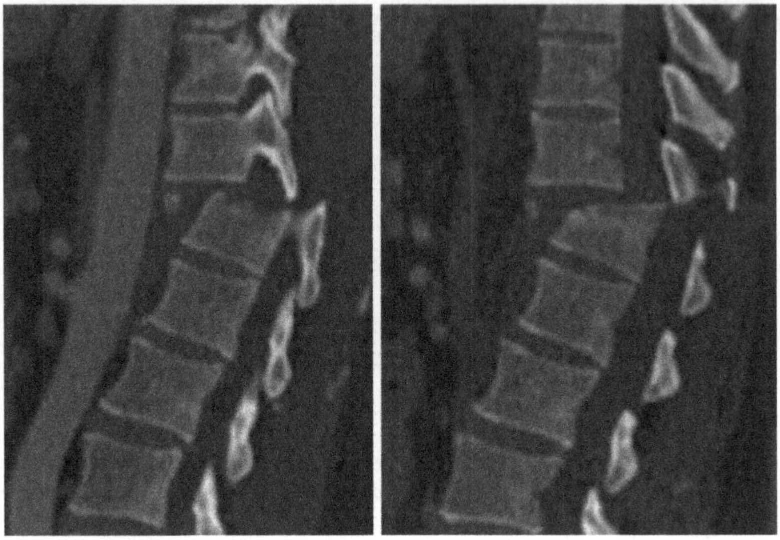

Fig. 1 Fracture-dislocation

Treatment Plan

Nonoperative

- Custom-fitted thoracic-lumbar-sacral orthosis (TLSO)
  - Critically ill or unstable patients

Surgical

- Percutaneous posterior instrumentation 1–2 levels above and below the injury site (damage control)
  - Patients with complete spinal cord injury
  - Goals of stabilization:
    - Facilitate nursing care and rehabilitation
    - Maintain alignment to prevent further decompensation
- Open posterior decompression, fusion, and instrumentation
  - For patients with incomplete spinal cord injury requiring decompression

References

Gelb D, Ludwig S, Karp JE, Chung EH, Werner C, Kim T, et al. Successful treatment of thoracolumbar fractures with short-segment pedicle instrumentation. J Spinal Disord Tech. 2010;23(5):293–301.

Wood KB, Li W, Lebl DS, Ploumis A. Management of thoracolumbar spine fractures. Spine J. 2014;14(1):145–64.

Sacral Fractures

Often occurring in conjunction with pelvic ring injuries, sacral fractures are often diagnosed late and can be associated with neurologic compromise.

Overview

- Usually high-energy (often MVA) trauma or low-energy insufficiency fractures
- 1/3 missed on initial evaluation, so need high suspicion *IMPORTANT*
- Associated with injuries to the pelvis, cauda equina, lumbosacral and sacral plexuses, sciatic nerve, iliac vessels

History

- Mechanism of injury? (Helps to aid in identifying other concomitant injuries)
- Other musculoskeletal injuries?
- Neurologic deficits, including bowel or bladder dysfunction?
- Other areas of pain along the spine?

Physical Exam

- Monitoring of hemodynamic status
- Trauma evaluation (Appendix A)
- Thorough pelvic, abdominal, and urologic examination (± gynecologic exam for women)

M.C. Makhni et al. (eds.), *Orthopedic Emergencies*,
DOI 10.1007/978-3-319-31524-9_25

- Presence of Morel-Lavallee lesion (lumbosacral degloving injury with palpable subcutaneous tissue)
- Complete neurologic assessment (including rectal tone, peri-anal wink and sensation, and bulbocavernosus reflex)
- ABIs (± angiogram if abnormal ABI)

Diagnosis

Imaging

- Trauma series (including AP Pelvis, pelvic inlet, and outlet views)
- Lumbosacral X-rays (Fig. 1)
- CT pelvis/sacrum
- MRI to visualize neural compromise

Classification

- Denis Classification (Fig. 2):
  - Zone 1: lateral to foramina
    - Most common
    - Least likely for nerve injury (to L5)

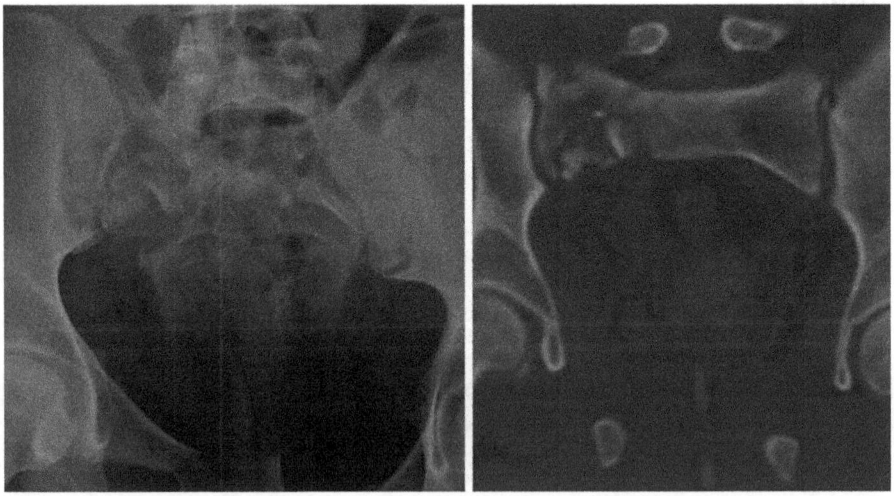

Fig. 1 Sacral fractures

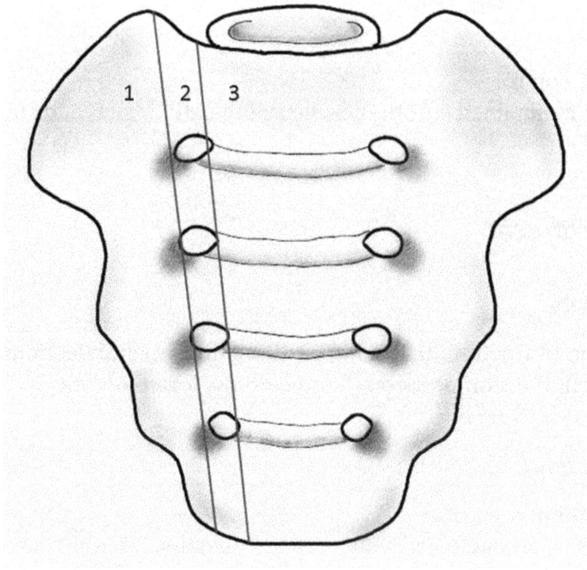

Fig. 2 Sacral fracture Denis classification

- Zone 2: through foramina
  - Unstable if shear component
  - Risk for nonunion and poor function
- Zone 3: medial to foramina
  - Most have neurologic deficit
  - Subcategories 1–4

- Classification by letter resembled by fracture (e.g.: H, U, T, lambda)
- H-shaped, U-shaped = spondylo-pelvic dissociation
  - Likely neurologic deficit
  - High mortality rate
- Transverse: likely neurologic deficit, especially if proximal sacrum affected

Treatment

- Management of associated pelvic ring injury (see Chapter "Pelvic Ring Injury")

Nonoperative Treatment

- WBAT, pain control
- Indications: maintained soft tissues, neurologically intact, and stable pelvis

Surgical Treatment

- Surgical Goals:
    - Reduction of fracture/dislocation, with indirect neural decompression
    - Direct neural decompression (laminectomy, foraminotomy)
    - Soft-tissue coverage
- Surgical Options:
    - Decompression
    - Open vs. percutaneous reduction/stabilization (e.g.: sacro-iliac, lumbo/sacral-pelvic)
- Indications:
    - Associated lumbosacral instability or unilateral facet dislocation
    - Lumbosacral spondylolisthesis
        - Bilateral facet dislocations
        - Unilateral facet fracture dislocations
        - Trans-sacral fractures
    - Neurologic deficit with compression
    - Sacral fractures with poor integrity soft-tissue envelope

References

Kuklo TR, Potter BK, Ludwig SC, Anderson PA, Lindsey RW, Vaccaro AR, et al. Radiographic measurement techniques for sacral fractures consensus statement of the Spine Trauma Study Group. Spine (Phila Pa 1976). 2006;31(9):1047–55.

Mehta S, Auerbach JD, Born CT, Chin KR. Sacral fractures. J Am Acad Orthop Surg. 2006;14(12):656–65.

Vertebral Osteomyelitis

Vertebral osteomyelitis is an infection of the disc and/or vertebral body of the spine. Patients are typically treated with 6 weeks of IV antibiotics. Patients with an abscess may require an open vs. percutaneous drainage.

History

- Have you had any fevers, night sweats, or chills?
- Do you have pain at night?
- Do you have any weakness, numbness, or tingling?
- ROS for infectious sources (i.e., PNA, UTI, immunosuppressed) Do you use IV drugs?

Physical Exam

- Complete Neurologic Exam (Appendix A)

Diagnosis

Imaging

- XRs—AP, lateral
- MRI with gadolinium contrast—hyperintensity seen on T2 sequence of disc and endplate. Sensitive and specific. MRI is preferred imaging following X-rays

M.C. Makhni et al. (eds.), *Orthopedic Emergencies*,
DOI 10.1007/978-3-319-31524-9_26

- Technetium Tc99m bone scan—Sensitive but not specific
- CT—Demonstrates osseous involvement

Workup

- If patient stable, hold antibiotics prior to drawing blood cultures
- If Blood Cultures Are Negative
  - Typically CT-guided biopsy
  - If CT-guided biopsy not readily available, open biopsy can be done

Treatment

Non-operative (Most Patients)

- Minimum 6 weeks of IV antibiotics
  - Consult with infectious disease team
  - If patient is critically ill, consider empiric antibiotics
- Bracing
  - For symptomatic improvement of pain and possible prevention of deformity
  - Lumbar spine—Molded contact brace
  - Cervical spine—Cervicothoracic orthosis or halo

Operative Management

- Necessary for abscess drainage
  - CT-guided drainage is often sufficient
- Structural instability
- Failure of medical management
- Surgical debridement necessary for patients with spinal instrumentation

Reference

Carragee EJ. Pyogenic vertebral osteomyelitis. J Bone Joint Surg Am. 1997;79(6):874–80.
Zimmerli W. Vertebral osteomyelitis. N Engl J Med. 2010;362(11):1022–9.

Part IV
Shoulder and Upper Arm

Manish Noticewala, David Trofa, Robert Parisien, Luke Nicholson, and Eric C. Makhni

Glenohumeral Dislocation 101

Proximal Humerus Fracture 111

Clavicle Fracture 117

Acromioclavicular (AC) Joint Injury 123

Sternoclavicular (SC) Joint Injury 127

Septic Arthritis of the Shoulder 131

Glenoid and Scapula Fracture 133

Humerus Shaft Fracture 137

Distal Humerus Fractures 145

Olecranon Fracture 151

Radial Head Fracture 157

Elbow Dislocation 163

Coronoid Fracture 169

Elbow Capitellar Fracture 173

Radius and Ulna Shaft Fractures 177

Part IV
Shoulder and Upper Arm

Glenohumeral Dislocation

Glenohumeral dislocation is one of the most commonly encountered dislocations in the body. These dislocations can be anteroinferior (most common), posterior, and even inferior.

Overview

- Should differentiate between *dislocation* and *subluxation.*
- Dislocation refers to complete separation of the glenohumeral joint (in any direction). Subluxation is a more subtle event in which there is glenohumeral laxity (without frank separation).
- Extremely high rate of recurrence in patients who have initial dislocation <30 years.
- Most dislocations are antero-inferior (abduction-external rotation).
- Posterior dislocations commonly found after seizure or electrocution (adduction—internal rotation).
- May be associated with axillary nerve injury, bony injury on humerus (Hill-Sachs) or glenoid (Bankart), or soft-tissue injury.

M.C. Makhni et al. (eds.), *Orthopedic Emergencies*,
DOI 10.1007/978-3-319-31524-9_27

History

- Mechanism of event?
- Did it get reduced (either spontaneously or with effort) or is it still dislocated?
- Prior dislocations? Frequency?
- History of electrocution or seizure?

Physical Exam

- Inspection.
  - Gross deformity.
  - Dimpling of lateral skin secondary to increased acromial-humeral space due to migration of the humeral head out of the glenoid fossa.
  - Anteriorly dislocated shoulders may have inability to adduct or internally rotate.
  - Posteriorly dislocated shoulders will be typically **locked in internal rotation**.
  - Arm locked in full abduction (luxatio-erecta).
- Neurovascular examination *prior* to any attempted manipulation.
  - Axillary nerve.
    - Deltoid function and sensation.
    - Most often injured.
  - Musculocutaneous nerve.
    - Biceps and brachialis function.
    - Lateral antebrachial cutaneous nerve sensation over lateral forearm.
  - Brachial, radial, and ulnar pulses examined and compared to contralateral.
- Range of motion (ROM) will be limited.
- Posterior dislocation is a very commonly missed diagnosis. Be aware of inability to externally rotate, or unsuccessful prior work-ups. * IMPORTANT *
- Post-reduction.
  - ROM testing is not advised as may cause another dislocation event.
  - Repeat neurovascular exam.

Diagnosis

Imaging

- XR: Orthogonal views mandatory—single views can miss dislocation, leading to significant morbidity. * IMPORTANT *
- XR: Grashey view.
  - "True AP" of the shoulder taken perpendicular to the plane of the scapula and parallel to the glenoid fossa, typically angled approx. 20–30° towards view of joint.
- XR: Scapular-Y.
- XR: Axillary or Velpeau axillary—orthogonal to true AP; integral in diagnosing dislocation.
- XR: West point axillary—for anterior-inferior glenoid rim defects.
- XR: Stryker notch—for Hill-Sachs defect of posterior-superior humeral head.
- CT: can provide further understanding of associated fracture morphology.
  - Size and location of associated glenoid fracture.
  - Presence of concomitant proximal humerus fracture.
  - Get if associated proximal humerus fracture or locked dislocation to better assess fracture and ensure that fracture won't propagate with reduction attempt (e.g.: turning non-displaced fracture into a displaced fracture). * IMPORTANT *
- MRI (limited utility in the acute setting).

Classification

- Anterior (most common) (Figs. 1 and 2).
  - Sub-coracoid (67 %)—humeral head located below coracoid process.
  - Sub-glenoid (33%)—humeral head located inferior to glenoid.
- Posterior (<10 %).
  - High-energy MVA, football players, seizures (ETOH withdrawal), and electric shock.
  - 30–40 % have associated fracture.
  - Nearly 50 % are missed on initial presentation.

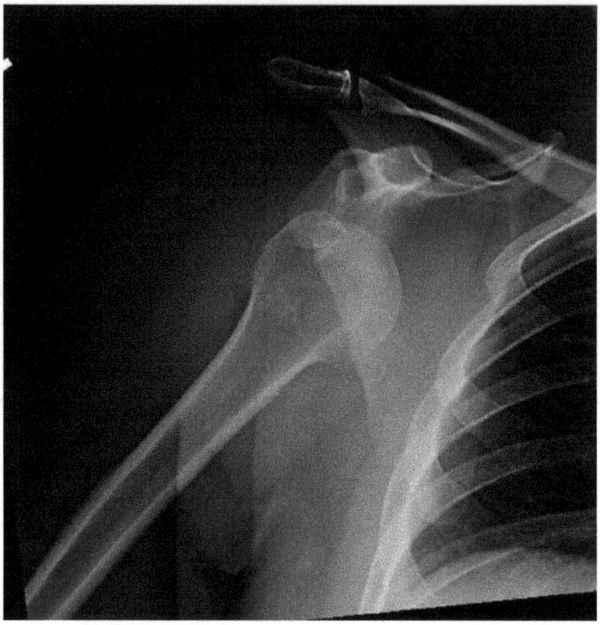

Fig. 1 Antero-inferior shoulder dislocation

- Inferior or *luxatio-erecta* (uncommon).
  - Humeral head directly inferior to glenoid.
  - Humerus locked in 100° to 160° of abduction.

Treatment

Closed Reduction

Closed Reduction of Anterior Dislocation

- Adequate analgesia, conscious sedation, and muscle relaxation are essential with careful monitoring of respiratory depression resulting from excessive sedation.
- Intra-articular gleno-humeral lidocaine injection for analgesia.

Traction-countertraction.

- *Patient:* supine.
- *Assistant:* countertraction is provided by a sheet wrapped around the waist of an assistant and around the upper patient's upper thorax.

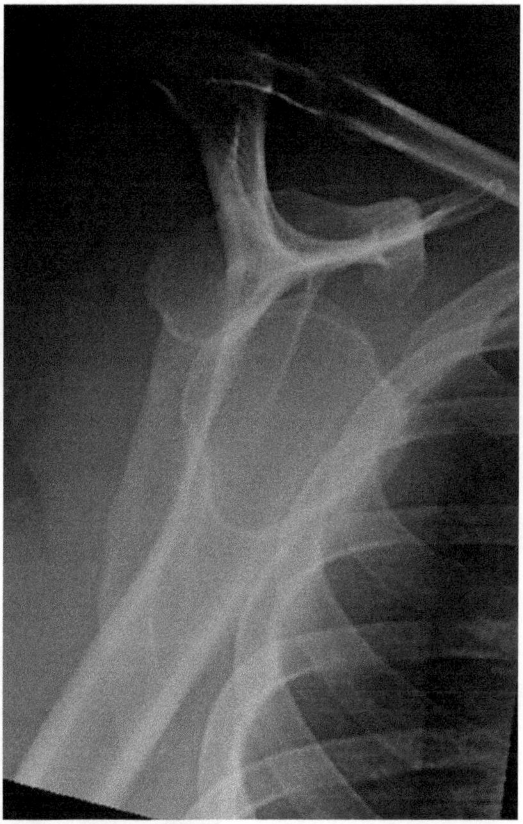

Fig. 2 Antero-inferior shoulder dislocation—*Scapular Y View*

- *Physician:* the physician stands on the side of the dislocated shoulder with a second sheet wrapped around his/her waist as well as the patient's forearm with the elbow flexed at 90°. Traction-countertraction is then applied with gentle IR, ER, abduction, and adduction of the arm by the physician.

Milch Technique.

- *Patient:* supine or prone.
- *Physician:* arm slowly abducted while stabilizing the humeral head with the other arm. Shoulder is then gently externally rotated to 90° with reduction of the humeral head into the glenoid fossa.

Stimson Technique.

- *Patient:* prone with affected arm hanging free over the table.
- *Physician:* slow, steady traction applied by attaching weights around the patient's wrist causing fatigue and relaxation of the shoulder musculature.
- May take up to 15–20 min.
- Prolonged period in this position may result in traction injury to the brachial plexus or a peripheral nerve.

Closed Reduction of Posterior Dislocation

- 30–40 % have an associated fracture - for these, closed reduction should only be attempted in the operating room.
- Requires complete muscle relaxation.
- May be achieved with adduction and internal rotation to "unlock" the shoulder.
- Arthroscopic vs. open reduction may be required if fixed dislocation or in chronic cases (Figs. 3 and 4).

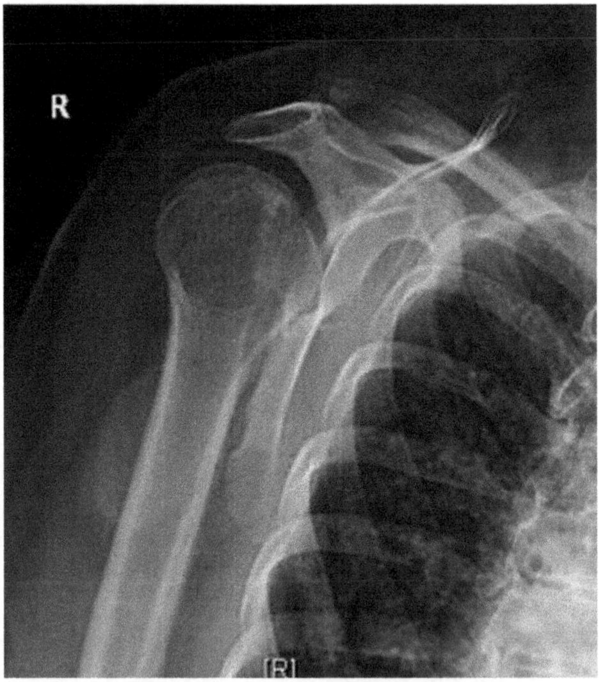

Fig. 3 Posterior dislocation—"lightbulb" sign

Fig. 4 Posterior dislocation—axillary view

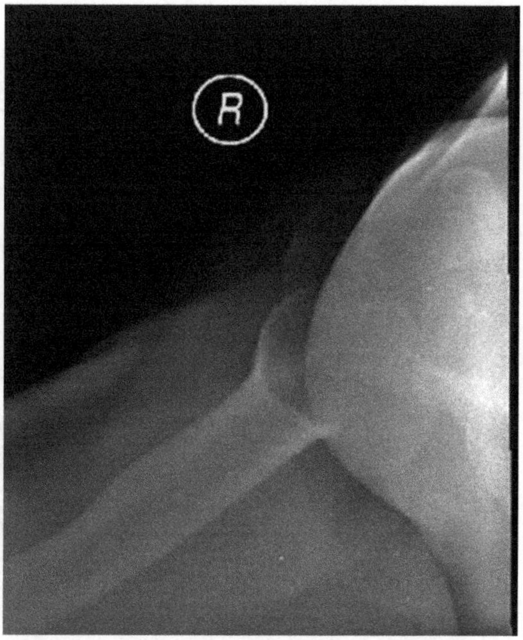

Closed reduction of luxatio-erecta (inferior dislocation)

- Adequate analgesia, conscious sedation, and muscle relaxation are essential with careful monitoring of respiratory depression resulting from excessive sedation.
- Intra-articular gleno-humeral lidocaine injection for analgesia.
- Two-step reduction converting inferior dislocation to anterior dislocation to reduction.
- *Patient:* supine.
- *Physician:* one hand on humeral shaft and the other on the medial condyle. The hand on the shaft initiates and anteriorly directed force rotating the humeral head from an inferior to anterior position. Adduct the humerus against the body. Humerus is then externally rotated reducing the humeral head into the glenoid fossa.

Post-reduction

- Obtain Grashey and axillary or Velpeau axillary views to confirm reduction (Fig. 5).
- Complete neurovascular examination to be compared to pre-reduction exam.
- Immobilize in a sling and swathe (for posterior dislocation immobilize in slight external rotation) (Fig. 6).
- Follow up with orthopedic surgeon within 1 week to discuss plan for early range of motion.

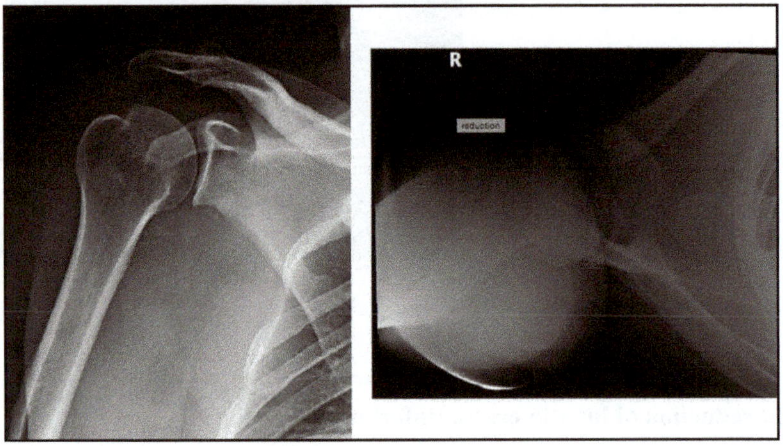

Fig. 5 AP and axillary view of reduced shoulder

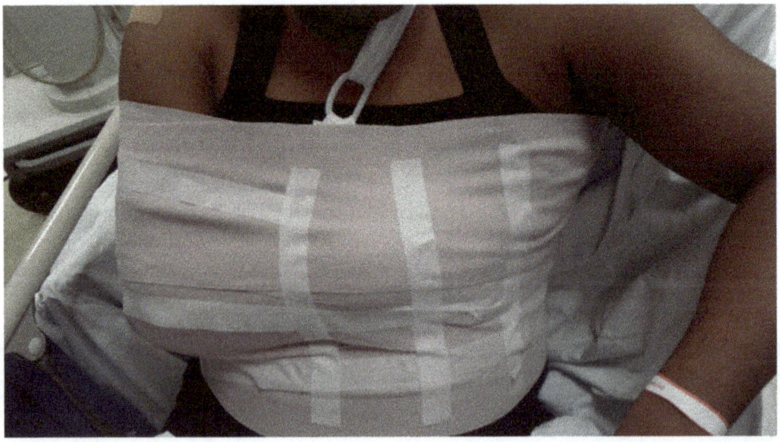

Fig. 6 Sling and swathe for shoulder immobilization

- Operative intervention in acute setting if dislocation is locked and irreducible OR fracture dislocation with possibility for further fracture propagation.
- Surgical intervention indicated in patients who may have recurrent instability, associated bone/soft-tissue loss.

References

Court-Brown CM, Heckman JD, McQueen MM, Ricci WM, Tornetta III P, editors. Rockwood and Green's fractures in adults. 8th ed. Philadelphia, PA: Wolter Kluwers Health/Lippincott Williams and Wilkins; 2015. McKee MD. (Assoc. Editor); Copyright © 2015.

Hovelius L, Olofsson A, Sandström B, Augustini BG, Krantz L, Fredin H, et al. Nonoperative treatment of primary anterior shoulder dislocation in patients forty years of age and younger. a prospective twenty-five-year follow-up. J Bone Joint Surg Am. 2008;90(5):945–52.

Nho SJ, Dodson CC, Bardzik KF, Brophy RH, Domb BG, MacGillivray JD. The two-step maneuver for closed reduction of inferior glenohumeral dislocation (luxatio erecta to anteriordislocation to reduction). J Orthop Trauma. 2006;20(5):354–7.

Orvets N, Parisien RL, Chung J, Murakami A, Li X. Acute versus delayed MRI imaging and associated pathology in traumatic shoulder dislocations.

Robinson CM, Howes J, Murdoch H, Will E, Graham C. Functional outcome and risk of recurrent instability after primary traumatic anterior shoulder dislocation in young patients. J Bone Joint Surg Am. 2006;88(11):2326–36.

Robinson CM, Jenkins PJ, White TO, Ker A, Will E. Primary arthroscopic stabilization for a first-time anterior dislocation of the shoulder. A randomized, double-blind trial. J Bone Joint Surg Am. 2008;90(4):708–21.

Proximal Humerus Fracture

Proximal humerus fractures often result from either high-energy injury in young patients or low-energy injury in older patients with osteopenia/osteoporosis. Treatment is often guided by displacement and angulation of fracture fragments. Most of these fractures in older patients can be treated nonoperatively in a sling.

Overview

- Occurring at or proximal to the surgical neck of the humerus.
- Second most common upper extremity fracture in patients over age 65 (more common in women).
- Over 90 % due to falls from standing height in patients >60 years of age.
- 90 % are isolated injuries (all age groups).

History

- What was the mechanism of trauma (low energy vs. high energy)?
- History of other prior fragility fractures indicating osteopenia/osteoporosis (distal radius, hip/IT, or vertebral compression fractures)?

Physical Exam

- Skin integrity (tenderness, ecchymosis—open fractures rare).
- Limited shoulder ROM due to pain.
- Distal UE neurovascular exam (Appendix A: UE neuro exam).

M.C. Makhni et al. (eds.), *Orthopedic Emergencies*,
DOI 10.1007/978-3-319-31524-9_28

- Axillary nerve function (most frequently affected nerve). * IMPORTANT *
  - Sensory: Hypoesthesia over deltoid suggests axillary nerve injury.
  - Motor: Deltoid function (shoulder abduction, or extension to test posterior deltoid).

Diagnosis

Imaging

- XR shoulder complete series:
  - Grashey view ("true AP" of the shoulder taken perpendicular to the plane of the scapula and parallel to the glenoid fossa).
  - Scapular-Y
  - Axillary (or Velpeau if unable to tolerate axillary).
- CT shoulder: often not necessary, but can assist with operative planning .

Classification

- Neer Classification (Fig. 1)
  - Four parts: greater tuberosity, lesser tuberosity, surgical neck, or anatomic neck.
  - Displacement defined as >1 cm or angulation ≥45° (.5 cm for greater tuberosity).
- Valgus impacted
- Risk factors of developing osteonecrosis (and therefore requiring arthroplasty in older patients):
  - >40–45° angulation.
  - 3–4-part fractures.
  - Head split component.
  - <8 cm of intact medial calcar (Figs. 2, 3, and 4).

Treatment Plan

Non-operative (Majority of Proximal Humerus Fractures)

- Indications
  - Stable, non-displaced, or minimally displaced fractures.
  - Elderly patients with low functional demand.

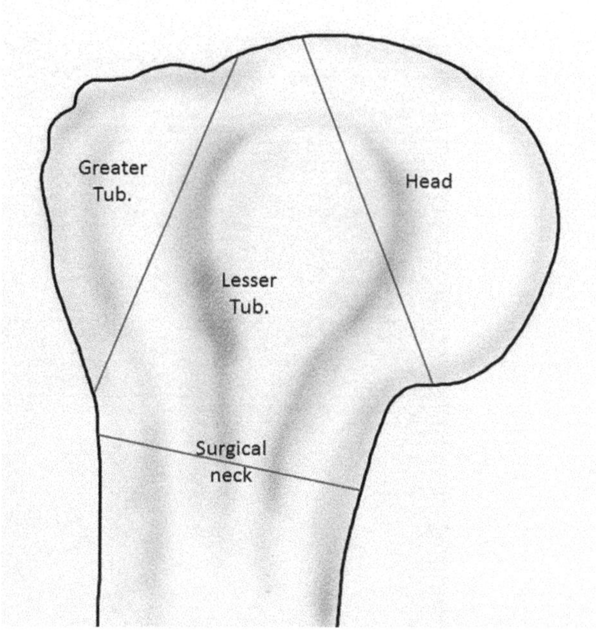

Fig. 1 Proximal humerus fractures

Fig. 2 Proximal humerus fracture—surgical neck

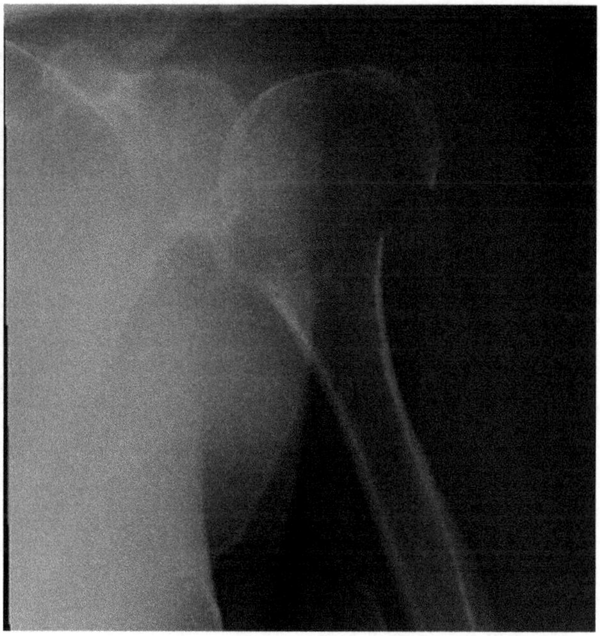

Fig. 3 Three-part proximal humerus fracture

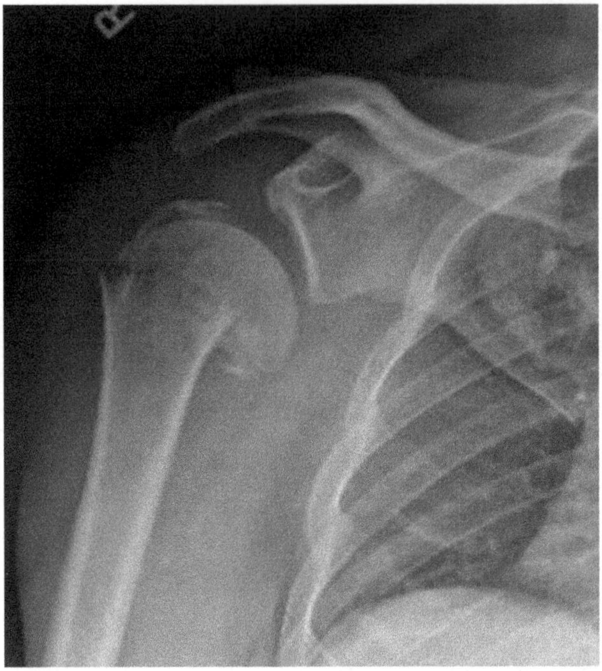

Fig. 4 Osteonecrosis after fixation of three-part proximal humerus fracture

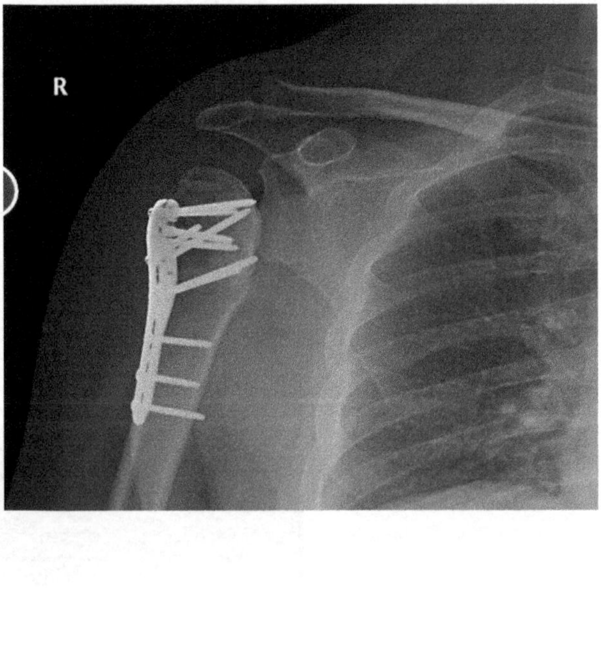

  - Valgus impacted.
    - Minimally displaced, two-part and three-part variants in the elderly.
- Treatment: Immobilization in sling for 4–6 weeks.
  - Frequent immediate active ROM of the elbow, wrist, and digits to prevent stiffness.
  - Periodic radiographs for the first 4 weeks.
  - Final radiographs at 3 months to confirm union.

Surgical (Majority Non-urgent, with Follow-Up Within 1 Week to Clinic)

- CRPP.
- ORIF.
  - Fractures in younger patients.
  - Greater tuberosity fractures that would heal above level of humeral head (and therefore cause impingement with abduction).
- Hemiarthroplasty (HA).
  - Three- and four-part fractures in older patients.
  - Head split fractures.
  - Requires anatomic reduction and healing of the tuberosities (to avoid impingement).
- Reverse total shoulder arthroplasty (RSA).
  - Complex three- and four-part fractures in the elderly, especially when tuberosity reduction and healing unlikely.

References

Court-Brown CM, Heckman JD, McQueen MM, Ricci WM, Tornetta III P, editors. Rockwood and Green's fractures in adults. 8th ed. Philadelphia, PA: Wolter Kluwers Health/Lippincott Williams and Wilkins; 2015. McKee MD. (Assoc. Editor); Copyright 2015.

Gupta AK, Harris JD, Erickson BJ, Abrams GD, Bruce B, McCormick F, et al. Surgical management of complex proximal humerus fractures-a systematic review of 92 studies including 4500 patients. J Orthop Trauma. 2015;29(1):54–9.

Jawa A, Yi PH, Boykin RE, Gardner MJ, Gerber C, Lorich DG, Walch G, Warner JP. The treatment of proximal humeral fractures: comparison of shoulder and trauma-trained surgeons. Am J Orthop. 2015.

Rangan A et al. Surgical vs. nonsurgical treatment of adults with displaced fractures of the proximal humerus: the PROFHER randomized clinical trial. JAMA. 2015;313(10):1037–47.

Clavicle Fracture

Following direct injury/blow to the clavicle or indirect through forces propagated through the shoulder girdle

Overview

Common injury in young, active patients
Can result from direct injury (blow to the lateral shoulder girdle) or from indirect injury (fall onto outstretched hand)

History

- Mechanism of injury? If high energy, will require full trauma survey to rule out any other internal or MSK injuries (i.e. ipsilateral shoulder girdle/scapula, chest/thorax/aortic root, etc.)
- Assess for any pain in neck, shoulder, or back

Physical Exam

- Assess for skin tenting, bony deformity, or open fracture
- Palpation: tenderness, crepitus/motion with gentle manipulation
- Limited shoulder ROM due to pain

M.C. Makhni et al. (eds.), *Orthopedic Emergencies*,
DOI 10.1007/978-3-319-31524-9_29

Diagnosis

Imaging

- XR: AP chest (showing bilateral clavicles to assess for shortening) and 45° cephalic tilt view of injured clavicle

Classification

- Allman classification with Neer modifications (based on anatomic location)
- **Group I:** Fracture of middle third (Fig. 1)
  - Most common (~80 %)
- **Group 2:** Fracture of distal third (~10–15 %) (Fig. 2–4)
  - Often displaced, higher rate of nonunion (28–44 %)
  - Subclassification based upon relative location of fracture to CC ligaments (conoid and trapezoid)
  - *Type 1*: Lateral to CC ligaments. Proximal fragment stabilized by CC ligaments
  - *Type 2*: Medial to CC ligaments. Proximal fragment no longer stabilized by CC ligaments (medial clavicle unstable)
    - *2A*: Fracture medial to conoid ligament
    - *2B*: Fracture lateral to conoid and medial to trapezoid

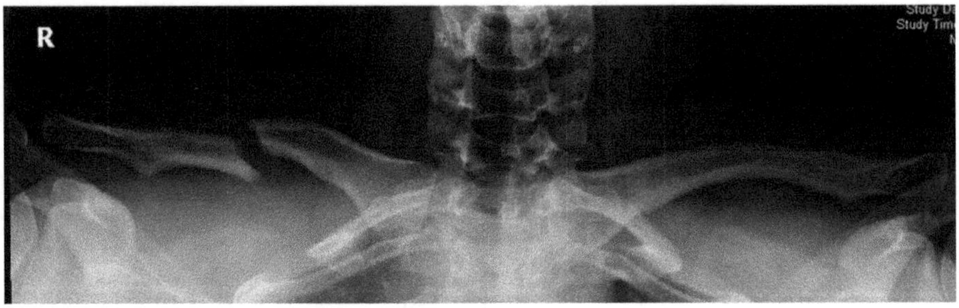

Fig. 1 Displaced right midshaft clavicle fracture

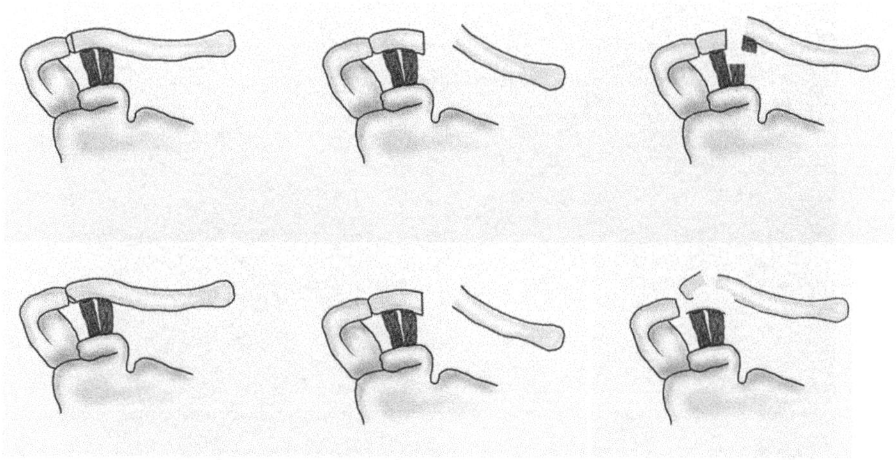

Fig. 2 Type 1, 2a, 2b, 3, 4, and 5 Clavicle Fractures

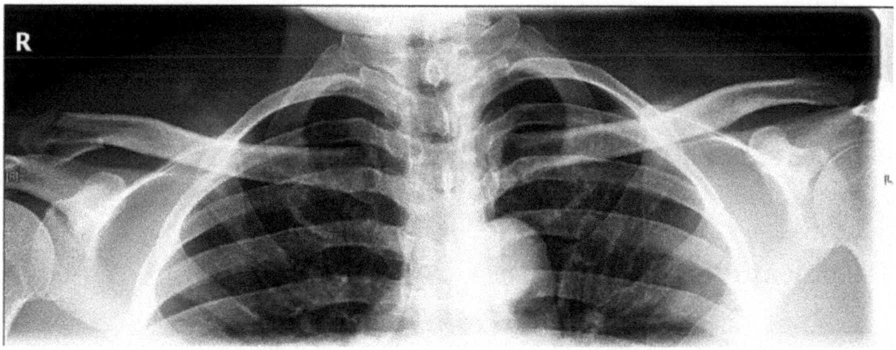

Fig. 3 Minimally displaced right distal clavicle fracture

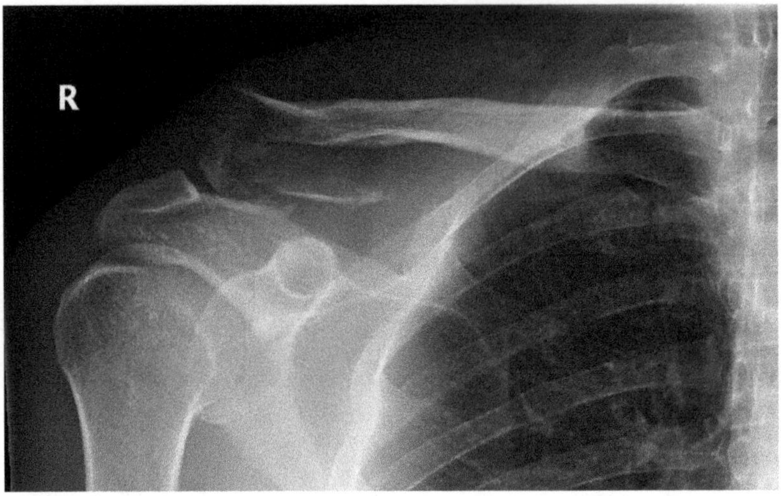

Fig. 4 Displaced right distal clavicle fracture

  - *Type 3*: Lateral to CC ligaments but extend into the AC joint
  - *Type 4*: Through physis (skeletally immature)
  - *Type 5*: Comminuted fracture, ligaments maintained to comminution (medial clavicle unstable)

- **Group 3:** Fracture of proximal third (~2–10 %)

Treatment Plan

Limited strength of evidence supporting operative treatment for displaced fractures. For displaced midshaft fractures, some studies suggest that surgery leads to improved endurance, as well as lower nonunion or symptomatic malunion, as well as quicker time to radiographic union and earlier return to function.

Non-operative

- Indications Group 2 (Types 1, 3, and 4), Group 3
- Treatment: Sling 2 weeks for comfort, NWB, with gentle ROM as tolerated
- Active ROM of elbow, wrist, and hand immediately to prevent stiffness

Surgical

- Urgent only if open fracture, threatened/tented skin, or a vascular injury
- Indications:
  - Group 1: Consider for >2 cm of shortening, 100 % displacement, or patient preference
    - Treatment: ORIF (most common) vs. intramedullary fixation
  - Group 2: Type 2 and type 5 are inherently unstable and may benefit from surgery (limited evidence proving superiority of surgical over non-operative treatment)
    - Treatment: ORIF and/or CC ligament reconstruction
    - Emergent operative reduction and stabilization for Group 3 injuries with posterior displacement with airway or vascular compromise (to be done with thoracic surgeon present)
- Relative indications: Floating shoulder, polytrauma, painful malunion/nonunion

References

Allman Jr FL. Fractures and ligamentous injuries of the clavicle and its articulation. J Bone Joint Surg Am. 1967;49:774–84.

Banerjee R, Waterman B, Padalecki J, Robertson W. Management of distal clavicle fractures. J Am Acad Orthop Surg. 2011;19(7):392–401.

Jeray K. Acute midshaft clavicle fracture. J Am Acad Orthop Surg. 2007;15(4):239–48.

Acromioclavicular (AC) Joint Injury

AC injuries are very common following a fall onto the superolateral shoulder. These injuries range from sprains of the joint to instability of the ligamentous complex.

Overview

Fall onto superolateral shoulder drives acromion inferior to clavicle with disruption of AC ligaments as body weight displaces clavicle superiorly (most common).

A fall on the outstretched hand or elbow translate force to the AC joint and capsule causing similar disruption.

History

- Mechanism of injury?

Physical Exam

- Skin tenting (types III, V)
- Tender at AC joint
- Painful cross-body adduction
- Assess SC joint for ipsilateral injury
- Palpate coracoid to r/o coracoid fracture
- Palpate other bony structures of upper extremity to rule out additional fractures

M.C. Makhni et al. (eds.), *Orthopedic Emergencies*,
DOI 10.1007/978-3-319-31524-9_30

Diagnosis

Imaging/X-rays

- True shoulder AP
- Axillary lateral (rule out type IV, evaluate coracoid)
- Bilateral Zanca view (10–15° cephalad) to evaluate C-C distance (normal 1.1–1.3 cm) and compare with contralateral

*Tip: An AC dislocation with an intact C-C distance represents a coracoid fracture with intact C-C ligaments. Imaging to better assess coracoid: Axillary lateral, Stryker notch, CT scan.

Classification

Rockwood Classification [*Mnemonic: 1,2,3 PSI*]

I: Sprain
II: CC distance <25 % longer than contra-lateral side.
III: CC distance 25–100% longer than contra-lateral side (Fig. 1)
IV: Posterior clavicle displacement through trapezius fascia
V: Superior clavicle displacement 100–300 %, *irreducible*
VI: Inferior clavicle displacement (rare)

Treatment Plan

Non-operative

- Type I, II. Type III (controversial)
- Immobilization for 1–2 weeks in sling or shoulder immobilizer followed by gradual rehabilitation

Surgical

- Types IV, V, VI. Type III (controversial)

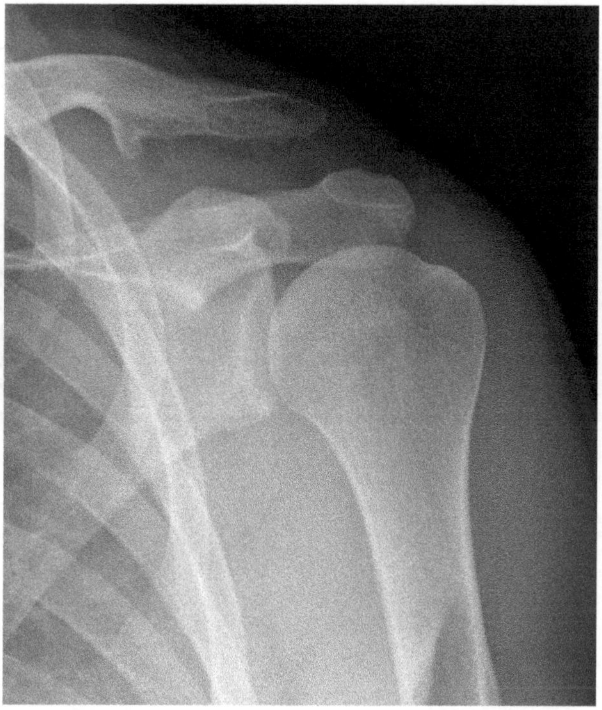

Fig. 1 Type III AC injury

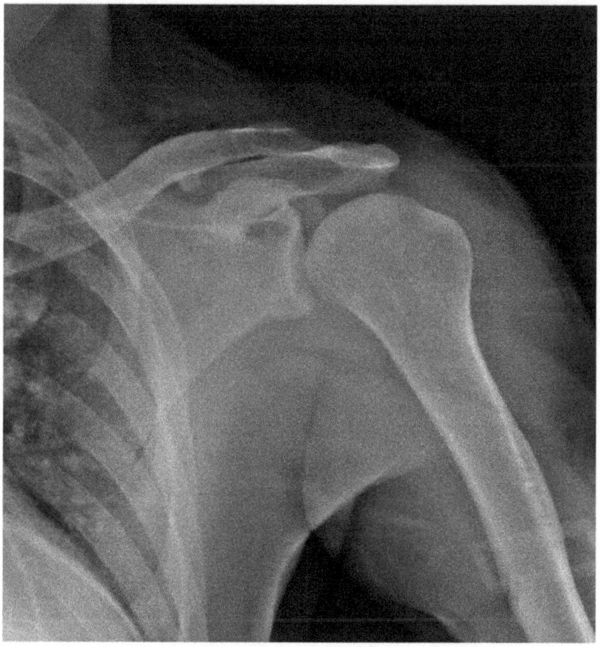

Fig. 2 CC ligament reconstruction for type III AC injury

- Multiple options for surgical fixation which entails CC ligament reconstruction. This includes allograft reconstruction, internal bracing constructs, and other modalities (Fig. 2)

References

Beitzel K, Mazzocca AD. Shoulder dislocations (acromioclavicular and sternoclavicular), Ch 49. In: The American Society for Surgery of the Hand textbook of hand and upper extremity surgery. Chicago: The American Society for Surgery of the Hand; 2011.

Simovitch R, Sanders B, Ozbaydar M, Lavery K, Warner JJ. Acromioclavicular joint injuries: diagnosis and management. J Am Acad Orthop Surg. 2009 Apr;17(4):207–19.

Williams Jr GR, Nguyen VD, Rockwood Jr CA. Classification and radiographic analysis of acromioclavicular dislocations. Appl Radiol. 1989;18:29–34.

Sternoclavicular (SC) Joint Injury

SC injuries can vary greatly in terms of clinical significance, with anterior dislocations often being well tolerated while posterior dislocations being life threatening.

Overview

In patients younger than 20–25 years, injury to the SC joint may actually represent a displaced physeal fracture and not a dislocation.

Commonly a high-energy injury with direct force to anteromedial clavicle (posterior dislocation) or an indirect lateral force to the shoulder (anterior or posterior dislocation).

History

- Mechanism of injury?
- Associated symptoms (particularly respiratory, difficulty swallowing, or neurovascular)?
- Prior occurrence?

Physical Exam

- Trauma eval (Appendix A)
  - A,B,Cs: posterior dislocation can result in life-threatening mediastinal injury. Dyspnea, dysphagia, or hoarseness suggest esophageal or tracheal injury

M.C. Makhni et al. (eds.), *Orthopedic Emergencies*,
DOI 10.1007/978-3-319-31524-9_31

while ipsilateral neck or upper extremity venous congestion indicates compression of the subclavian vessels.
  - Thorough neurovascular exam of ipsilateral upper extremity to evaluate for vascular and brachial plexus injury.

- UE eval (Appendix A).
- Significant swelling often makes clinical assessment of anterior or posterior displacement difficult.
- Assess AC joint to rule out ipsilateral injury.

Diagnosis

Imaging /X-rays

- Serendipity view (40° cephalic centered at sternum) to assess displacement.
- CT scan: indicated to differentiate sprains from dislocations and assess for mediastinal injury.
- MRI: in children if suspected physeal injury.

Classification

- I: Mild sprain. Ligaments intact.
- II: Moderate sprain. Disruption of sternoclavicular ligaments, intact costoclavicular ligament. Asymmetry on exam.
- III: Dislocation. Disruption of sternoclavicular and costoclavicular ligaments.

Treatment

- Anterior dislocations—generally treated non-operatively. Consider surgery in patients with chronic disease and unable to tolerate cosmetic deformity or in those with persistent pain. May need shoulder sling in acute period with early transition out of sling and to ROM/rehab.
- Posterior dislocation—Needs reduction (emergently if any airway or neurovascular compromise).
  - Reduction should be attempted in operating room.
  - Should be performed with thoracic surgeon in the room.

- Can try non-operative with arm abduction and traction and usually towel clip at clavicle to assist with reduction of the posterior SC joint.
- If irreducible, may require open reduction.

References

Allman Jr FL. Fractures and ligamentous injuries of the clavicle and its articulation. J Bone Joint Surg Am. 1967;49:774–84.

Beitzel K, Mazzocca AD, Shoulder dislocations (acromioclavicular and sternoclavicular). The American Society for Surgery of the Hand Textbook of Hand and Upper Extremity Surgery, Ch 49.

Groh GI, Wirth MA. Management of traumatic sternoclavicular joint injuries. J Am Acad Orthop Surg. 2011;19:1–7.

Septic Arthritis of the Shoulder

The shoulder is a rare site for septic arthritis, which may affect the glenohumeral, acromioclavicular, or sternoclavicular joints. Hosts often have multiple medical comorbidities and present with pain, fevers, and local signs of inflammation.

History

- Risk Factors:
  - Immunocompromised (HIV, immunosuppressant medications, chemotherapy)
  - IV drug abuse
  - Renal dialysis
  - Infected subclavian central lines

Physical Exam

- Inability to tolerate range of motion (particularly glenohumeral septic joint)
- Local erythema, warmth, swelling, tenderness
- Incisions from recent surgery

Diagnosis

Imaging

- XR: often normal
- MRI/ultrasound: assess for effusion

M.C. Makhni et al. (eds.), *Orthopedic Emergencies*,
DOI 10.1007/978-3-319-31524-9_32

Labwork/Aspiration

- Elevated systemic labs (WBC, ESR, CRP)
- Joint Aspiration (gold standard for diagnosis). * IMPORTANT *
  - Total cell count (#WBC>50,000 along with PMN shift)
  - Gram stain/culture

Treatment Plan

- Almost always require urgent/emergent operative washout (arthroscopic versus open)
- Consider serial bedside aspiration/lavage for:
  - Critically ill patients (i.e., widespread sepsis, significant medical comorbidities)
  - Smaller joint sepsis (e.g., AC)
- Thoracic consultation for SC joint septic arthritis
- Ideally begin antibiotics AFTER aspiration
  - Begin with broad coverage and then tailor as sensitivities return

References

Auerbach CE, Klingenstein GG, Flatow EL. Septic arthritis of the glenohumeral joint: a review of 23 cases. J Surg Orthop Adv. 2005;14(2):102–7.

Bossert M, Prati C, Bertolini E, Toussirot E, Wendling D. Septic arthritis of the acromioclavicular joint. Joint Bone Spine. 2010;77(5):466–9.

Ross JJ, Shamsuddin H. Sternoclavicular septic arthritis: a review of 180 cases. Medicine. 2004;83(3):139–48.

Glenoid and Scapula Fracture

Fractures of the scapula are uncommon and usually the result of high-energy injury. Fracture sites can include the scapular body, scapular neck, and glenoid, along with the acromion or coracoid (Fig. 1).

Overview

Often the result of high-energy injury and localized to scapular body and spine.

Commonly associated with rib, spine, and clavicle fractures, along with injury to the chest wall.

History

- Injury mechanism
- Concomitant respiratory, neurovascular symptoms
- Other sites of pain

M.C. Makhni et al. (eds.), *Orthopedic Emergencies*,
DOI 10.1007/978-3-319-31524-9_33

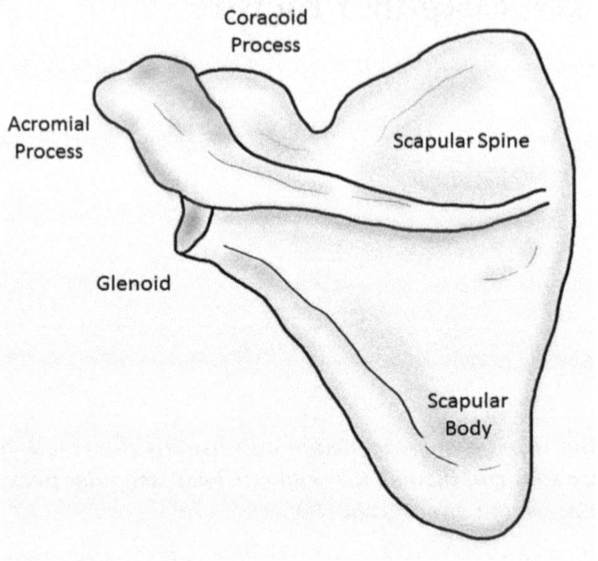

Fig. 1 Osteology of the scapula

Physical Exam

- Comprehensive trauma survey to rule out concomitant injury to the chest wall, spine, head, abdomen
- Perform thorough upper extremity neurovascular exam to rule out associated ipsilateral injury

Diagnosis

Imaging/XRs

- XR: Dedicated scapular views to assess body/neck
- XR: Full trauma X-rays to rule out associated injury (Fig. 2)
- CT: Often requires thin-slice CT with 3-D reconstruction to adequately assess and characterize the extent of the fracture (Fig. 3)
  - Of particular importance is extent into, and displacement of, articular surface of the glenoid

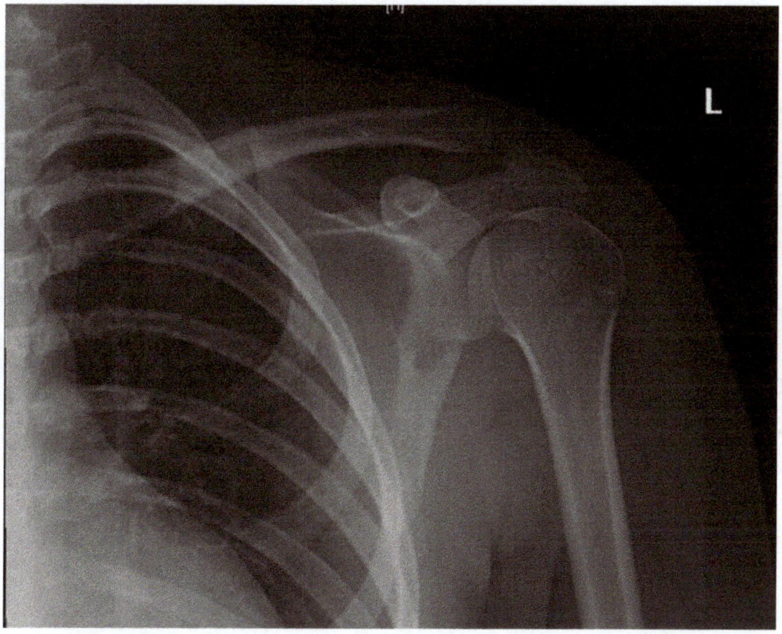

Fig. 2 Scapula fracture

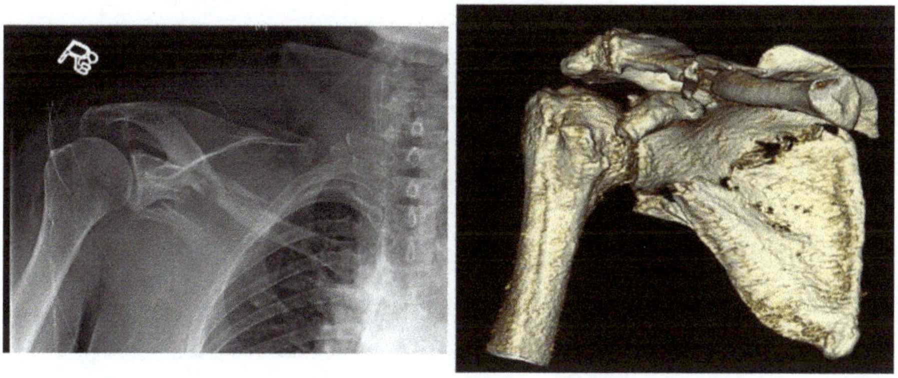

Fig. 3 Scapula/clavicle fracture (floating shoulder)

Treatment Plan

Non-operative

- Hallmark of treatment
- Sling usually sufficient while bone heals

Surgical

- If significant displacement of articular surface or of scapular body
  - Usually done after acute phase of injury
- Consider for floating shoulder, brachial plexus injury

References

Cole PA, Gauger EM, Schroder LK. Management of scapular fracture. J Am Acad Orthop Surg. 2012;20:130–41.

Goss TP. Scapular fractures and dislocations: diagnosis and treatment. J Am Acad Orthop Surg. 1995;3:22–33.

Humerus Shaft Fracture

Humeral shaft fractures can often initially be treated non-operatively given that the humerus can tolerate a large amount of deformity without a loss of function.

Overview

Radial nerve entrapment with spiral fractures at distal 1/3 humerus shaft (Holstein-Lewis).

History

Injury mechanism?
Associated neurologic symptoms?
If low energy, history of other prior fragility fractures indicating osteopenia/osteoporosis (distal radius, hip, or vertebral compression fractures)?

Physical Exam

Examine skin for open wounds consistent with open fracture.
UE neurologic exam (Appendix A), special attention to radial nerve examination.

M.C. Makhni et al. (eds.), *Orthopedic Emergencies*,
DOI 10.1007/978-3-319-31524-9_34

Diagnosis

Imaging

XR humerus: AP and transthoracic lateral (Figs. 1 and 2)
XR shoulder: AP and axillary
XR elbow: AP and lateral

Classification

By location (proximal, middle, and distal third) and fracture pattern (spiral, oblique, transverse)

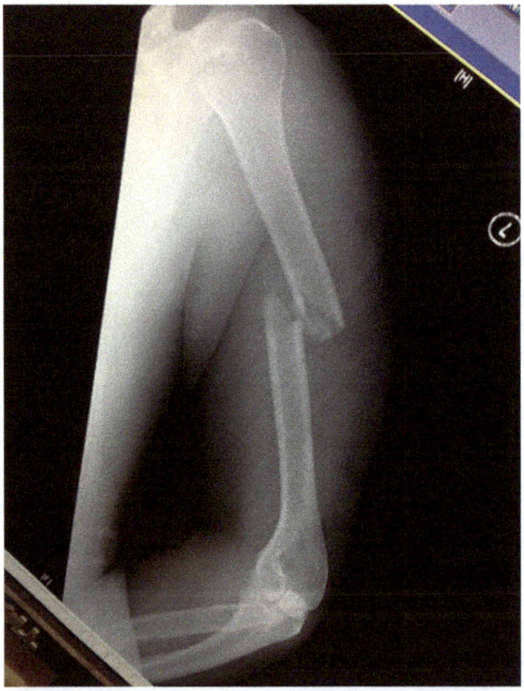

Fig. 1 AP of humerus shaft fracture

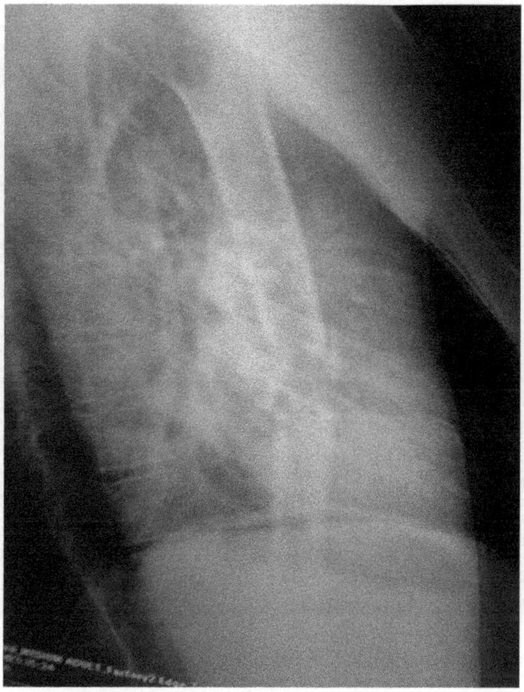

Fig. 2 Trans-thoracic lateral of humerus shaft fracture

Treatment Plan

Non-operative

Indications:

Maximum acceptable displacement (based on historical criteria) (Fig. 3):

3 cm shortening.
20° anterior angulation.
30° varus angulation.

Risk of nonunion higher with gapping at fracture site, transverse fracture, or proximal ⅓ shaft fracture.

Technique:

Immobilization in a coaptation splint (Fig. 4).

Valgus mold (typical deformity is varus).
Allow gravity to align fracture.

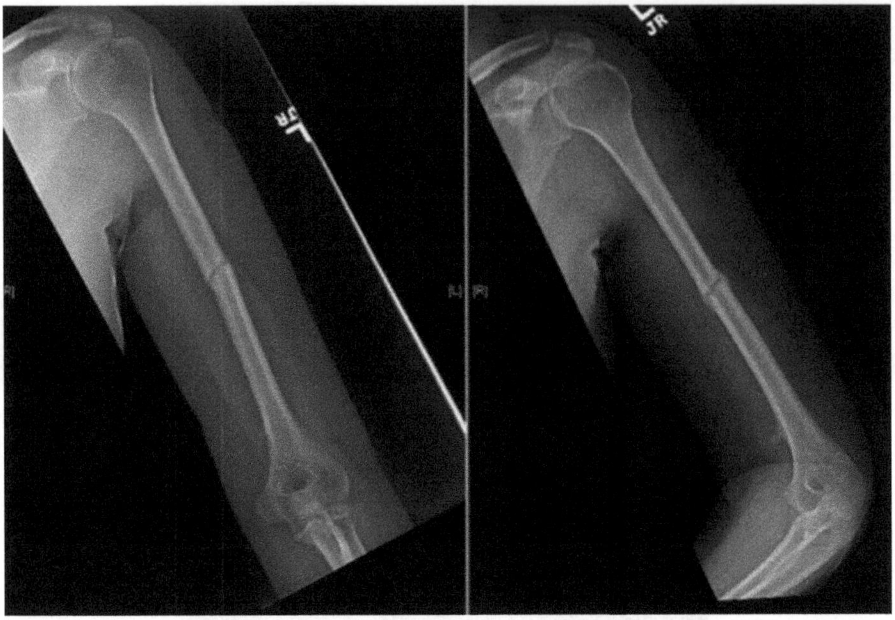

Fig. 3 Progressive healing of humeral shaft fracture

Fig. 4 Humerus shaft fracture in coaptation splint

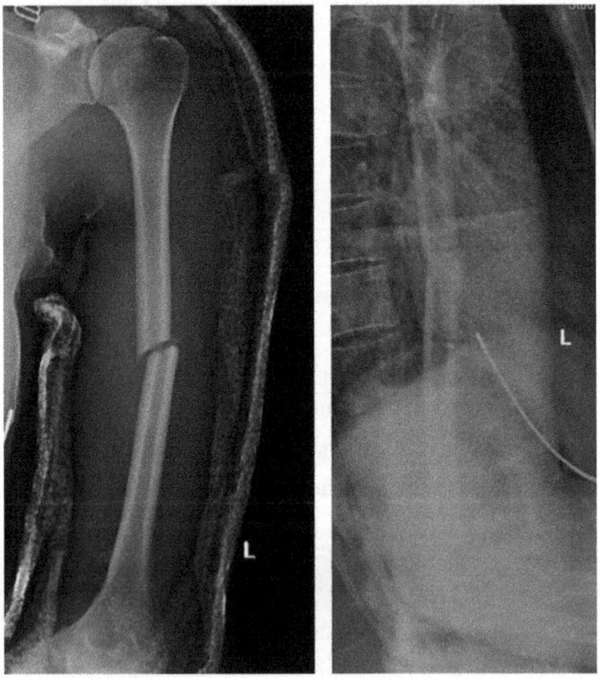

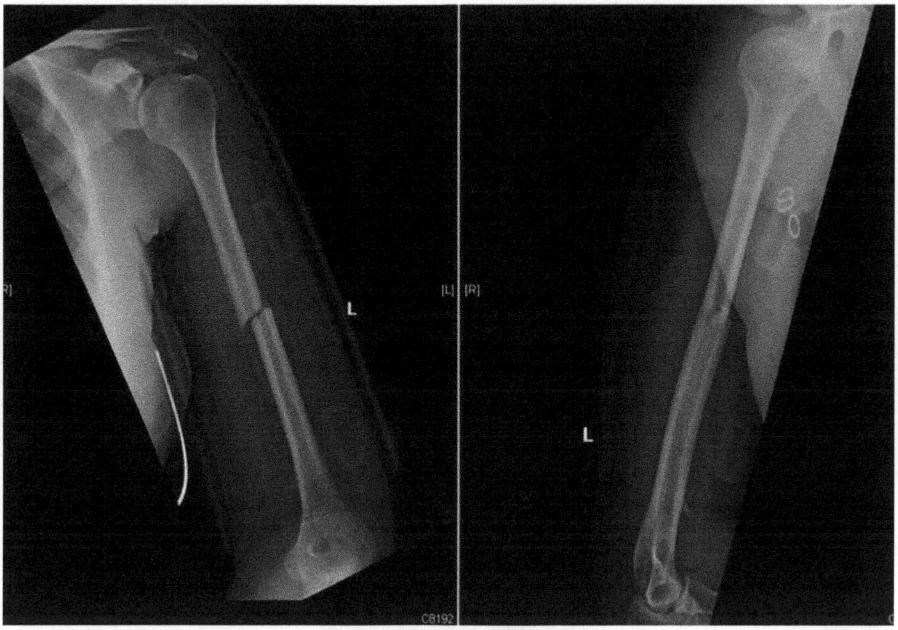

Fig. 5 Humerus shaft fracture transitioned into Sarmiento brace

Transition to functional brace (e.g.: "Sarmiento brace") in 5–7 days when swelling improves (Fig. 5).

Time to union: average 3mo for closed fractures, but can take up to 40 weeks.

Surgical

Treatment options: external fixation, intramedullary nailing, and open reduction internal fixation with plating.

ORIF with lower complication and reoperation rate, and lower shoulder impingement that IMN.

Consider IMN for pathologic fracture, or patient with morbid obesity or soft tissue compromise.

Absolute Indications:

- Open fracture.
- Vascular injury.

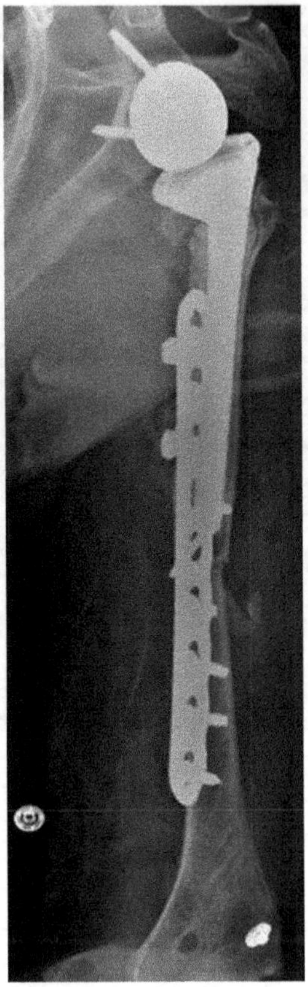

Fig. 6 ORIF of peri-prosthetic humerus shaft fracture

  - Brachial plexus injury.
  - Ipsilateral forearm fracture (floating elbow).

Relative Indications:

  - Bilateral humerus fractures or polytrauma patient.
  - Soft-tissue injuries that prevent non-operative management.
  - Failure of non-operative management.
- Pathologic fracture

*Note: nerve palsy alone is NOT an indication for surgery.

References

Carroll EA, Schweppe M, Langfitt M, Miller A, Halcorson JJ. Management of humeral shaft fracture. J Am Acad Orthop Surg. 2012;20:423–33.

Distal Humerus Fractures

Very often intra-articular, these fractures present clinical challenges when they occur in young patients. When in elderly patients, options range from non-operative treatment to internal fixation and even arthroplasty.

Overview

Bimodal incidence—common in young males secondary to high-energy trauma and elderly women secondary to low-energy fall.
Position of elbow at the moment of impact determines fracture type:

Elbow flexed <90° → transcolumnar extra-articular fracture
Elbow flexed >90° → intercondylar fracture
Direct posterior blow → olecranon fracture +/− distal humeral involvement

Must rule out associated injuries: elbow dislocation, terrible triad elbow injury, floating elbow, forearm compartment syndrome.
Full return of pre-injury elbow AROM unlikely.
Goal of treatment is to restore elbow AROM to perform daily functional activities (comb hair, brush teeth, feed oneself)—need to flex elbow 30–130°.

History

- Injury mechanism?
- Pre-existing elbow pain or arthritis?
- Prior elbow trauma?

M.C. Makhni et al. (eds.), *Orthopedic Emergencies*,
DOI 10.1007/978-3-319-31524-9_35

Physical Exam

UE neurovascular exam (Appendix A)
Avoid ROM testing given gross instability of fracture and potential for neurovascular injury
Compartment checks

Diagnosis

Imaging

- XR: humerus, elbow, and forearm (Fig. 1)
  - For comminuted fractures, traction view is especially helpful in delineating fracture pattern (Fig. 2)
- CT: helpful for surgical planning (Fig. 3)

Classification

Descriptive:

1. Comminution
2. Extra-articular versus intra-articular
3. Supracondylar, distal single-column (radial or ulnar), or distal both-column
4. If intra-articular extension, identify fragments for operative planning: capitellum/lateral trochlea, lateral epicondyle, posterolateral epicondyle, posterior trochlea, and medial trochlea/epicondyle.

Milch classification (single-column fractures)

1. Intact lateral trochlear ridge
2. Fractured lateral trochlear ridge

Jupiter classification (two-column fractures)

High T (transverse proximal to olecranon fossa)
Low T (transverse proximal to trochlea)
Y (bilateral exit of proximal fractures)
H (free trochlea fragment)
Medial lambda (medial exit of proximal fracture)
Lateral lambda (lateral exit of proximal fracture)

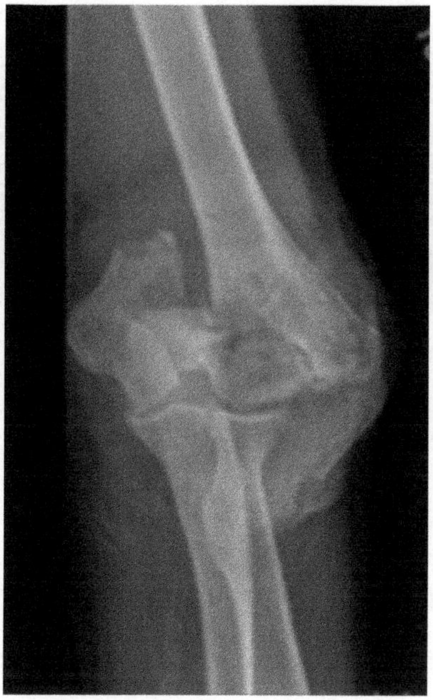

Fig. 1 Comminuted distal humerus fracture

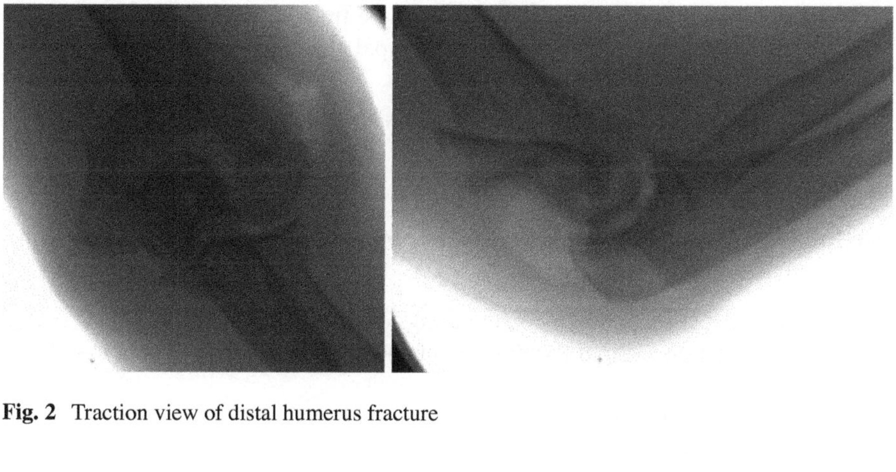

Fig. 2 Traction view of distal humerus fracture

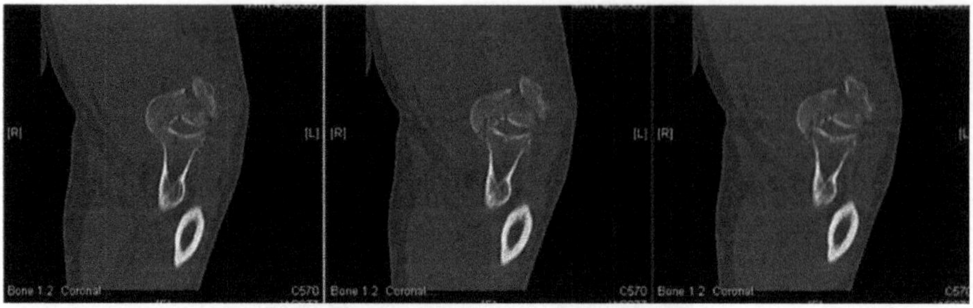

Fig. 3 CT scan—distal humerus fracture

Treatment Plan

Non-operative

Indication: non-displaced single-column fracture with intact lateral trochlea ridge (Milch I)
Treatment: long-arm cast and sling

1. Flex elbow 70–90°, forearm in neutral rotation
2. Well padded around bony prominences of elbow
3. Immobilize in supination for lateral condyle fracture
4. Immobilize in pronation for medial condyle fracture
5. Ensure cast does not extend past metacarpal heads volarly

Operative (Most Common)

Indication: supracondylar, displaced Milch I, Milch II, and both-column (Fig. 4)
Treatment: depends on fracture type

1. Closed reduction percutaneous pinning for displaced Milch I
2. Open reduction internal fixation for supracondylar, Milch II, and both-column (Fig. 5)
3. Consider total elbow arthroplasty for both-column fractures in elderly patients with poor bone stock

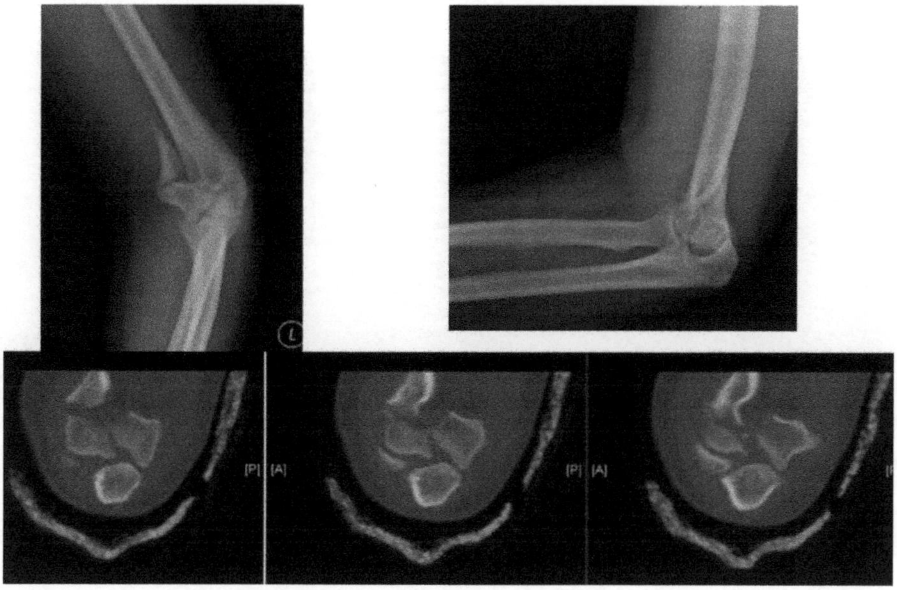

Fig. 4 Bicolumnar distal humerus fracture in a young patient

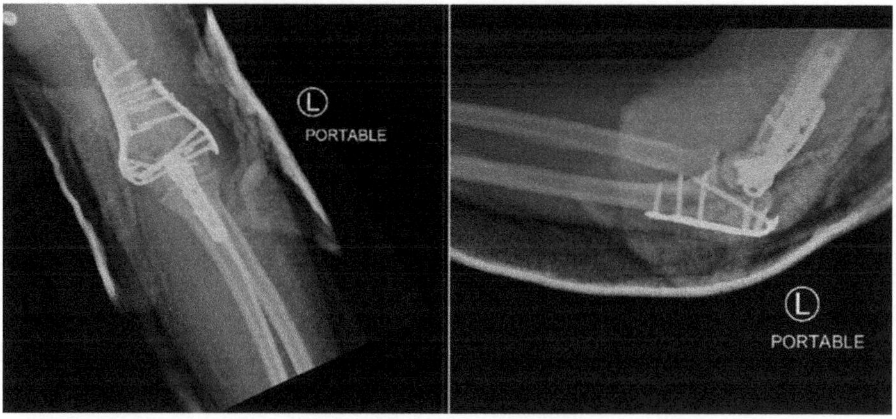

Fig. 5 Surgical fixation of bicolumnar distal humerus fracture

References

Galano GJ, Ahmad CS, Levine WN. Current treatment strategies for bicolumnar distal humerus fractures. J Am Acad Orthop Surg. 2010;18(1):20–30.

Olecranon Fracture

Olecranon fractures usually result from a direct trauma to the elbow. They may result in a variety of different fracture patterns that ultimately govern treatment strategy.

Overview

The fracture pattern often dictates the ultimate treatment rendered. Four common types of olecranon fractures are: transverse, oblique, comminuted, and trans-olecranon fracture dislocation.

History

Injury mechanism?

Physical Exam

Visualize for gross deformity.
Thorough skin evaluation—rule out open fracture given subcutaneous location. * IMPORTANT *
Ability to actively extend elbow against gravity (vs. just passively extending with gravity).
UE neurovascular exam (Appendix A).

M.C. Makhni et al. (eds.), *Orthopedic Emergencies*,
DOI 10.1007/978-3-319-31524-9_36

Diagnosis

Imaging

Elbow XR: AP and lateral (true lateral most important to determine fracture pattern (Fig. 1).

Classification

Multiple classification schemes exist. However, the following three descriptive factors are most important and will guide treatment:

1. Displacement
2. Comminution
3. Fracture pattern: Avulsion, transverse, or oblique

Be wary of the trans-olecranon fracture-dislocation, in which the distal humerus is driven through the olecranon (this is different from a simple transverse fracture and impacts type of fixation needed during surgery) (Fig. 2).

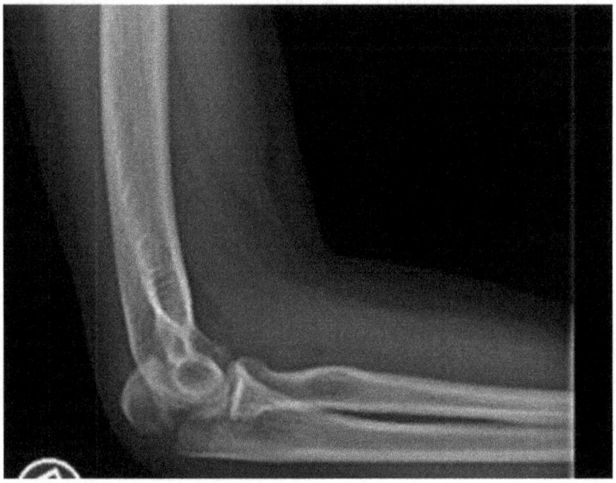

Fig. 1 Transverse olecranon fracture

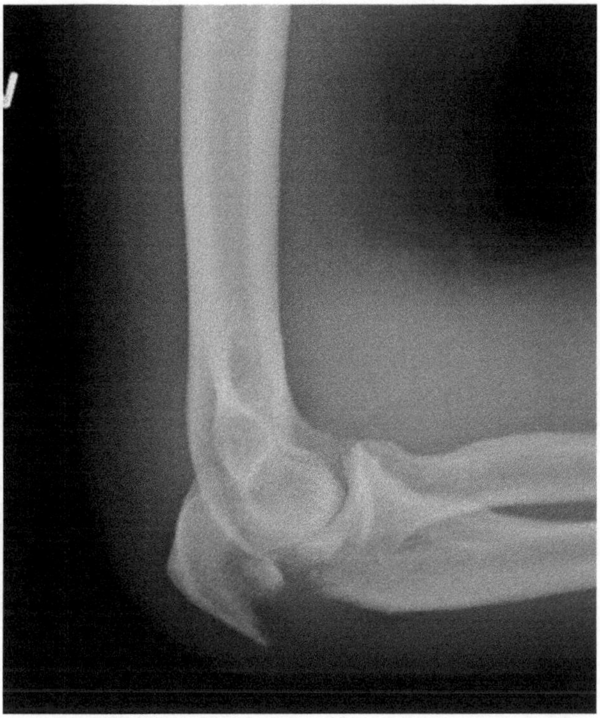

Fig. 2 Trans-olecranon fracture-dislocation

Treatment

Non-operative

Indication

1. Non-displaced fracture
2. Displaced fracture in low-demand elderly patient

Treatment: Long-arm well-padded posterior plaster splint in neutral rotation and sling immobilization

1. Immobilize in 60–90° of flexion for 4 weeks then begin ROM

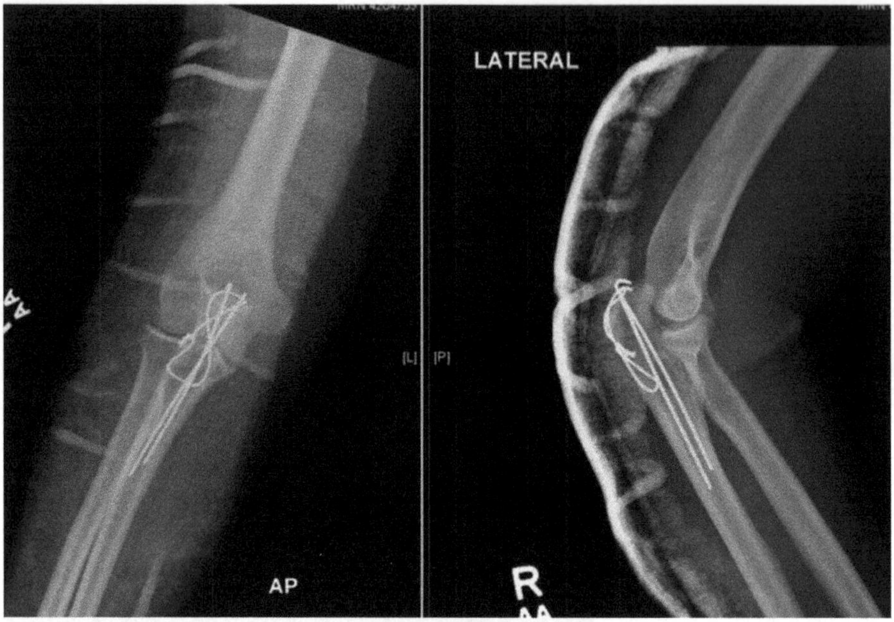

Fig. 3 Olecranon fracture treated with tension-band technique

Surgical

Treatment: Tension band technique (Fig. 3)
Indication: Transverse fracture with no comminution

Indication: Oblique fracture, comminuted fracture, or fracture dislocation (e.g.: trans-olecranon)
Treatment: Open reduction internal fixation with plate and screws

Indication: Non-union, elderly patient with osteoporotic bone (Fig. 4)
Treatment: Fragment excision with triceps advancement (fracture must involve <50 % of joint surface)

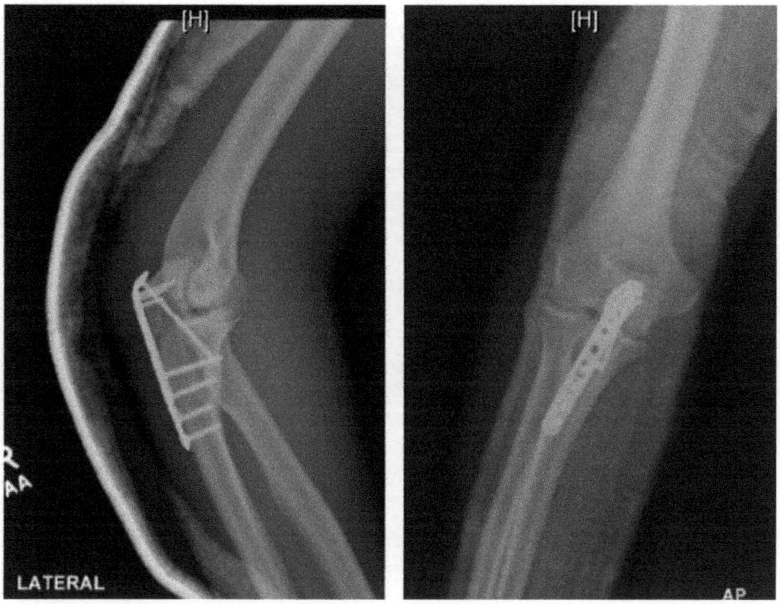

Fig. 4 Olecranon fracture treated with plate and screws

References

Hak DJ, Golladay GJ. Olecranon fractures: treatment options. J Am Acad Orthop Surg. 2000;8(4):266–75.

Rouleau DM, Sandman E, van Riet R, Galatz LM. Management of fractures of the proximal ulna. J Am Acad Orthop Surg. 2013;21(3):149–60.

Duckworth AD, Bugler KE, Clement ND, Court-Brown CM, McQueen MM. Nonoperative management of displaced olecranon fractures in low-demand elderly patients. J Bone Joint Surg Am. 2014;96(1):67–72.

Radial Head Fracture

A fracture of radial head is the most common fracture around the elbow and is often non-operative if there is no dislocation and no block to motion. A key to treatment success is early motion.

Overview

- Often due to fall onto outstretched pronated hand with axial force directed across elbow.
- Isolated or with associated injuries (complex elbow dislocation, coronoid fracture, MUCL or LUCL injury, interosseous membrane disruption, DRUJ injury, carpal fractures).

History

- Did you feel that your elbow dislocated or "popped back in"?
- Do you have pain in your forearm, wrist, or shoulder?
- Dominant elbow/ability to care for self?

Physical Exam

- Skin integrity, assess for deformity.
- Likely effusion.
- Tenderness, often lateral elbow or throughout.

M.C. Makhni et al. (eds.), *Orthopedic Emergencies*,
DOI 10.1007/978-3-319-31524-9_37

- AROM.
  - Flexion/extension (90° arc).
  - Pronation/supination (100° arc). *IMPORTANT*
- If limited due to pain, and swelling, consider aspiration/injection prior to ROM to assess if true mechanical block to motion.
- Varus/valgus stress test.
- Thorough UE assessment as well as distal neurovascular exam (Appendix A: UE neuro exam).

Diagnosis

Imaging

- Elbow XR: AP, lateral
  - If posterior fat pad sign on lateral with no visualized fracture, treat as non-displaced fracture.
- Elbow XR: optional radiocapitellar "radial head" view.
  - Neutral forearm rotation, 45° cephalad beam angle.
  - Better visualization of radial head.
- XR forearm, r/o elbow fx/dislocation (coronoid, ligamentous).
- CT Elbow: if comminuted/displaced fracture, for surgical planning

Mason Classification

1. Minimally displaced articular surface <2 mm (nonsurgical); Mason I (Fig. 1).
2. Partial articular, displaced >2 mm; Mason II.
3. Comminuted, displaced, mechanical block to motion (surgical); Mason III (Figs. 2, and 3)

Aspiration/Injection

- If displacement/block to ROM.
  - Difficult to assess due to pain and effusion.
  - Can aspirate joint under sterile conditions and inject with local anesthetic to facilitate range of motion during exam.

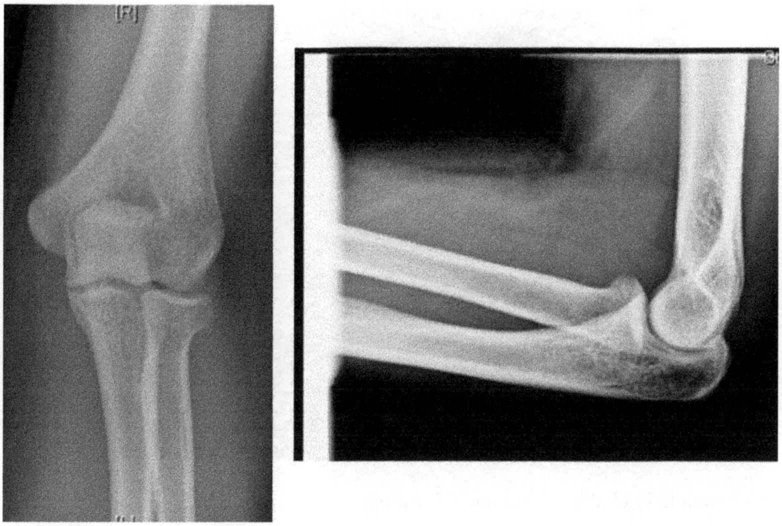

Fig. 1 Minimally displaced radial head fracture

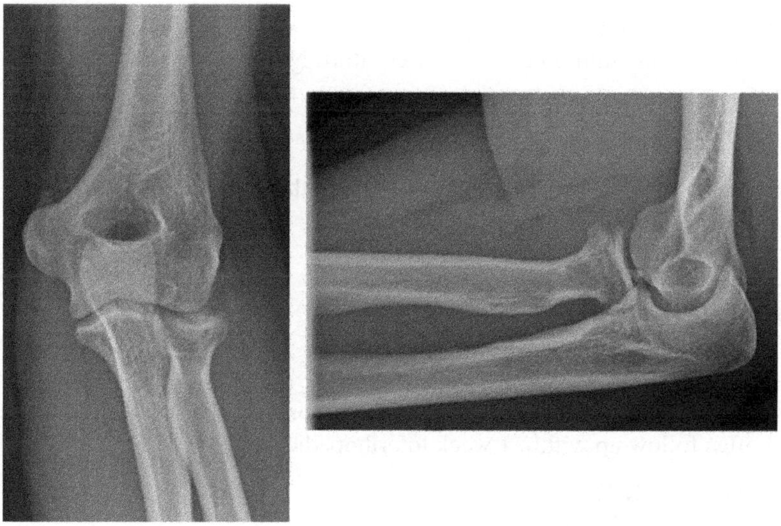

Fig. 2 Comminuted radial head fracture

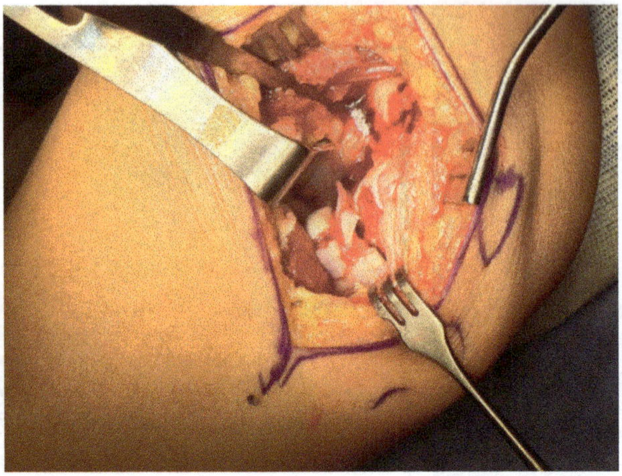

Fig. 3 Comminuted radial head fracture—intra-op

Treatment

Non-operative

- Indications: Mason type 1.
- Treatment: Sling immobilization for comfort, NWB.
  - 3–5 days then initiate ROM.
  - Stiffness if longer.
- Hematoma aspiration ± injection of local anesthetic.

Surgical

- Indication: Mason 3 (Mason 2 debatable).
- Usually non-urgent (unless open fx or other concerning associated injuries) and can often follow up within 1 week to orthopedic surgeon.
  - 2 parts → ORIF.
  - 3+ parts → radial head arthroplasty (Fig. 4).
  - Mason type 2 fragment with <25 % surface area of radial head → fragment excision.
  - Low-demand, sedentary patient with persistent pain from isolated fracture → head resection (rare).

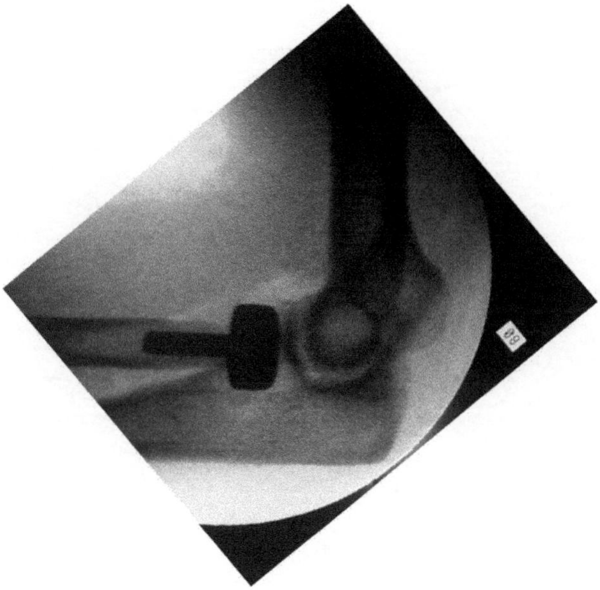

Fig. 4 Radial head replacement

References

McGuigan FX, Bookout CB. Intra-articular fluid volume and restricted motion in the elbow. J Shoulder Elbow Surg. 2003;12 (5).

Pike JM. Radial head fractures – an update. J Hand Surg Am. 2009;34(3).

Ring D, Quintero J, Jupiter JB. Open reduction and internal fixation of fractures of the radial head. J Bone Joint Surg Am. 2002;84-A(10):1811–5.

Tejwani NC, Mehta H. et al. Fractures of the radial head and neck: current concepts in management. J Am Acad Orthop Surg, 2007;15(7).

Elbow Dislocation

Elbow dislocation is the second most common type of joint dislocation (following shoulder dislocation). They can commonly occur with simultaneous bony and ligamentous injury and prompt, concentric reduction is paramount.

Overview

Named according to direction of displacement of distal fragment
Most common type is posterolateral dislocation, resulting from axial, valgus, and supination at the elbow
Posterolateral dislocations result from lateral to medial injury (LCL → MCL)
A "terrible triad" describes an elbow dislocation with concomitant radial head fracture and coronoid fracture

History

Injury mechanism?
Did the elbow reduce?
Any other sites of pain/discomfort?

Physical Exam

Visualize skin integrity and evaluate for gross deformity (Fig. 1)
UE neurovascular exam (Appendix A)
Avoid ROM testing given gross instability of fracture and potential for neurovascular injury

M.C. Makhni et al. (eds.), *Orthopedic Emergencies*,
DOI 10.1007/978-3-319-31524-9_38

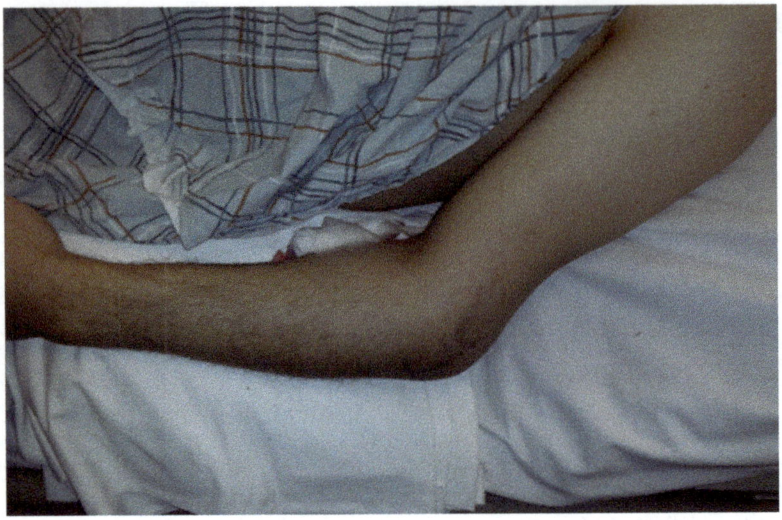

Fig. 1 Physical appearance—posterior elbow dislocation

Diagnosis

Imaging

XR elbow: AP and lateral (AP helps identify congruency of radiocapitellar joint and true lateral needed to assess ulnohumeral congruity) (Fig. 2)
XR elbow: oblique views optional (help assess fractures)

Classification

There are two components to describing elbow dislocations.

1. Describe direction of dislocation (relative position of ulna to olecranon)
2. Determine whether it is simple (no associated fracture) or complex (has associated fracture)
3. Terrible triad injuries consist of elbow dislocation, radial head fracture, and coronoid fracture

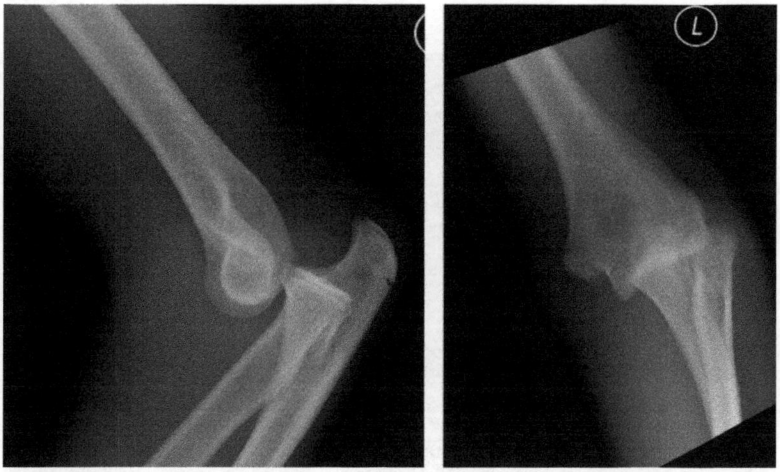

Fig. 2 X-ray of posterior elbow dislocation

Treatment

Initial Management

1. Sterile intra-articular block
2. Many different types of reduction maneuvers, e.g., longitudinal traction, extension at elbow, followed by subsequential manipulation at olecranon
3. Posterior mold splint
4. Post-splint X-ray to confirm concentric reduction and assess for associated fractures (Fig. 3)

Non-operative Treatment

Indication: acute simple dislocation with no instability after reduction
Treatment: long-arm posterior plaster splint in 70–90° of flexion

1. Splint elbow in pronation if only LCL complex disrupted. Splint elbow in supination if LCL complex and MCL disrupted
2. Only immobilize for 7–10 days
3. Initiate early supervised physical therapy/occupation therapy to work on ROM

Indication: acute simple dislocation with varus-valgus instability after reduction
Treatment: hinged elbow brace 90° of flexion

1. Immobilize elbow in pronation if only LCL complex disrupted. Immobilize elbow in supination if LCL complex and MCL disrupted
2. Immobilize for 2–3 weeks

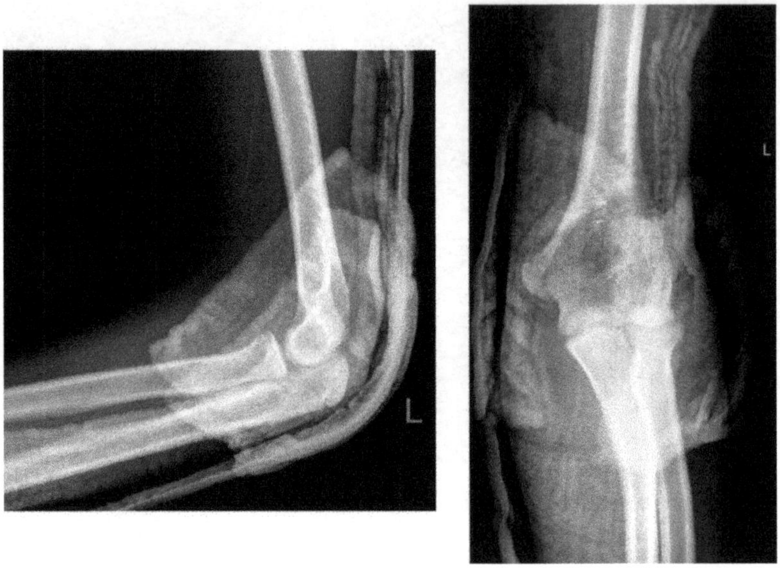

Fig. 3 X-ray of reduced elbow dislocation

Operative Treatment

Indications:

1. Mechanical block to closed reduction
2. Persistent instability following closed reduction
3. Acute complex dislocation

Treatment:

1. Open reduction internal fixation of coronoid, olecranon, or radial head as needed, LCL complex repair, +/− MCL repair (for terrible triad injuries)

   Approach(es) dictated associated elbow injuries that need to be addressed (options include posterior, lateral, and medial approaches; combinations of approaches may also be needed).

   LCL complex may be repaired or reconstructed. Common extensor tendon origin may also be avulsed and require repair.

   Elbow should be examined with valgus stress intraoperatively following LCL repair/reconstruction. If valgus instability persists, then MCL repair/reconstruction is needed (Figs. 4 and 5).

Indication: chronic elbow dislocations
Treatment: open reduction + capsular release + dynamic hinged elbow fixator

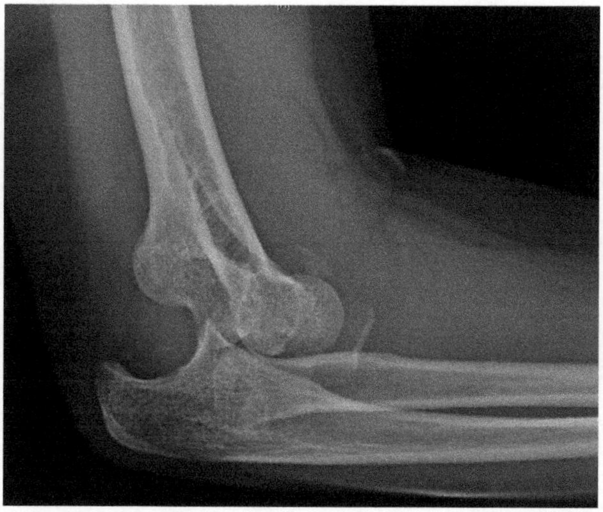

Fig. 4 Terrible triad injury: posterior elbow dislocation, coronoid fracture, and radial head fracture

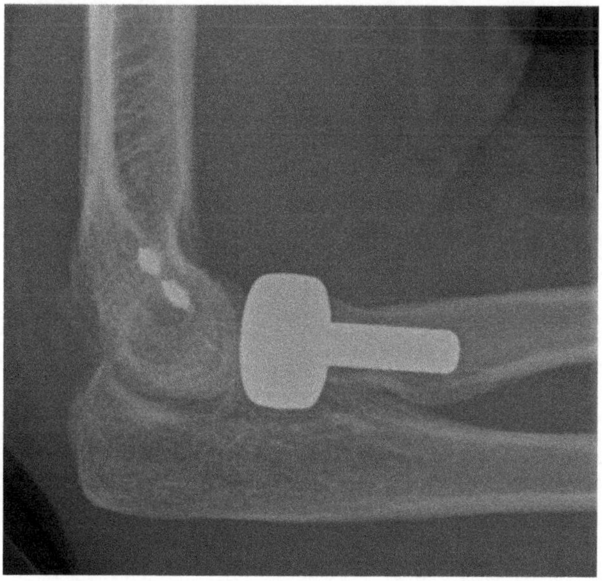

Fig. 5 Terrible triad injury treatment: radial head replacement and LCL repair

Reference

Mathew PK, Athwal GS, King GJ. Terrible triad injury of the elbow: current concepts. J Am Acad Orthop Surg. 2009 Mar;17(3):137–51.

Coronoid Fracture

These fractures usually present with elbow instability. The precise location of the fracture corresponds to specific types of instability.

Overview

Osteology of Coronoid

1. Coronoid tip: Intra-articular structure; fracture may contribute to instability.
2. Coronoid process: Serves as anterior buttress to prevent posterior dislocation; anteromedial facet: critical for varus and posteromedial rotatory stability; site of sublime tubercle (= insertion of medial UCL) (Fig. 1).
3. Coronoid base: Fracture through this area would remove anterior buttress function.

Injury Combinations:

Terrible triad elbow injury: Elbow dislocation + radial head fracture + transverse coronoid fracture.

Posterolateral rotatory instability: LCL Injury + radial head fracture + coronoid tip fracture.

Posteromedial rotatory instability: LCL injury + anteromedial facet coronoid fracture.

Olecranon fracture-dislocation: Elbow dislocation + trans-olecranon fracture + basal coronoid fracture.

M.C. Makhni et al. (eds.), *Orthopedic Emergencies*,
DOI 10.1007/978-3-319-31524-9_39

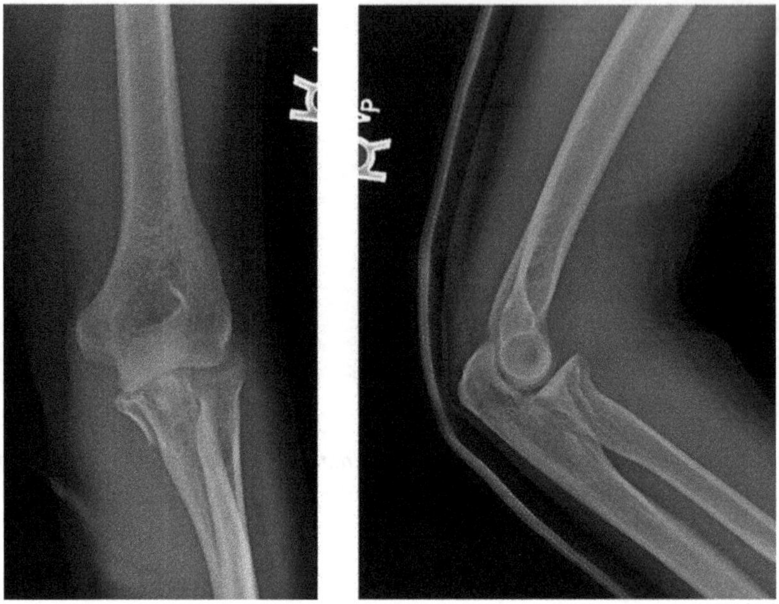

Fig. 1 Anteromedial coronoid fracture

History

Injury mechanism?
Was there a dislocation event?
Any other sites of pain/discomfort?

Physical Exam

Inspect for skin integrity and gross deformity.
UE neurovascular exam (Appendix A).
Avoid ROM testing given gross instability of fracture and potential for neurovascular.

Diagnosis

Imaging

XR elbow: AP and lateral.
CT elbow: If suspicious for coronoid fracture but indeterminate XRs, evaluate extent of injury for surgical planning.

Classification

Although other classification systems exist (notably O'Driscoll), Regan and Morrey Classification is used most often (Table 1). Usually the best way to classify these fractures (and also indicate the level of instability involved) would be descriptive based on location (tip, process, anteromedial facet, bases).

Treatment

Non-operative

Indication: Minimally displaced coronoid fracture (<2 mm) with no elbow instability.
Treatment: Long-arm posterior plaster splint in neutral rotation and sling immobilization. Only immobilize for 3–5 days, then discontinue splint/sling, and begin elbow ROM.

Operative

Indication: Displaced fracture at any level, associated elbow instability.
Treatment: Open reduction internal fixation.

Initial management with long-arm plaster splint with sling. Typically, single posterior slab splint with forearm in neutral rotation is applied.
Encourage wrist and finger of ROM.
Elective surgical fixation.

Table 1 Regan and Morrey classification

Type	Description
I	Coronoid process tip fracture
II	Coronoid fracture 50 % or less of height
III	Coronoid fracture greater than 50 % of height

Reference

Steinmann SP. Coronoid process fracture. J Am Acad Orthop Surg. 2008;16:519–29.

Elbow Capitellar Fracture

These rare fractures often require surgical fixation in order to restore elbow motion and function.

Overview

Fracture at the lateral distal humerus and in the coronal plane
Result often from fall onto outstretched hand

History

Injury mechanism?
Any other sites of pain/discomfort?

Physical Exam

UE neurovascular exam (Appendix A)

M.C. Makhni et al. (eds.), *Orthopedic Emergencies*,
DOI 10.1007/978-3-319-31524-9_40

Diagnosis

Imaging

XR elbow: AP and Lat of elbow (look for "double bubble" sign) (Fig. 1)
CT: further evaluation of fracture, and for surgical planning

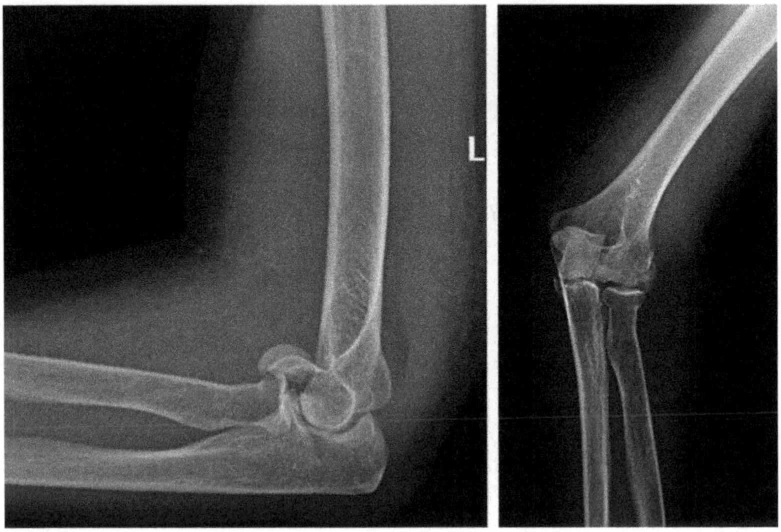

Fig. 1 Capitellum fracture "double bubble sign"

Classification (Table 1)

*Although multiple eponyms involved, this fracture classification does determine treatment.

Treatment

Non-operative

Indication: minimally displaced (<2 mm) type I or type II fractures
Treatment: long-arm posterior plaster splint in neutral rotation and sling immobilization

Immobilize 2–3 weeks then begin elbow ROM

Table 1 Capitellum fracture classification

Type	Description
I	Single large fragment that may include trochlea
II	Kocher-Lorenz fracture: Shear fracture of articular cartilage
III	Broberg-Morrey fracture: Severely comminuted capitellum fracture
IV	McKee fracture: Coronal shear fracture of capitellum and trochlea

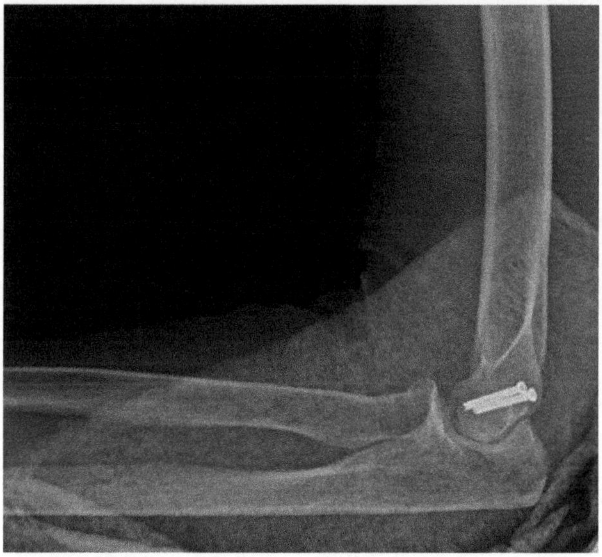

Fig. 2 Fixation of capitellum fracture

Operative

Initial management still consists of long-arm well-padded posterior plaster splint

Indication: Displaced (>2 mm) type I fracture, type IV fracture

Treatment: Open Reduction Internal Fixation (Fig. 2)

Indication: Displaced (>2 mm) type II or type III fractures

Treatment: Fragment Excision

Indication: Inability to reconstruct capitellar fracture in elderly patient with concurrent medial column instability

Treatment: Total Elbow Arthroplasty

Reference

Ruchelsman DE, Tejwani NC, Kwon YW, Egol KA. Coronal plane partial articular fractures of the distal humerus: current concepts in management. J Am Acad Orthop Surg. 2008;16(12):716–28.

Radius and Ulna Shaft Fractures

The radius and ulna articulation is treated as an articular joint; therefore, anatomic reduction is necessary in order to restore pro/supination.

Overview

Can occur in isolation or together as a "both-bone fracture."
Must rule out injury at the elbow (radial head fracture/dislocation) and wrist (DRUJ).
Radial bow must be restored for proper joint kinematics (pro/supination).

History

- Injury mechanism?
- Pre-existing elbow pain or arthritis?
- Prior elbow trauma?

Physical Exam

High-energy injuries should be evaluated for compartment syndrome.
Rule out associated nerve injury.

M.C. Makhni et al. (eds.), *Orthopedic Emergencies*,
DOI 10.1007/978-3-319-31524-9_41

Diagnosis

Imaging

- XR: forearm, elbow, and wrist.
  - Galeazzi fracture—distal 1/3 radial shaft fracture with DRUJ disruption.
  - Monteggia fracture—proximal ulna shaft fracture with radial head dislocation.
  - "Nightstick" fracture is isolated fracture of ulna diaphysis.
- Advanced imaging not routinely utilized (Figs. 1 and 2).

Treatment Plan

Non-operative

Indication: non-displaced or minimally displaced isolated ulna shaft fracture.
Treatment: in acute setting, may place in ulnar gutter short-arm splint.

Definitive treatment in functional brace (which can also be applied in acute setting provided no concerns for skin injury or significant swelling, etc.).

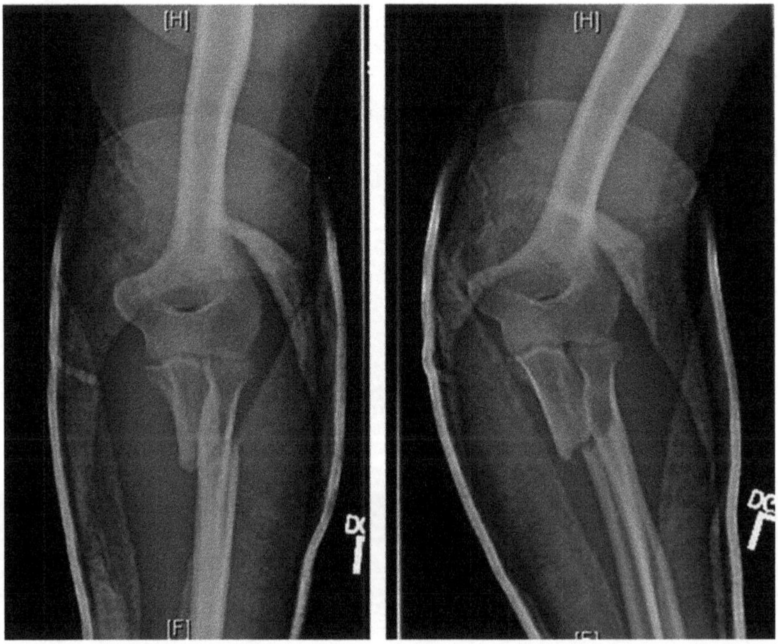

Fig. 1 Proximal ulnar fracture

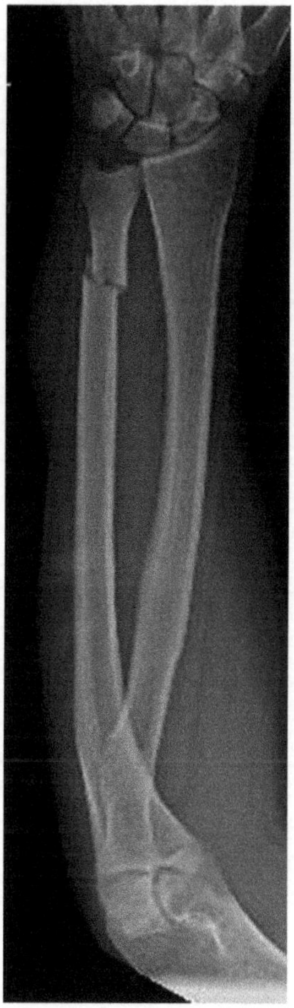

Fig. 2 Distal ulna fracture

Operative

Indication: displaced ulna shaft fractures, proximal 1/3 ulna fractures, all radial shaft fractures (in order to restore radial bow), both-bone fractures.
Treatment: ORIF.

Reference

Sarmiento A, Latta LL, Zych G, McKeever P, Zagorski JP. Isolated ulnar shaft fractures treated with functional braces. J Orthop Trauma. 1998;12(6):420–3.

Part V
Wrist and Hand

Stephanie Gancarzyk, Robert Parisien, and Joseph Lombardi

Distal Radius Fracture 183

DRUJ Injury 189

Carpal Fracture (Excluding Scaphoid) 193

Scaphoid Fracture 201

Scapholunate Instability 205

Perilunate Dislocation 209

Tendon Lacerations 215

Finger Fractures and Dislocations 221

Digit Amputations 231

Foreign Bodies in the Hand and Wrist 237

Hand Infections 239

Distal Radius Fracture

Distal radius fractures are one of the most common fragility fractures in patients who are elderly or osteopenic. They also occur in high-energy injuries in younger patients.

Overview

May have associated injuries that warrant further investigation (DRUJ, radial styloid)

Many fracture classifications exist, but main radiographic measurements focus on involvement of ulnar styloid, presence of dorsal cortical comminution, articular incongruity (gap, step-off), radial inclination, and ulnar variance

Several studies have shown that nonoperative management of displaced, dorsally angulated distal radius fractures (Colles type) is equivalent to surgical management; however, articular shear fractures, complex intra-articular fractures, and those in younger patients warrant consideration for surgery

Mainstay of management in the ER is closed reduction and sugar-tong splinting

History

FOOSH (fall onto outstretched hand) in elderly or osteopenic patients

Higher energy injury in younger patients

Must rule out concomitant carpal tunnel syndrome

Prior fragility fractures?

M.C. Makhni et al. (eds.), *Orthopedic Emergencies*,
DOI 10.1007/978-3-319-31524-9_42

Physical Exam

Visual inspection for alignment and open fracture presence
Detailed neurovascular hand examination, must rule out acute carpal tunnel syndrome

Diagnosis

Imaging/Wrist X-Rays

AP wrist X-rays will demonstrate degree of articular incongruity, radial inclination, and ulnar variance (Fig. 1).
Lateral wrist X-rays will demonstrate tilt in the sagittal plane (dorsal angulation), along with dorsal comminution (Fig. 2).

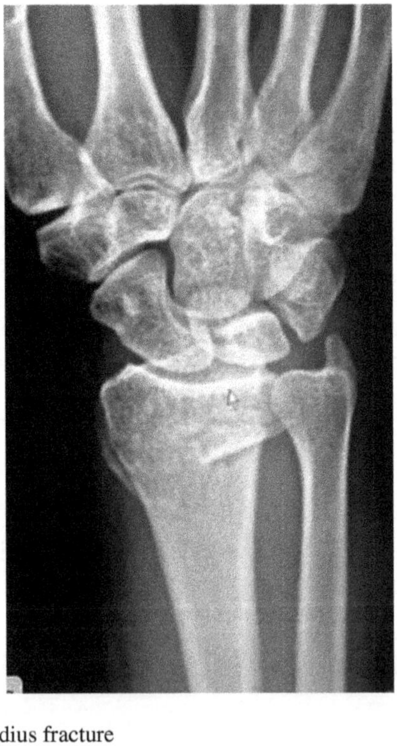

Fig. 1 AP view—distal radius fracture

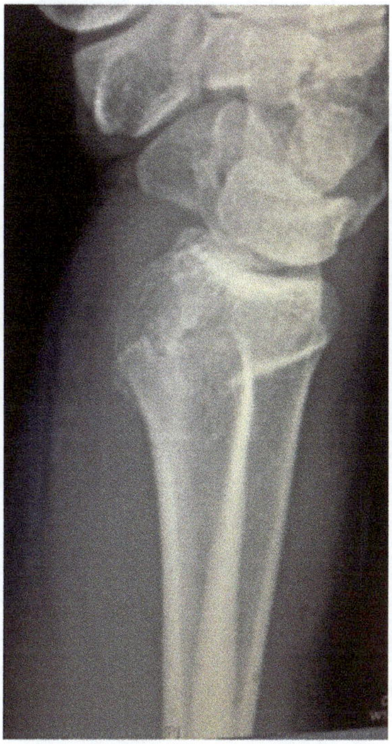

Fig. 2 Lateral view—distal radius fracture

Classification Systems

Several different types of classification systems, but ability to describe fracture is most important

Adequate description includes presence or absence of ipsilateral bony injuries (radial styloid, ulnar styloid, trans-scaphoid injuries), ligamentous injuries (DRUJ disruption), and fracture characteristics (comminution? Alignment of carpus on radius? Shear component? Displacement with respect to articular incongruity, tilt, and inclination?)

Treatment

Nonoperative

Indication:

- Fractures with acceptable post-reduction alignment (dorsal tilt <10°, radial shortening <3 mm, and intra-articular step-off and displacement <2 mm)

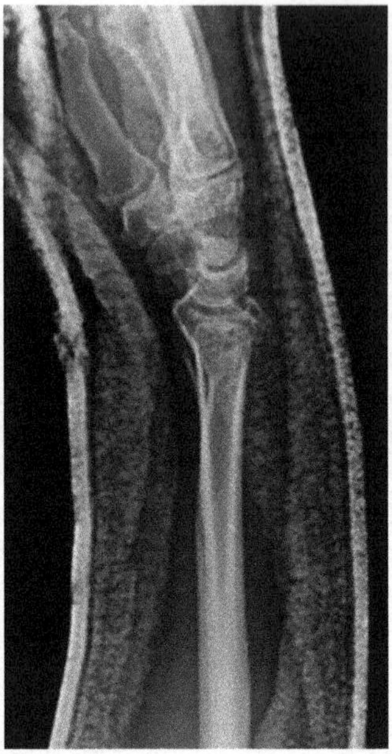

Fig. 3 Sugar tong splint—distal radius fracture

- Fracture in patient >55yrs old (ample literature suggesting that fracture reduction in dorsally angulated fractures do not correlate to functional outcomes in these patients)

Treatment:

Closed reduction (hematoma block, exaggeration of deformity, maintenance of reduction with sugar tong splint, support with sling). Curved immobilization helps maintain alignment (Fig. 3)

For non-displaced fractures in older patients (with minimal risk of subsequent swelling), can consider short arm cast

Surgical

Indication:

- Acute surgery for evolving neurological symptoms, carpal tunnel syndrome
- Open injury
- Extensive soft tissue injury/fracture comminution/displacement
- Displaced fracture in younger patient
- Unstable shear fracture

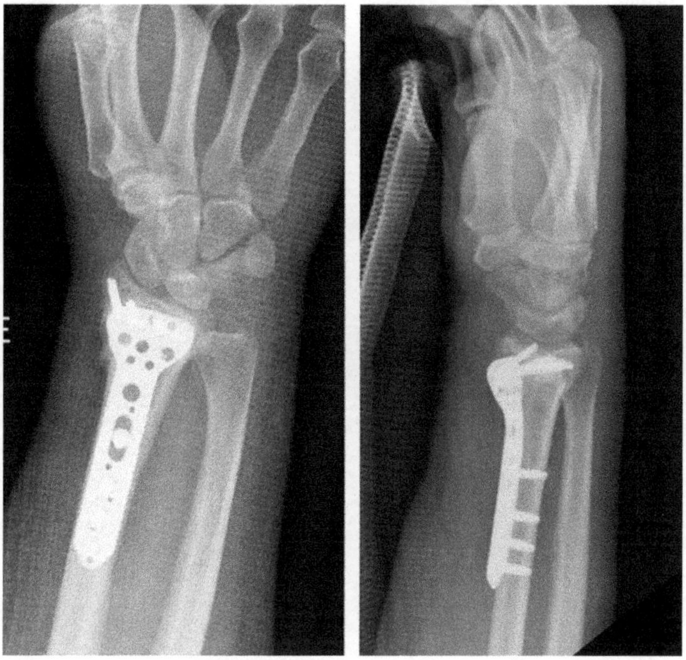

Fig. 4 Plate fixation—distal radius fracture

Treatment:

- Initial ER management consists of closed reduction and splinting
- Most common treatment is open reduction, internal fixation using a plate and screw construct (Fig. 4)
- Can be performed as outpatient, unless evolving neurological symptoms or open fracture
- External fixation may be required for extensive soft-tissue injury or as adjunct for fixation

References

Koval K, Haidukewych GJ, Service B, Zirigbel BJ. Controversies in the management of distal radius fractures. J Am Acad Orthop Surg. 2014;22:566–75.

Lichtman DM, Bindra RR, Boyer MI, Putnam MD, Ring D, Slutsky DJ, et al. AAOS clinical practice guideline summary: treatment of distal radius fractures. J Am Acad Orthop Surg. 2010;18:180–9.

DRUJ Injury

DRUJ injury: the distal radioulnar joint (DRUJ) is a complex forearm articulation that involves the interosseous membrane, triangular fibrocartilage complex (TFCC), and proximal radioulnar joint (PRUJ). As a result, trauma can result in many associated injuries both near and far.

Overview

The DRUJ is stabilized by several soft tissue structures, such as the dorsal and palmar radioulnar ligaments, as well as the TFCC (triangular fibrocartilage complex which includes the articular disk, the meniscal homologue, the ulnocarpal ligaments, the ulnar collateral ligament, and the external carpi ulnaris subsheath).

History

Especially common in setting of radial shaft fracture, but can exist with other types of fractures as well (e.g., ulna fractures).

Physical Exam

Point tenderness at DRUJ (palpated directly ulnar to Lister's tubercle)

"Shuck test"—hold the distal ulna and displace it anteriorly and posteriorly from the distal radius

May have crepitus with motion in cases of chronic injury/arthritis of the DRUJ

M.C. Makhni et al. (eds.), *Orthopedic Emergencies*,
DOI 10.1007/978-3-319-31524-9_43

Diagnosis

Imaging/X-Rays

Complete hand and wrist series

- In particular, will see malalignment of the radius and ulnar on the true lateral
- On AP, may see widening of the joint

Dynamic CT may aid in the diagnosis (assess DRUJ in neutral, pronation, and supination)

MRI for soft tissue assessment of DRUJ complex

DRUJ injuries may be seen as part of combined injuries:

- Galeazzi fracture (fracture distal 1/3 radial shaft along with DRUJ injury) (Figs. 1 and 2)
- Essex-Lopresti injuries (radial head fracture along with DRUJ injury)

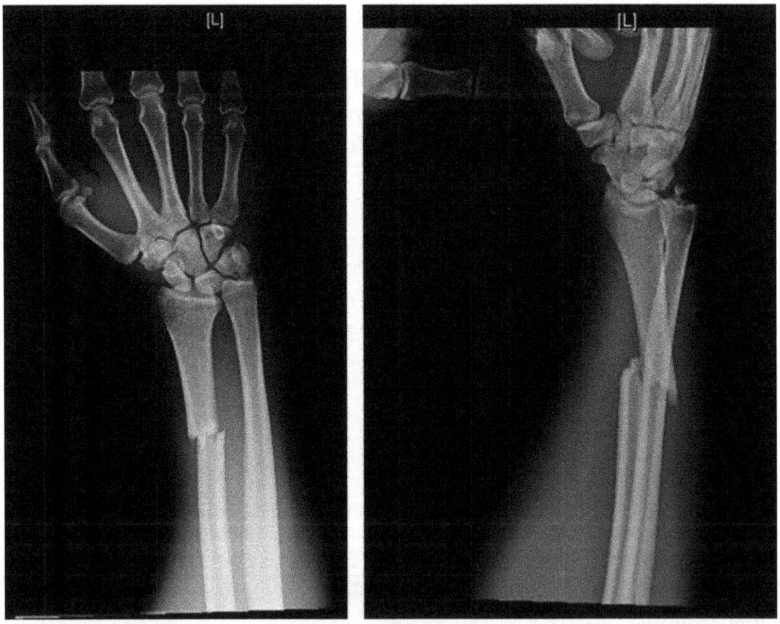

Fig. 1 Galeazzi fracture: note DRUJ injury

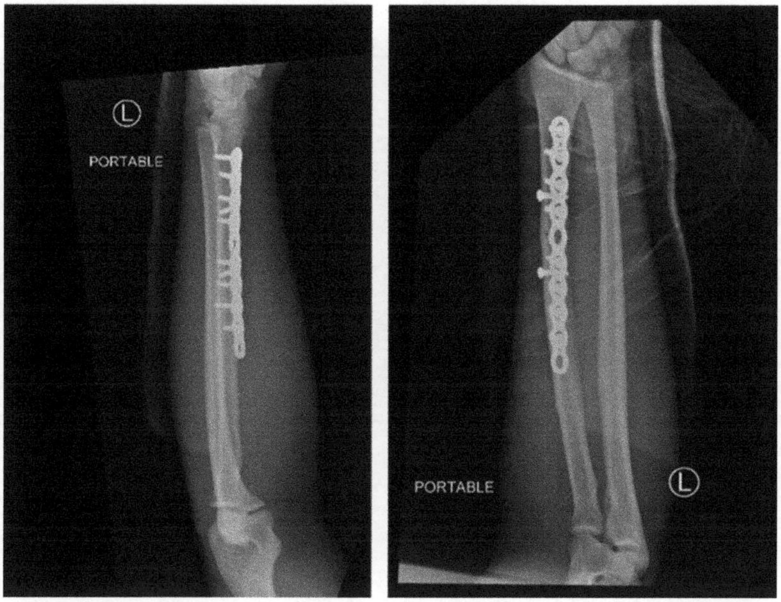

Fig. 2 Fixation of Galeazzi injury

Treatment Plan

Non-operative

Indication:

1. For most injuries, provided no other indication for surgical intervention (i.e., open fracture, poly-trauma, etc.)

Treatment:

1. Splint for comfort (sugar tong versus short arm cast)
2. Outpatient follow-up the following week

Surgical

Indication:

1. DRUJ instability or arthritis
2. Rarely performed in acute setting unless other prevailing factors

Treatment:

Fixation of associated injury with sugar tong splinting
Closed reduction percutaneous pinning may be necessary

Carpal Fracture (Excluding Scaphoid)

Injuries to the carpus range from purely bony injuries to ligamentous and dislocation events. Often these injuries are missed due to lack of clinical suspicion or inadequate physical exam and imaging.

Overview

The carpus consists of the scaphoid, lunate, triquetrum, pisiform, hamate, capitate, trapezoid, and trapezium.

Of these, the scaphoid is most commonly injured.

In addition to bony injuries, inter-carpal ligamentous injuries should also be evaluated.

Especially in polytrauma patients, these injuries may be overlooked, and a diligent secondary exam may aid in diagnosis.

History

Injury mechanism?

Associated neurovascular complaints (i.e., carpal tunnel compression symptoms with lunate dislocation)?

Physical Exam

Comprehensive hand exam (sites of tenderness, deficits in motion, visual abnormalities).

M.C. Makhni et al. (eds.), *Orthopedic Emergencies*,
DOI 10.1007/978-3-319-31524-9_44

Comprehensive neurovascular exam (rule out nerve entrapment, vascular injury).

Rule out carpal tunnel in perilunate/lunate dislocation.
Rule out ulnar tunnel for hook of the hamate fracture.

Diagnosis and Treatment

Imaging

- Standard hand X-ray series which includes PA, lateral, pronation (vs. supination) oblique.
- Special views include ulnar deviation, carpal tunnel views.
- CT may be warranted when suspicious of occult fracture or to assess size of fragment.
- MRI indicated to detect occult fracture and assess ligamentous injury.

Triquetrum Fracture (Fig. 1)

Classification

- **Dorsal cortical fracture (avulsion injury)**
  - Most common representing over 90 % of all triquetral fractures.
  - Fall on dorsiflexed and ulnarly deviated wrist.
  - Avulsion, shear forces, and impaction.
- **Triquetral body fracture**
  - Second most common triquetral fracture.
  - High energy.
  - Commonly associated ligamentous injury with 12%-25% incidence of perilunate fracture-dislocation.
- **Volar avulsion fracture (rare)**

  Avulsion of the palmar ulnar triquetral ligament and the LTIO ligament.

Treatment

- Dorsal Cortical Fracture/Avulsion fracture
  - **Nonoperative**
    - Up to 4–6 weeks of immobilization in removable wrist splint.
    - Can typically treat as a "wrist sprain" with return to activity as tolerated.

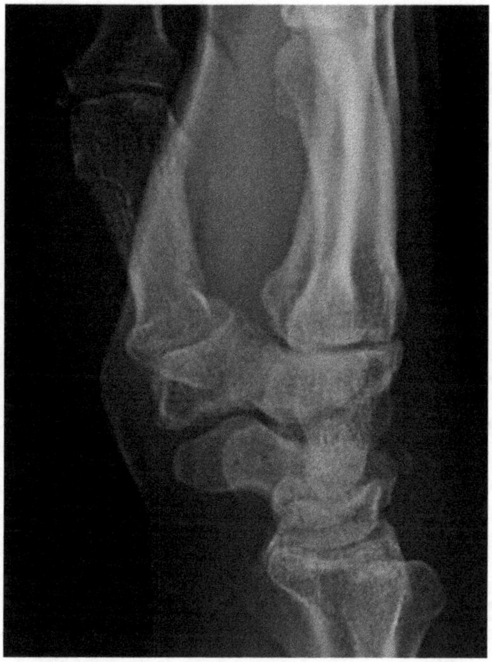

Fig. 1 Dorsal triquetral fracture

- **Operative**
  - Symptomatic nonunion.
  - Excision of fragment.

– **Triquetral Body Fracture**

- **Nonoperative**
  - 4–6 weeks immobilization in short arm cast.
  - Close orthopedic follow-up.
- **Operative**
  - Associated perilunate fracture-dislocation or scapho-lunate instability.
  - ORIF ± ligamentous repair.

– **Volar Avulsion Fracture**

- **Nonoperative**
  - 4–6 weeks of immobilization if carpus is stable.
- **Operative**
  - Restoration of carpal stability rather than treating the small avulsion fragment.

Trapezium Fracture

Classification

- Vertical trans-articular fracture (most common).
- Horizontal fractures.
- Fractures of the dorsal-radial tuberosity.
- Fractures of the anterior medial ridge.
- Comminuted.

Treatment

- **Nonoperative**
  - 4–6 weeks of immobilization in thumb spica cast if fracture is stable and non-displaced.
  - Close orthopedic follow-up.
- **Operative**
  - Displaced fracture.
  - Excision of fracture fragment when indicated.
  - ORIF ± bone grafting.

Capitate Fracture

Most commonly incurred as part of a trans-scaphoid perilunate fracture-dislocation. High-energy with wrist hyperextended and radially deviated.

Classification (transverse patterns most common, wrist hyperextended and radially deviated at time of injury)

- Transverse fracture of the proximal pole.
- Transverse fracture of the body.
- Vertical-coronal fracture.
- Parasagittal fracture.

Treatment

- **Nonoperative**
  - Non-displaced fractures.
  - 4–6 weeks of immobilization in short arm cast.
  - Close orthopedic follow-up.

- **Operative**
  - Displaced fractures, delayed diagnosis of non-displaced fractures and trans-scaphoid trans-capitate perilunate fracture-dislocations.
  - ORIF with headless compression screws ± bone grafting, ligamentous repair or scaphoid repair as indicated.

Hamate Fracture

Classification

- Hook of hamate fracture (seen mostly in athletes and following direct/repetitive trauma i.e., from baseball bat or golf club) (Fig. 2).
- Hamate body fracture (seen after trauma/direct blow or shear injury).

Treatment

- **Nonoperative**
  - Acute, non-displaced fractures.
  - 4–6 weeks of immobilization in short arm cast.
  - Close orthopedic follow-up.
- **Operative**
  - Displaced, symptomatic or chronic hook fractures.
  - Open excision of fragment.
  - Consider acutely in high-level athletes.

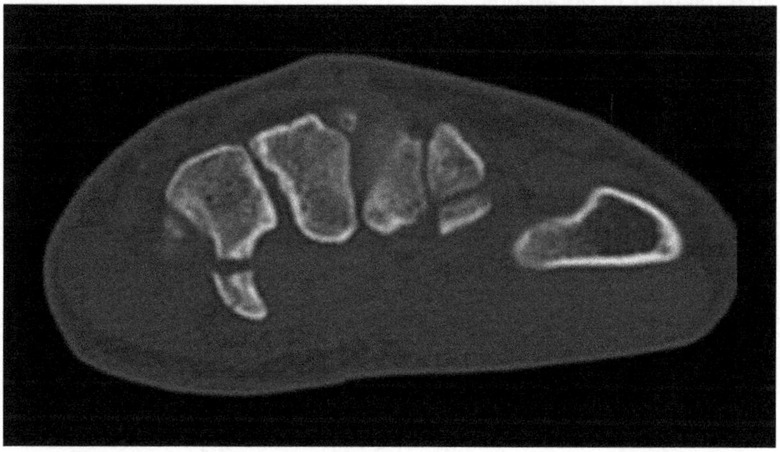

Fig. 2 Hook of the hamate fracture seen on axial CT

Pisiform

Classification (uncommon injuries, may result from direct trauma/impaction to ulnar hand/wrist)

- Transverse.
- Parasagittal (better prognosis).
- Comminuted.
- Pisiform-triquetral impaction.

Treatment

- **Nonoperative**
  - Acute, non-displaced fractures.
  - 4–6 weeks of immobilization in short arm cast.
  - Close orthopedic follow-up.
- **Operative**
  - Comminuted, displaced transverse and symptomatic nonunions.
  - Open pisiformectomy.

Lunate

Classification (usually the result of direct compression injury)

- Frontal fractures of the palmar pole.
- Osteochondral fractures of proximal articular surface.
- Frontal fractures of dorsal pole.
- Transverse body fractures.
- Transarticular frontal body fractures (most common).

Treatment

- **Nonoperative**
  - Isolated, non-displaced fractures.
  - 4–6 weeks of immobilization in short arm cast.
  - Close orthopedic follow-up.
- **Operative**
  - Displaced fractures.
  - ORIF.

Trapezoid Fracture

Classification

Least commonly injured carpal bone.

Treatment

- **Nonoperative**
  - Isolated, non-displaced fractures.
  - 4–6 weeks of immobilization in short arm cast.
  - Close orthopedic follow-up.
- **Operative**
  - Displaced fractures.
  - ORIF.

References

Botte MJ, Gelberman RH. Fractures of the carpus, excluding scaphoid. Hand Clin. 1987;3:49–161.
Garcia-Elias M. Carpal bone fractures (excluding scaphoid fractures). In: Watson HK, Weinberg J, editors. The wrist. Philadelphia, PA: Lippincott Williams & Wilkins; 2001. p. 174–81.
Milch H. Fracture of the hamate bone. J Bone Joint Surg Am. 1934;16:459–62.
Wolfe, SW (Editor-in-Chief), Hotchkiss RN, Pederson, WC, Kozin, SH. (Editors) Greens operative hand surgery. 6th edn. Copyright © 2011. Elsevier/Churchill Livingstone. Philadelphia, PA.

Scaphoid Fracture

Scaphoid fractures typically result from a fall on an outstretched and extended wrist. Because of its tenuous blood supply, these fractures are notorious for developing nonunion and subsequent degenerative disease.

Overview

Most commonly fractured carpal bone, usually following FOOSH. Patients will often have characteristic "snuff box tenderness." Because of retrograde blood supply from radial artery, proximal pole fractures exhibit high rates of nonunion.

Missed or chronic scaphoid fractures that lead to nonunion develop SNAC (scaphoid nonunion advanced collapse) wrist, with degenerative changes and progression similar to that found in SLAC wrist.

History

- Typically via FOOSH mechanism
- Also present after high-energy fall

Physical Exam

- Snuffbox tenderness (dorsal tuberosity of the scaphoid)
- Tenderness at volar scaphoid tuberosity as well

M.C. Makhni et al. (eds.), *Orthopedic Emergencies*,
DOI 10.1007/978-3-319-31524-9_45

Diagnosis

Imaging/Wrist X-Rays

- Should obtain full wrist and hand X-rays (Fig. 1)
- Important to order **ulnar deviation view**

Advanced Imaging

Growing body of literature suggesting increased cost-effectiveness in obtaining advanced imaging in the acute setting

MRI—high sensitivity, may be challenging to obtain in some EDs
CT—excellent sensitivity. Thin cut protocol focused on scaphoid necessary to have high sensitivity

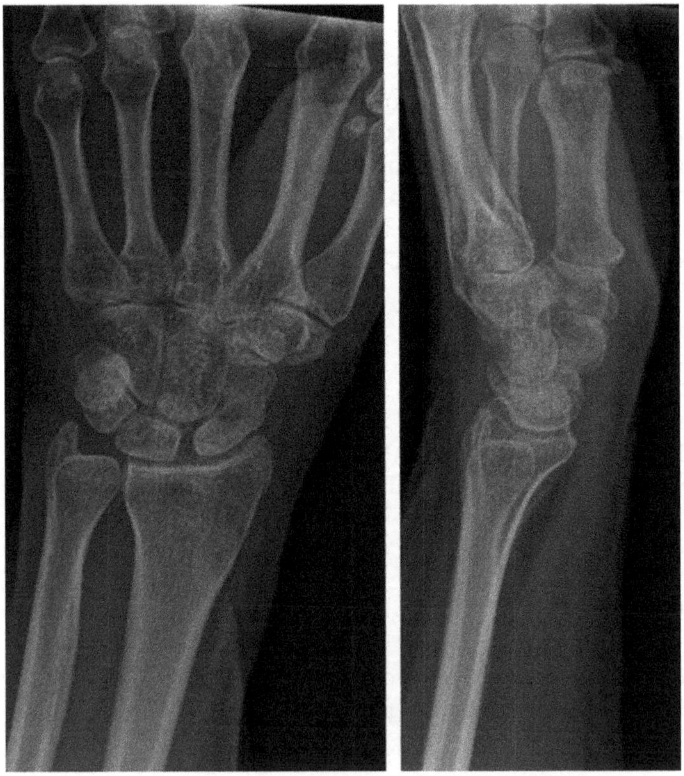

Fig. 1 Scaphoid fracture

Classification Systems

- Location of fracture (along with displacement) most important consideration for decision to undergo surgical fixation
- Should be able to describe fracture location as proximal, waist (middle), or distal pole
- Should also note amount of displacement
- Chronic injuries will have evidence of marginal sclerosis and may affect type of surgical technique

Treatment Plan: Discharge

Nonoperative

Indications:

1. Nondisplaced waist, distal pole fractures
2. <1 mm displacement waist, distal pole fractures (controversial)
3. Nondisplaced proximal pole fractures (controversial)

Technique:

1. In acute setting (assuming no other dislocation or injuries that require treatment), thumb-spica cast or splint is sufficient
    - Cast if likely to be treated nonoperative
    - Splint if high likelihood for surgery
    - Consider splinting if risk for soft tissue swelling and compartment syndrome
    - Recent evidence suggesting cast without thumb immobilization might be sufficient for nondisplaced or minimally displaced waist fractures

Surgical

Indications:

1. Usually as outpatient, unless significant morbidity/polytrauma
2. Displaced scaphoid fractures
3. Any fracture of the proximal pole, due to high risk of nonunion

Technique:

1. Mainstay is reduction and screw fixation (Fig. 2)
2. Chronic injuries may require bone grafting if nonunion present

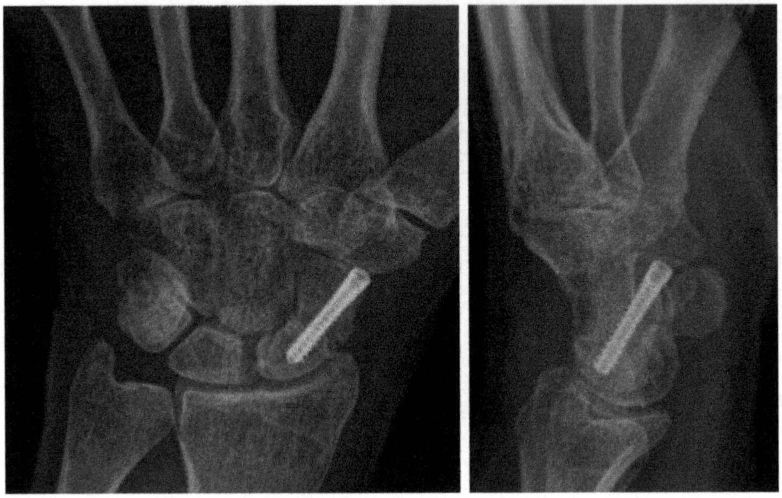

Fig. 2 Screw fixation of scaphoid fracture

3. Chronic injuries with resultant arthritis are treated on basis of degenerative severity, similar to SLAC (scapho-lunate ligament advanced collapse) wrist

References

Gutow AP. Percutaneous fixation of scaphoid fractures. J Am Acad Orthop Surg. 2007;14: 474–85.

Karl JW, Swart E, Strauch RJ. Diagnosis of Occult Scaphoid Fractures: A Cost-Effectiveness Analysis. J Bone Joint Surg Am. 2015 Nov 18;97(22):1860–8. doi:10.2106/JBJS.O.00099.

Moon CS, Dy CJ, Derman P, Vance MC, Carlson MG. Management of nonunion following surgical management of scaphoid fractures: current concepts. J Am Acad Orthop Surg. 2013;21: 548–57.

Buijze GA, Goslings JC et al. Cast immobilization with and without immobilization of the thumb for nondisplaced and minimally displaced scaphoid waist fractures: a multicenter, randomized, controlled trial. J Hand Surg Am. 2014;39(4):621–7.

Scapholunate Instability

Disruption of the scapholunate ligament commonly results from a fall onto the outstretched wrist. Disruption of the ligament can cause acute symptoms of pain and instability, and can lead to degenerative wrist disease if left untreated.

Overview

The scapholunate ligament complex consists of three different structures (dorsal, volar, and proximal), with the dorsal ligamentous structure being the strongest.

Injury occurs following axial load to a wrist that is extended and in ulnar deviation. A SLAC (scapholunate advanced collapse) wrist is a chronic, degenerative condition in patients with untreated S-L injuries.

Arthritis progresses from involving the articulation between the radial styloid and the scaphoid, to the scaphoid and its facet, and then between the capitate and the lunate.

History

Fall onto outstretched hand

Subjective instability

Standard upper extremity history (dominant side, baseline function, prior trauma/nerve injury, comprehensive medical and surgical history)

S-L disruption may result in carpal instability with the scaphoid hyperflexed and the lunate hyperextended

M.C. Makhni et al. (eds.), *Orthopedic Emergencies*,
DOI 10.1007/978-3-319-31524-9_46

Physical Exam

Pain over S-L interval (approximately 1 cm distal and ulnar to the radial styloid)
+ Watson shift test (place finger on scaphoid tuberosity from volar wrist, and range wrist from ulnar to radial deviation; will experience pain as scaphoid dislocates out of facet (and reduces after relieve the pressure)

Diagnosis

Imaging/Wrist X-Rays

Gapping between the scaphoid and the lunate
Patients with chronic injury will display degenerative changes affecting the articulations described above (Fig. 1)

Watson Stages of SLAC Wrist

Stage I: radial styloid/scaphoid arthritis
Stage II: scaphoid/scaphoid facet (on radius) arthritis
Stage III: capitate/lunate arthritis
Stage IV: pan-carpal disease

Treatment Plan: Discharge

Nonoperative

Indications:

1. Non-displaced injuries (S-L reduced)
2. Initial management prior to definitive reduction and fixation in the operating room

Treatment:

1. Short arm cast versus thumb spica cast, well padded
2. If significant swelling, can consider thumb spica splint

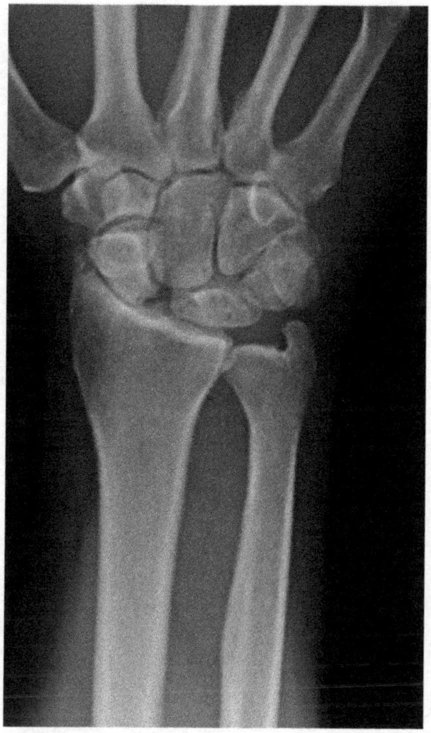

Fig. 1 Scapholunate injury with early degenerative changes at radio-scaphoid joint

Surgical

Indication:

1. Disruption of the S-L ligament (widened S-L interval)
2. Can be acute or chronic injury

Treatment:

1. For acute injury, consists of reduction and fixation (Fig. 2)
2. Chronic injury treatment depends on degree of corresponding arthritis, with multiple options available including bony resection and selective fusion.

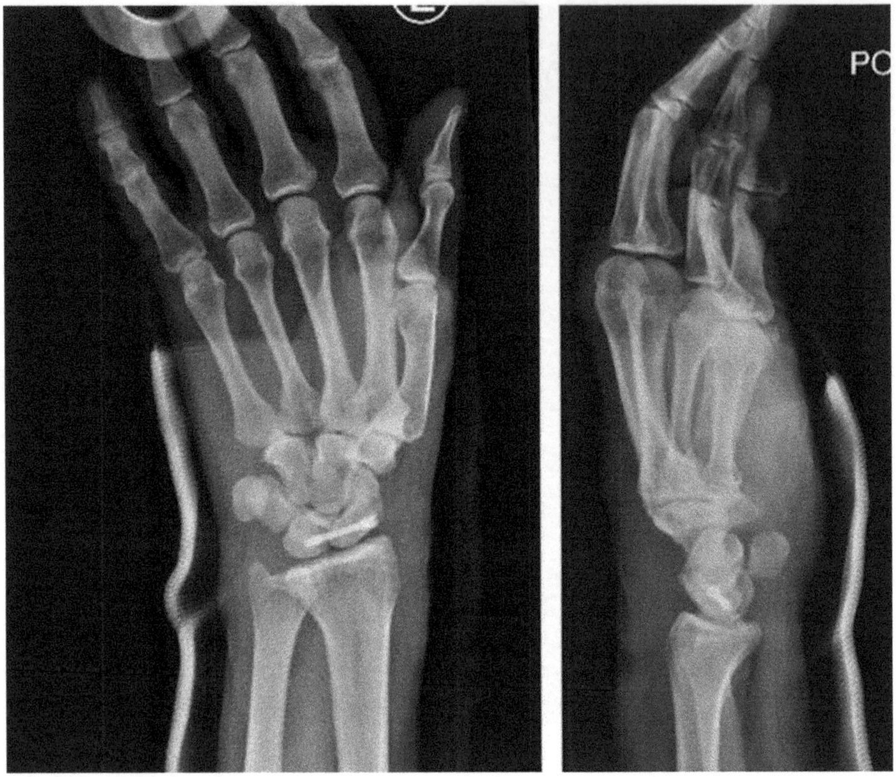

Fig. 2 Screw stabilization of acute S-L injury

References

Walsh JJ, Berger RA, Cooney WP. Current status of scapholunate interosseous injuries. J Am Acad Orthop Surg. 2002;10:32–42.

Perilunate Dislocation

These dislocations follow high-energy events and can easily be missed in the emergency room setting. Proper diagnosis requires a comprehensive history and physical examination, along with scrutiny of all imaging of the hand and wrist. Concomitant neurovascular injury should be ruled out.

Overview

High-energy trauma to the wrist usually in extension, ulnar deviation, and carpal supination

History

Mechanism of injury
Associated neurovascular complaints (i.e., carpal tunnel compression symptoms)

Physical Exam

Comprehensive hand exam (sites of tenderness, deficits in motion, visual abnormalities)
Comprehensive neurovascular exam (rule out nerve entrapment, vascular injury)

- Rule out carpal tunnel in perilunate/lunate dislocation

M.C. Makhni et al. (eds.), *Orthopedic Emergencies*,
DOI 10.1007/978-3-319-31524-9_47

Diagnosis

Imaging/Hand X-Rays

- PA
- Lateral
  - Evaluate colinearity of radius–lunate–capitate
- Traction radiograph
- CT
  - For operative planning
  - Identify occult fractures, degree of comminution, and fragment morphology
- MRI
  - Sensitive and specific for ligamentous injury and occult fractures (Fig. 1)

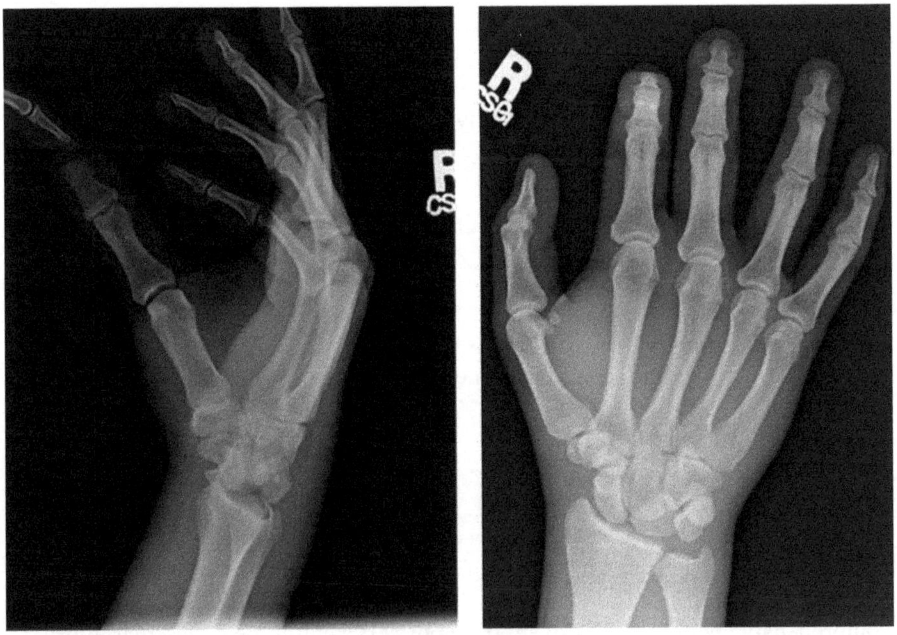

Fig. 1 Lunate dislocation (transradial fracture)

Classification

Carpal Instability Complex Categories (dissociative and non-dissociative)

1. Dorsal perilunate dislocations (lesser arc)
2. Dorsal perilunate fracture-dislocations (greater arc)
3. Palmar perilunate dislocations (lesser or greater arc)

Mayfield Classification (lesser arc injury pattern)

1. Scapholunate
2. Scapholunate–capitolunate
3. Scapholunate–capitolunate–triquetrolunate
4. Scapholunate–capitolunate–triquetrolunate–radiolunate

Treatment

Nonoperative

Indication:

1. Definitive nonoperative intervention typically reserved for patients with too many medical comorbidities to tolerate surgery
2. In acute setting, focus is on reducing the dislocation and stabilizing/immobilizing the wrist in a comfortable position

Technique:

1. Need adequate sedation for reduction, as these can be very challenging. If unable to reduce with local anesthesia and sedatives, may require formal anesthesia to achieve necessary relaxation for reduction
2. With dorsal dislocation, wrist extension, traction, and subsequent wrist flexion
3. With transscaphoid injuries, immobilize with thumb spica splint

Surgical

Indications

1. Perilunate dislocations and fracture-dislocations typically require surgical intervention due to the extensive soft tissue and ligamentous disruption involved

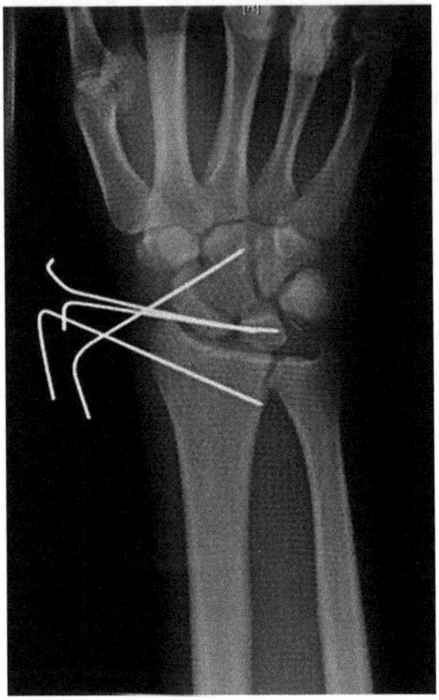

Fig. 2 Pin stabilization of transradial lunate dislocation

2. If reduction is achieved in the emergency room setting, surgery may be performed as an outpatient and by a hand surgeon
3. Inability to achieve reduction with general anesthesia may warrant emergent open reduction and fixation

Technique:

1. May be achieved with pin fixation and immobilization for acute injuries, along with ligamentous repair as warranted
2. Chronic injury treatment options governed by extent of degenerative changes (Fig. 2)

References

Court-Brown CM, Heckman JD, McQueen MM, Ricci WM, Tornetta III P editors, McKee MD Assoc. editor. Rockwood and Green's fractures in adults. 8th ed. Philadelphia, PA: Wolter Kluwers Health/Lippincott Williams and Wilkins; 2015.

Herzberg G, Comtet JJ, Linscheid RL, et al. Perilunate dislocations and fracture-dislocations: a multicenter study. J Hand Surg Am. 1993;18:768–79.

IWIW. Terminology Committee: Wrist: terminology and definitions. J Bone Joint Surg Am. 2002;84 Suppl 1:1–69.

Mayfield JK, Johnson RP, Kilcoyne RK. Carpal dislocations: pathomechanics and progressive perilunar instability. J Hand Surg Am. 1980;5:226–41.

Stanbury SJ, Elfar JC. Perilunate dislocation and perilunate fracture-dislocation. J Am Acad Orthop Surg. 2011;19(9):554–62.

Wolfe SW editor-in-chief, Hotchkiss RN, Pederson WC, Kozin SH editors. Green's operative hand surgery. 6th ed. Philadelphia, PA: Elsevier/Churchill Livingstone; 2011.

Tendon Lacerations

Tendon lacerations are extremely common in the hand and wrist. Detailed neurovascular examination is crucial in identifying concomitant injuries. While flexor tendons require reapproximation in the operating room, extensor tendon repairs can be performed in the emergency room.

Overview

Flexor and extensor tendons are organized into zones

Flexor Tendon Zones

Zone I—distal to the FDS insertion (jersey finger)
Zone II—FDS insertion to distal palmar crease ("no man's land")
Zone III—palm
Zone IV—carpal tunnel
Zone V—wrist to forearm

Extensor Tendon Zones

Zone I—disruption of the terminal extensor tendon at the level of the DIP joint of the finger (mallet finger) or interphalangeal (IP) joint of the thumb
Zone II—disruption over the middle phalanx of the finger or proximal phalanx of the thumb

M.C. Makhni et al. (eds.), *Orthopedic Emergencies*,
DOI 10.1007/978-3-319-31524-9_48

Zone III—disruption over the PIP joint of the finger (central slip injury/boutonniere deformity) or MCP joint of the thumb
Zone IV—disruption over the proximal phalanx of the finger or metacarpal of the thumb
Zone V—disruption over the MCP joint of the finger and CMC joint of the thumb
Zone VI—disruption over the metacarpal of the finger
Zone VII—disruption at the level of the wrist joint
Zone VIII—disruption at the distal forearm

History

- Injury mechanism
- Timing/chronicity of injury
- Tetanus and immunization record
- Associated neurovascular complaints

Physical Exam

- Detailed neurovascular examination
- Irrigation, debridement of open wound
- Detailed tendon examination—must isolate each extensor, superficial flexor, and deep flexor as appropriate (Fig. 1)

Diagnosis

- May require irrigation, probing, as skin laceration may not coincide with location for tendon laceration (e.g., if occurs during a clenched fist in a fight)
- If fight bite, rule out concomitant fracture and joint seeding

Treatment Plan:

Nonoperative

Indications:

1. For flexor tendon injuries, ER management goal to do thorough irrigation and debridement, manage skin wounds (suture for acute injuries or plan for secondary intention in chronic injuries)

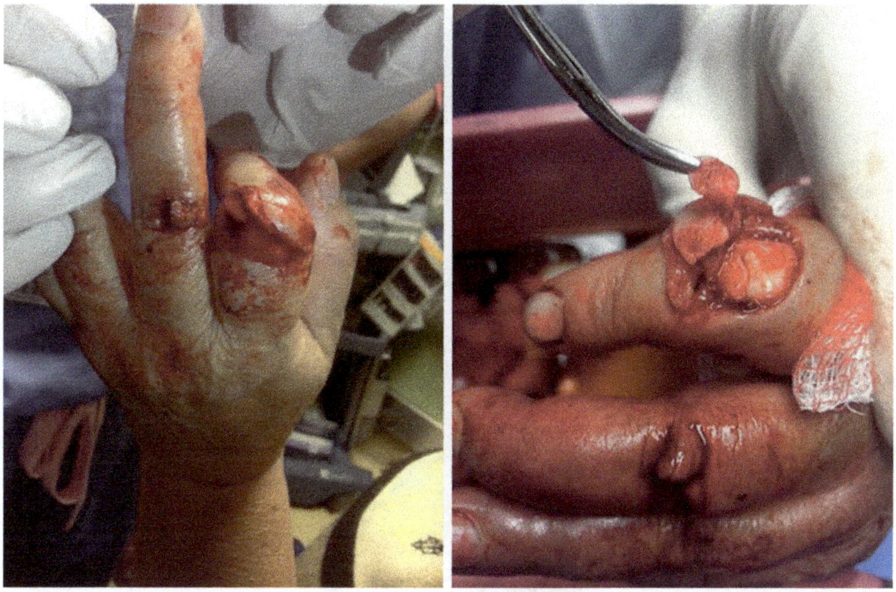

Fig. 1 Extensor tendon laceration

2. Soft dressing with finger splint or volar plaster splint as required in order to rest the soft tissues
3. Extensor tendon injuries comprising <50 % of the tendon may be left alone and treated with management of the skin laceration
4. Injuries that are chronic (>7 days) or infected should not undergo tendon repair. The skin ends may be loosely sutured together with nylon sutures, and the patient may be referred to a hand surgeon for definitive management.

Technique:

1. For extensor tendon tip avulsions (mallet finger), need to do extension splinting continuously with outpatient ortho hand evaluation. Bony mallet injuries may require operative fixation under certain circumstances (Figs. 2–4)
2. For jersey finger (FDP avulsions) at the finger tip, can provisionally splint and manage wound and arrange for close ortho follow-up (within 3–5 days)
3. Otherwise, ER management of these injuries consists of copious irrigation (can use dilute Betadine), and if acute injury with clean cut edges, can provisionally suture with loose nylon sutures.
4. If wound is contaminated, poor margins (e.g., crush injury), consider soft dressing until definitive management
5. "Fight bite" injuries at MC head/neck (can be associated with fracture) must be thoroughly irrigated and treated as an open fracture/injury, and patient must be placed on antibiotics.

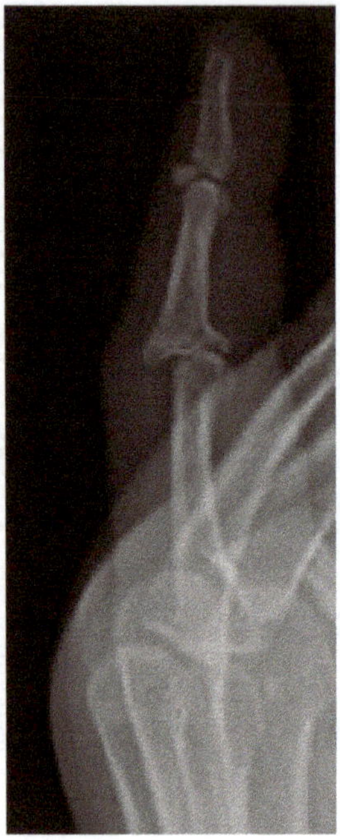

Fig. 2 Bony mallet injury at distal phalanx

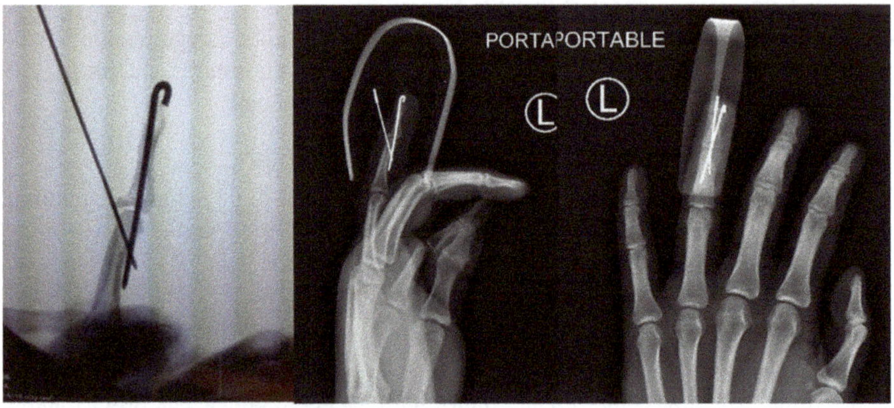

Fig. 3 Pin fixation of bony mallet

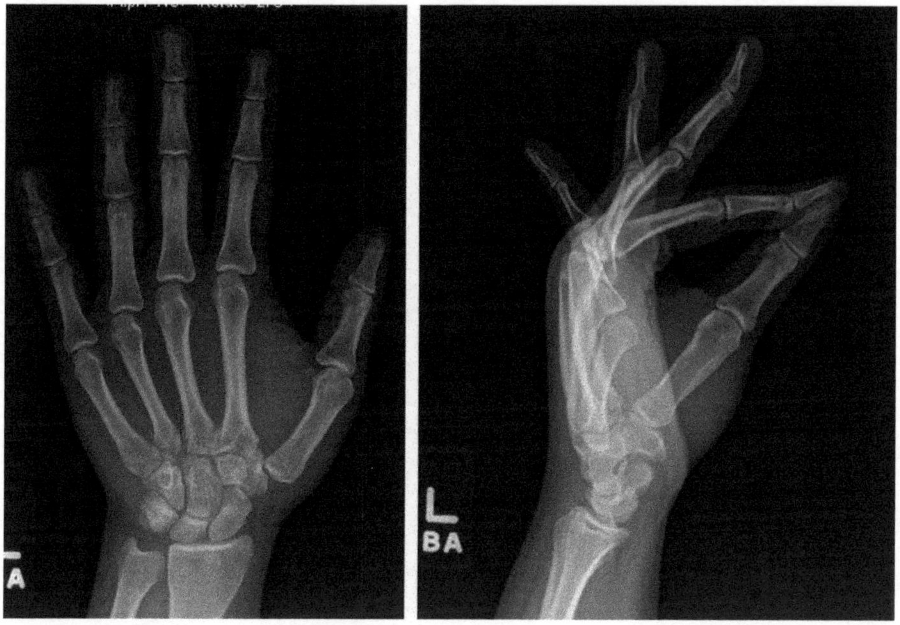

Fig. 4 Bony mallet after pin removal

Surgical

Indication:

1. Extensor tendon repair may be safely performed in the emergency room setting, provided free tendon ends are readily visible and >50–60 % of the tendon is torn
2. If the injury occurred during digit flexion, the tendon ends may be proximal to the skin wound.
3. If unable to mobilize tendons or otherwise unable to repair in ER, can refer to hand surgeon that week for early repair

Technique:

1. A variety of techniques exist, but in general can use figure-of-eight stitches or a running horizontal mattress configuration, with 4-0 nonabsorbable suture, along with epitendinous repair if possible.

Reference

Newport ML. Extensor tendon injuries in the hand. J Am Acad Orthop Surg. 1997;5:59–66.

Finger Fractures and Dislocations

Treatment of finger injuries depends on integrity of bony and soft tissue structures.

Overview

Metacarpal Fractures

Categories include metacarpal head, neck, shaft, and base fractures

Metacarpal neck fractures will typically present apex dorsal deformity secondary to pull of intrinsics

Fracture of the fifth metacarpal neck is referred to as a "boxer's fracture"

Fractures of the base of the metacarpal are often associated with dislocations (Bennett fracture dislocation for base of first digit, along with "Reverse Bennett" for base of fifth digit)

Obtain oblique hand X-rays to better identify these injuries

Phalanx Fractures

Deformity is dependent on fracture location

Proximal phalanx fracture typically exhibit apex volar deformity because of intrinsic pull

M.C. Makhni et al. (eds.), *Orthopedic Emergencies*,
DOI 10.1007/978-3-319-31524-9_49

Middle phalanx fractures proximal to FDS insertion display apex dorsal deformity, while those fracture distal to the FDS insertion display apex volar deformity

Malrotation and extensor lag are typical findings in displaced fractures of the digit

History

Mechanism and timing of injury
Presence of open or contaminated (e.g., bite to finger) injury

Physical Exam

- Must assess for presence of open fracture
- Detailed neurovascular exam
- Visual inspection to assess alignment
- Malrotation must be assessed—can assess when asking patient to flex hand and compare to contralateral side, or assess orientation of the fingernails in comparison to other digits on the ipsilateral or contralateral hand
- Assess active and passive range of motion where indicated

Diagnosis

Imaging/Hand X-Rays

Obtain full series of X-rays including hand and involved digit (AP, lateral, and oblique)
Ensure that true lateral of the isolated digit is taken
MC base fractures and CMC dislocations, often require oblique views to identify fracture

Treatment Plan (According to Particular Injury)

First CMC Dislocation

Reduce, place in thumb spica splint

First MC Fracture/Dislocation

Reduce, immobilize in thumb spica splint

First Digit UCL Sprain ("Game Keeper"/"Skiier's Thumb")

Injury to the ulnar collateral ligament at the first digit MCP joint (Fig. 1)
Diagnosed with pain at origin, along with ligamentous laxity upon stress testing

Increased laxity to ulnar stress at MCP in flexed position when compared to contralateral

Treat acutely with thumb spica splint/cast

2nd–5th MC Fractures (Figs. 2–4)

Following reduction (hematoma block), can immobilize in intrinsic plus short arm splint

Can also consider metacarpal mitt splint

10, 20, 30, 40° angulation acceptable with 2nd, 3rd, 4th and 5th MC shaft fractures, with up to an additional 10° acceptable at each digit for neck fractures. About 7° extensor lag expected for every 2 mm MC shortening, but some shortening is often well tolerated.

Consider surgery for poly-trauma patient, multiple fractures in the same hand or rotated, or severely angulated fractures

MCP Dislocation (Simple If No Interposed Tissue or Associated Fracture)

Dorsal/volar dislocation: reduction and immobilization with buddy tape and intrinsic plus splint
For complex dislocations or with interposed tissue (volar plate for irreducible dorsal MCP dislocation), will need to go to operating room on urgent basis

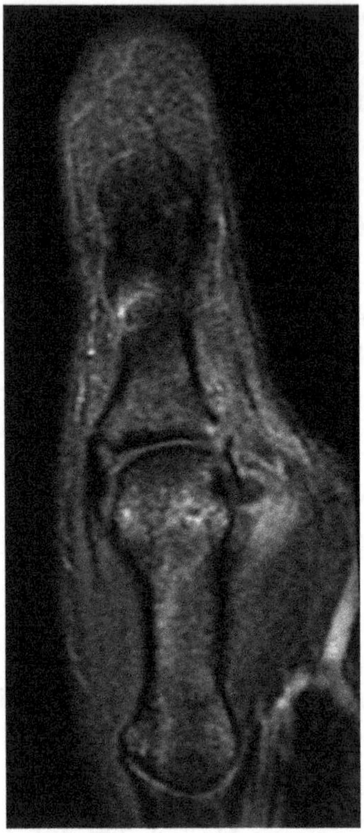

Fig. 1 Thumb UCL injury (MRI)

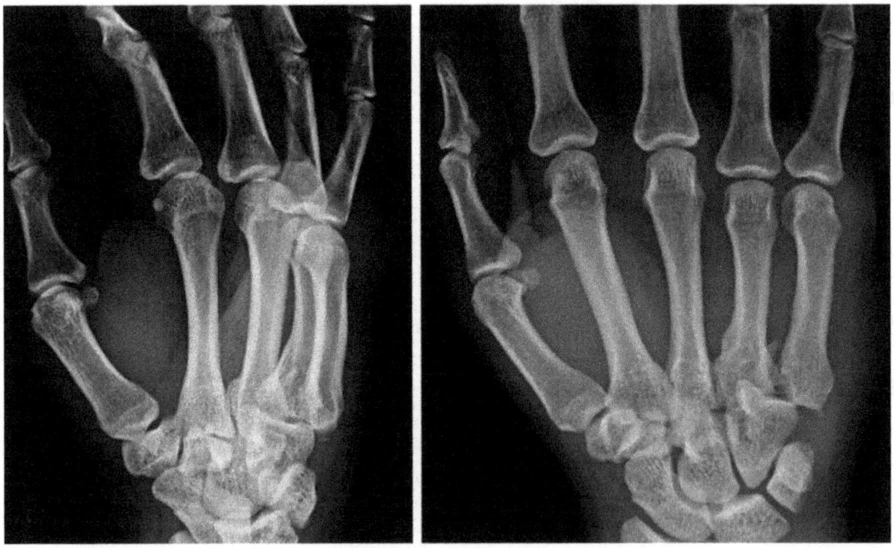

Fig. 2 Fracture dislocation of base of fifth MC ("reverse Bennett's fracture")

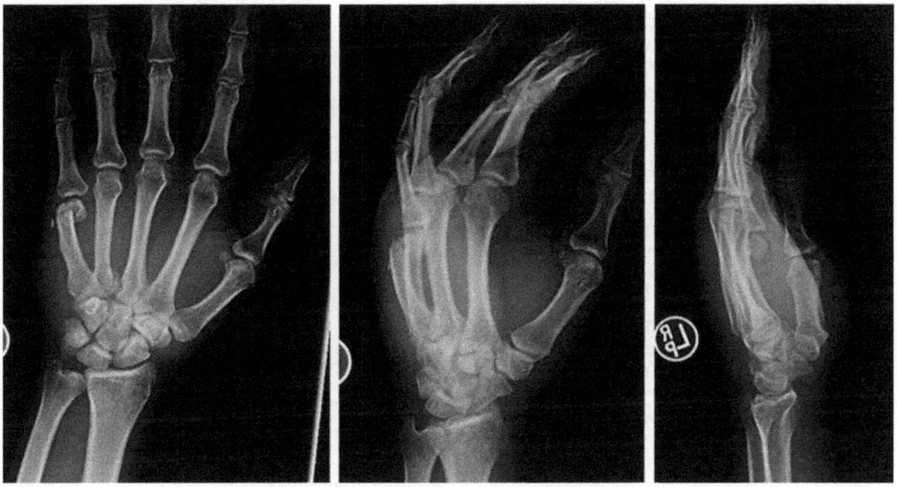

Fig. 3 Metacarpal fracture (fifth MC head/neck and fourth MC base)

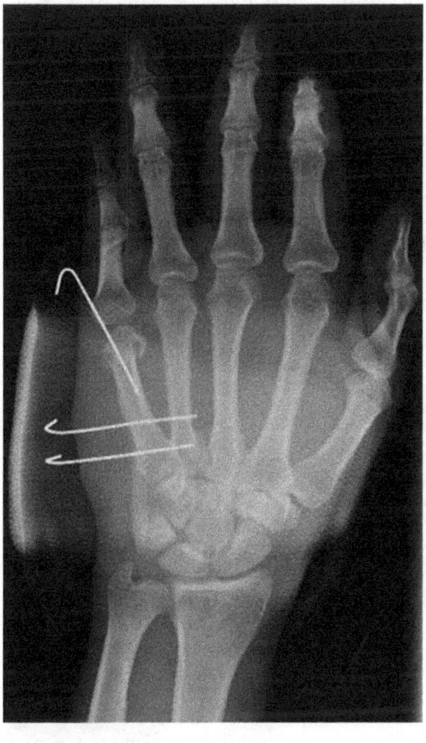

Fig. 4 Pin stabilization of multiple metacarpal fractures

Phalanx Fractures

Reduction (can lever with pen in between adjoining digits) followed by buddy taping
Should buddy tape to adjacent fingers to help maintain reduction
AlumaFoam splinting generally sufficient
Acceptable non-operative treatment sufficient for proximal and middle phalanx fractures if able to maintain stable reduction in extra-articular fractures with less than 10° angulation without rotational overlap and <50 % overlap with the adjacent finger. About 10–12° extensor lag expected for every 1 mm phalangeal shortening. Distal phalanx fractures rarely require surgical intervention, although displaced transverse fractures can be considered for closed reduction and percutaneous pinning.

PIP Dislocations (Simple)

Dorsal dislocations most common (Fig. 5)—disruption of volar plate. Axial traction for reduction, buddy taping, and early ROM after 3–4 days immobilization. Missed injury leads to volar plate attenuation, which can lead to swan neck deformity.

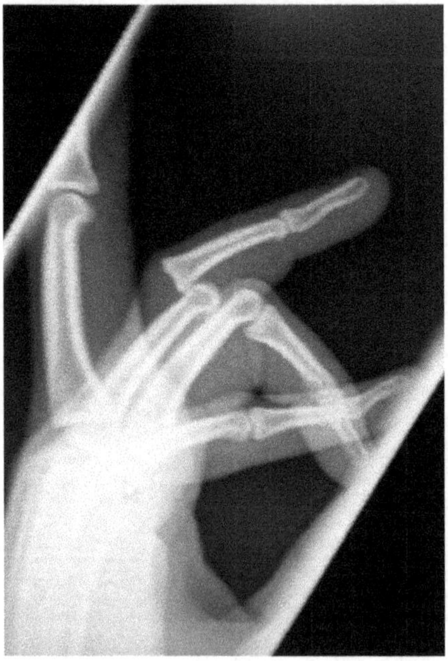

Fig. 5 Simple PIP dorsal dislocation

Volar dislocation—rupture of the central slip. Following reduction, will need to be immobilized in extension for 4–6 weeks for central slip repair. Missed/chronic central slip injury leads to boutonniere deformity

PIP Fracture Dislocations

If >40 % joint surface involved, usually requires surgical fixation; provisionally splint in ER

Technique dependent on amount of bone preserved (Figs. 6, 7, and 8)

In general, nonoperative interventions listed above used in emergency room setting.

Surgical management reserved for irreducible fractures/fracture dislocations, open injuries, those with neurovascular compromise (not always), and digit injuries with malrotation.

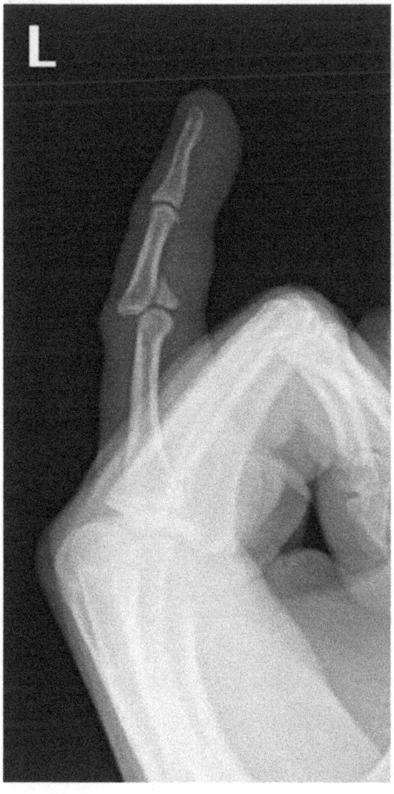

Fig. 6 Dorsal PIP fracture dislocation

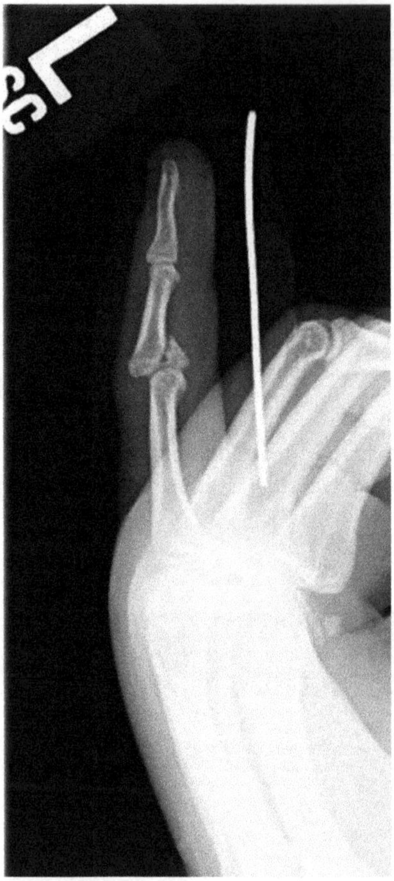

Fig. 7 Persistent dislocation despite extension splinting

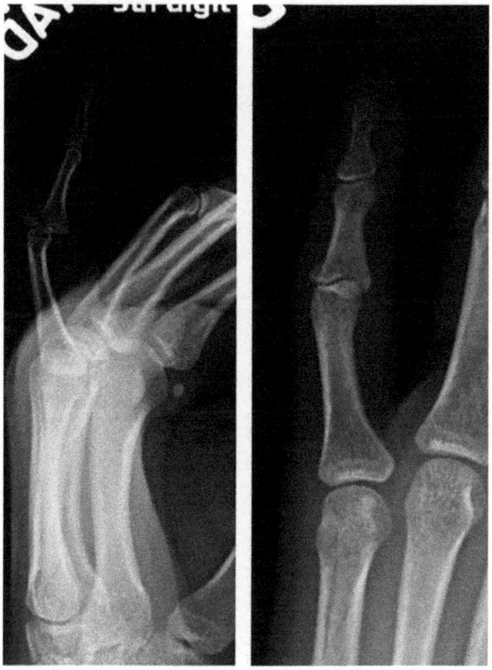

Fig. 8 Volar PIP fracture dislocation

Digit Amputations

The goal of management of digital amputations in the emergency room is to safely secure the digit for either discharge to home or reimplantation in the operating room. For most fingertip amputations, local wound care is sufficient in the emergency room situation, with definitive care performed by a hand surgeon.

Overview

Ultimate goal of treatment in fingertip amputation is restoration of a functional, sensate, and painless digit

Most fingertip amputations can be managed with local soft tissue and bony management in the emergency room

Bony involvement warrants immediate antibiotic administration continued for 24 h

History

- Mechanism of injury
- Timing of injury
- Transport of amputated digit (if applicable)
- Other associated upper extremity injuries

Physical Exam (Figs. 1 and 2)

- Detailed neurovascular examination to determine extent of injury
- Presence of exposed bone?

M.C. Makhni et al. (eds.), *Orthopedic Emergencies*,
DOI 10.1007/978-3-319-31524-9_50

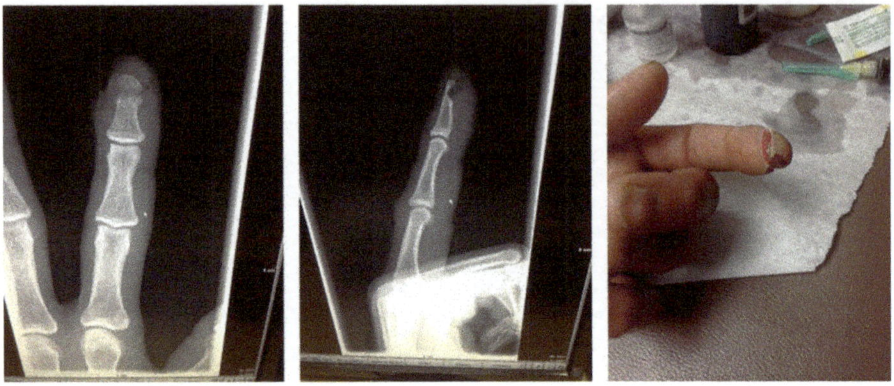

Fig. 1 Partial fingertip amputation

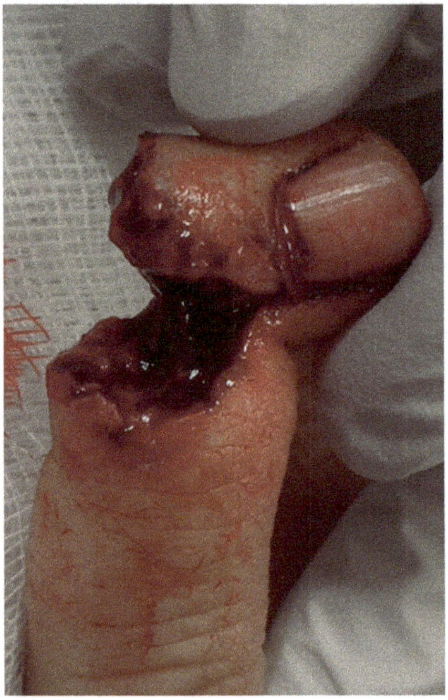

Fig. 2 Fingertip near complete amputation

- Size, quality, character of soft tissue and bony defect
- Tetanus and immunization history

Diagnosis

Imaging/Hand X-Rays

- Full series of films for affected limb (AP, lateral, oblique)

Treatment Plan

General Principles

- Many fingertip injuries can be managed in the emergent care setting; however, more extensive amputations involving wound flaps are better served to be done in an operating room setting.
- For replantation, amputated digits may tolerate up to 12 h of warm ischemia time and 24 h of cold ischemic time (while amputations proximal to the wrist can tolerate 6 and 12 h of warm and cold ischemic time, respectively).
- Whenever bony involvement is present, the patient should be administered IV antibiotics in the emergency room. It is also essential to ensure that tetanus booster shots are up to date.
- Analgesia can be achieved through a digital block at the level of the metacarpal head. One can also consider a wrist block or ulnar nerve block in instances of more extensive amputations.
- The hand and forearm should be prepped and draped in a typical sterile fashion.
- A bloodless field is essential for thorough inspection of the wound. Hemostasis can be achieved through use of Penrose drain clamped around the base of the finger, a pneumatic digital sleeve, a wrist tourniquet, or a blood pressure cuff placed around the forearm. ***Do not forget to remove this tourniquet at the end of the procedure! Patient will be insensate and may not realize a tourniquet is in place.***
- The wound should be thoroughly irrigated with at least 2L of NS and then undergo close inspection and debridement of nonviable tissue.
- For those injuries with no soft tissue loss, the wound can be closed primarily. Viable native skin flaps should be loosely sutured and an AlumaFoam splint applied for bony support in instances of fracture.

Soft Tissue Loss Without Exposed Bone

- These injuries should be treated by either secondary intention or through use of skin flaps.
- It is typically recommended that if the soft tissue defect is 1 cm^2 or less, successful treatment can be achieved by leaving the wound open and allowing for secondary healing.
- Complete healing usually takes 3–5 weeks and occurs by reepithelialization and wound contracture.
- Patients should begin warm water/peroxide soaks 7–10 days after the injury.
- Larger skin defects (>1 cm^2) that are treated nonoperatively are at danger of healing with a very thin epithelial layer that is not durable.
- These instances may require tissue flaps to achieve a more durable, functional digit.

Soft Tissue Loss with Exposed Bone (Fig. 3)

- When bone is exposed, the primary goal should be to provide adequate soft tissue coverage.
- This can be accomplished in the ED by shortening the bone with rongeur (3–5 mm) just below the level of the skin and then attempting a primary closure over the remaining bone or pursuing healing by secondary intention.
- Reattachment of the fingertip as a composite graft is usually not recommended as the literature demonstrates poor outcomes with such approaches. Removing the fat from the distal tip with a rongeur then suturing the amputated skin back to cover the exposed bone may serve as a temporary biologic dressing until the patient returns to the OR for flap coverage; this may allow the patient to retain some of the bone as compared to shortening it in the ER.

Revision Amputation

- Revision amputation refers to the shortening and closure of fingertip amputations when not enough sterile matrix remains (under 5 mm) to produce an adherent, stable nail.
- This can be done on an outpatient basis by a hand surgeon; the technique depends on the nature of the injury.
- These involve amputations through the level of the eponychium. If 25 % or greater of the nail bed distal to the eponychium remains intact, the patient would benefit from maintaining that nail. If less than 25 % of nail bed remains, it is

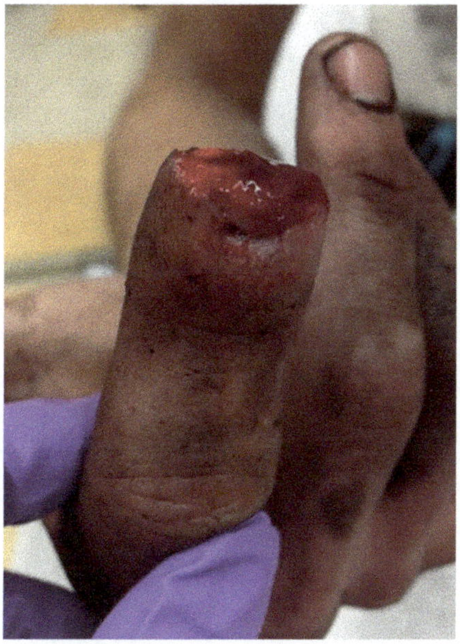

Fig. 3 Soft tissue loss with exposed bone

recommended that the remainder be resected which requires removal of the dorsal roof and ventral floor of the nail fold.

- Revision amputation can also be considered in patients with advanced age or a systemic condition where local flaps offer low success rates.

References

Boulas HJ. Amputations of the fingers and hand: indications for replantation. J Am Acad Orthop Surg. 1998;6:100–5.

Lee DH, Mignemi ME, Crosby SN. Fingertip injuries: an update on management. J Am Acad Orthop Surg. 2013;21:756–66.

Foreign Bodies in the Hand and Wrist

Foreign bodies in the hand and wrist from penetrating injuries and can usually be safely removed if large and visible enough; retained foreign bodies rarely cause problems and can be often removed later if needed unless medically warranted (i.e., nidus of infection).

History

Nature/mechanism of injury
How contaminated was the object that entered your hand?
Do you have worse pain over the site of the foreign body?
Are you having numbness or tingling?
When was your last tetanus shot?

- Signs/symptoms of infection

Physical Exam

Tenderness at site of foreign body
Assess if foreign body visible or easily accessible without dissection
Comprehensive hand physical exam

M.C. Makhni et al. (eds.), *Orthopedic Emergencies*,
DOI 10.1007/978-3-319-31524-9_51

Diagnosis

Imaging

XR hand/wrist
Can consider advanced imaging if unable to localize foreign body

Treatment Plan

Nonoperative

Remove in ER if visible and does not require dissection to obtain

- Do not "search" the hand in the ER regardless of access to fluoroscopy
- If need to look for object, then safer and more sterile to do so in OR

Most foreign bodies (in estimated 71 % of patients) left in hand

- Average particle size smaller when retained (3 mm) than when removed (6 mm)
- Few (4 %) with retained foreign bodies experienced persistent symptoms
- Rarely required subsequent surgical removal (2 %)

Consider MRI if suspect foreign body but unable to visualize with plain XR

Surgical Treatment

Remove emergently if causing neurovascular compromise
Remove urgently if grossly infected
Remove on elective basis if causing persistent pain or discomfort

Reference

Potini VC, Francisco R, Shamian B, Tan V. Sequelae of foreign bodies in the wrist and hand. HAND. 2013;8:77–81.

Hand Infections

Hand infections may be treated as an outpatient or need to be admitted, depending on the clinical course and disease course. Nearly all infections require antibiotics, and some require irrigation and debridement in the ED or in the operating room.

Overview

- *Staphylococcus aureus* is the most common pathogen
- Other common bacteria—*Pasteurella multocida* (dog/cat bite), *Eikenella* (human bite)
- In addition to providing local wound care and systemic antibiotic treatment, important to consider need for tetanus prophylaxis, rabies treatment

History

- Do you have a history of recent trauma to the site?
- Have you had infections in your hand before?
- Recent fevers or chills?
- Do you have diabetes or any type of immune deficiency?
- Have you noticed pus or fluid coming out of the site?
- Do you have any decrease in movement or sensation in the hand?
- History of IV drug use?

M.C. Makhni et al. (eds.), *Orthopedic Emergencies*,
DOI 10.1007/978-3-319-31524-9_52

Physical Exam

- Note any acute or subacute lacerations, puncture wounds, or other signs of swelling, tenderness, or purulence
- Distal neurovascular exam (Appendix A) including 2-pt sensation on radial and ulnar aspects of involved digits
- Note for hallmark Kanavel signs of flexor tenosynovitis (fusiform swelling of digit, flexed resting position of digit, pain with passive extension of digit, tenderness to palpation along flexor tendon sheath in digit and palm)
- Purulence, tenderness, or fullness at nail fold
- Rule out compartment syndrome by assessing passive range of motion throughout hand and wrist
- Assess function of all flexors/extensors to digits, especially if laceration, puncture, or bite wound

Diagnosis

Imaging

- XR: affected region (digit/hand/wrist) to assess for bony injury or foreign body

Treatment Plan

Elevate and treat with antibiotics (PO vs. IV) all hand infections
After I&D, can pack for 1–2 days then remove and begin regular soaks and dry dressing changes

Cellulitis

Depending on severity and progression, either outpatient PO antibiotic course versus inpatient admission for monitoring, IV antibiotics and elevation. Can mark borders of erythema to track progression

Paronychia (Fig. 1)

I&D in ER then dispo on PO antibiotics
Usually do not need to remove nail
Use curved blunt clamp to lift nail fold, spread to release purulence

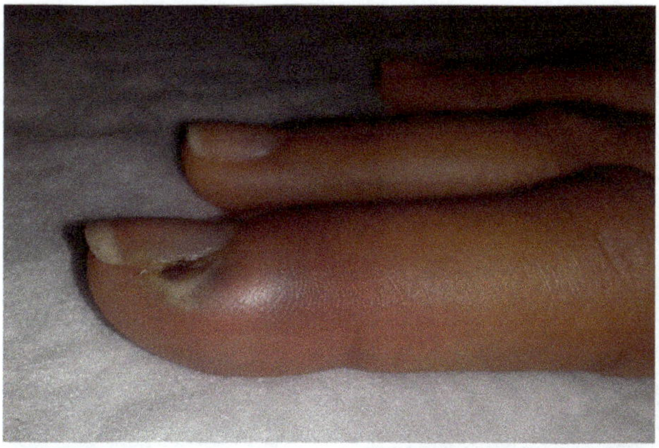

Fig. 1 Paronychia

Can curve around to lateral aspect of distal digit if needed
Often may appear to have associated felon, but usually is just extension of paronychia

Felon

I&D in ED then dispo most common
Can approach through longitudinal incision volar or lateral (ulnar aspect of digits 2–4 or radial of digit 5)—however, the best method of approach is through center of lesion

Bite Wounds (Fig. 2)

If acute, consider I&D, primary closure, and dispo with PO antibiotics
If subacute and worsening, consider admission, IV antibiotics, and strict elevation
Assess for "fight bite" over MCP (requires joint debridement)

Deep Space Infection

Less common, but requires I&D in addition to IV antibiotics

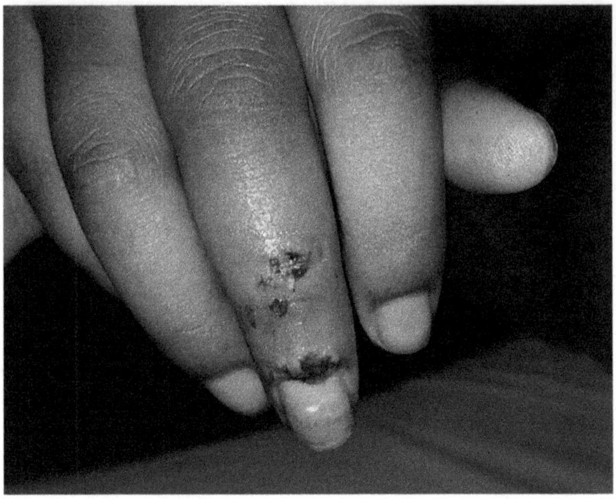

Fig. 2 Human bite wound

Flexor Tenosynovitis

Nearly all cases should be treated urgently/emergently with I&D in OR
Can consider initial admission with close monitoring/antibiotics/elevation

References

Abrams RA, Botte MJ. Hand infections: treatment recommendations for specific types. JAAOS. 1996;4(4):219–30.

Draeger RW, Bynum DK. Flexor tendon sheath infections of the hand. JAAOS. 2012;20(6): 373–82.

Shafritz AB, Coppage JM. Acute and chronic paronychia of the hand. JAAOS. 2014;22(3): 165–74.

Part VI
Pelvis and Lower Extremity

Eric F. Swart and Joseph Laratta

Acetabular Fractures 245

ACL Rupture 251

Distal Femur Fracture 253

Femoral Head Fracture 257

Femoral Shaft Fracture 259

Hip Dislocation (Native) 265

Hip Dislocation (Total Hip Arthroplasty) 269

Impending Fractures 273

Intertrochanteric/Subtrochanteric Fracture 277

Femoral Neck Fracture 283

Knee Dislocation 289

Meniscus Tear 293

Quadriceps or Patellar Tendon Rupture 295

Patella Fractures 299

Patella Dislocation 303

Pelvic Ring Injuries 307

Periprosthetic Hip Fracture 311

Periprosthetic Knee Femur Fracture 315

Tibia-Fibula Shaft Fracture 319

Tibial Plateau Fracture 325

Acetabular Fractures

High energy intra-articular injuries to the weight-bearing portion of the pelvis. Frequently require operative fixation in younger patients. Low energy elderly patients sometimes nonoperatively treated.

History

- High energy in younger patients, frequently MVC/MCC's. Older patients can be from ground level falls.

Physical Exam

- Full trauma exam (Appendix A: Trauma exam)
- Check pelvis stability to confirm no associated pelvic ring injury

Diagnosis

Imaging

- AP pelvis should be part of initial trauma series
- Judet views of pelvis: obturator oblique and iliac oblique
- CT usually required to help better classify fracture and determine treatment plan (Fig. 1)

M.C. Makhni et al. (eds.), *Orthopedic Emergencies*,
DOI 10.1007/978-3-319-31524-9_53

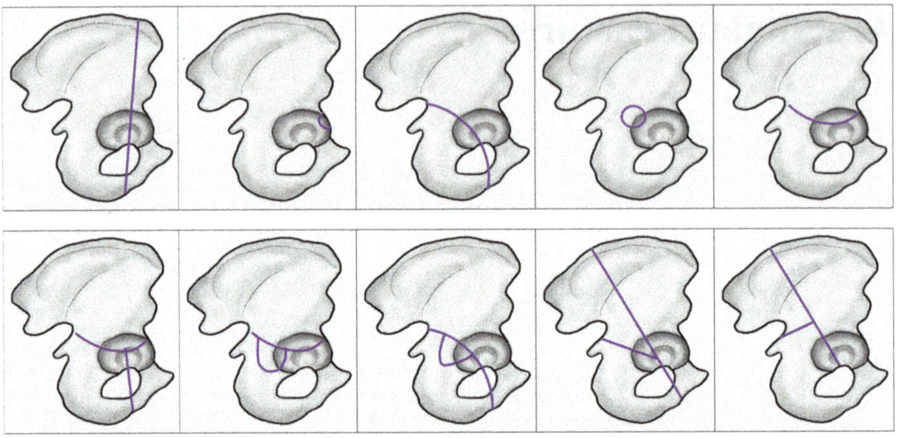

Fig. 1 Acetabulum fractures

Classification

Letournel classification (Judet R. J Bone Joint Surg Am. 1964;46:1615–38) based on injuries to defined posterior wall, anterior wall, posterior column, and anterior column.

Elementary types:

- Posterior wall (Fig. 2)
- Anterior wall
- Posterior column
- Anterior column
- Transverse

Associated types:

- Posterior column + posterior wall
- Transverse + posterior wall (Fig. 3)
- T-type
- Anterior column + posterior hemistransverse
- Associated both columns

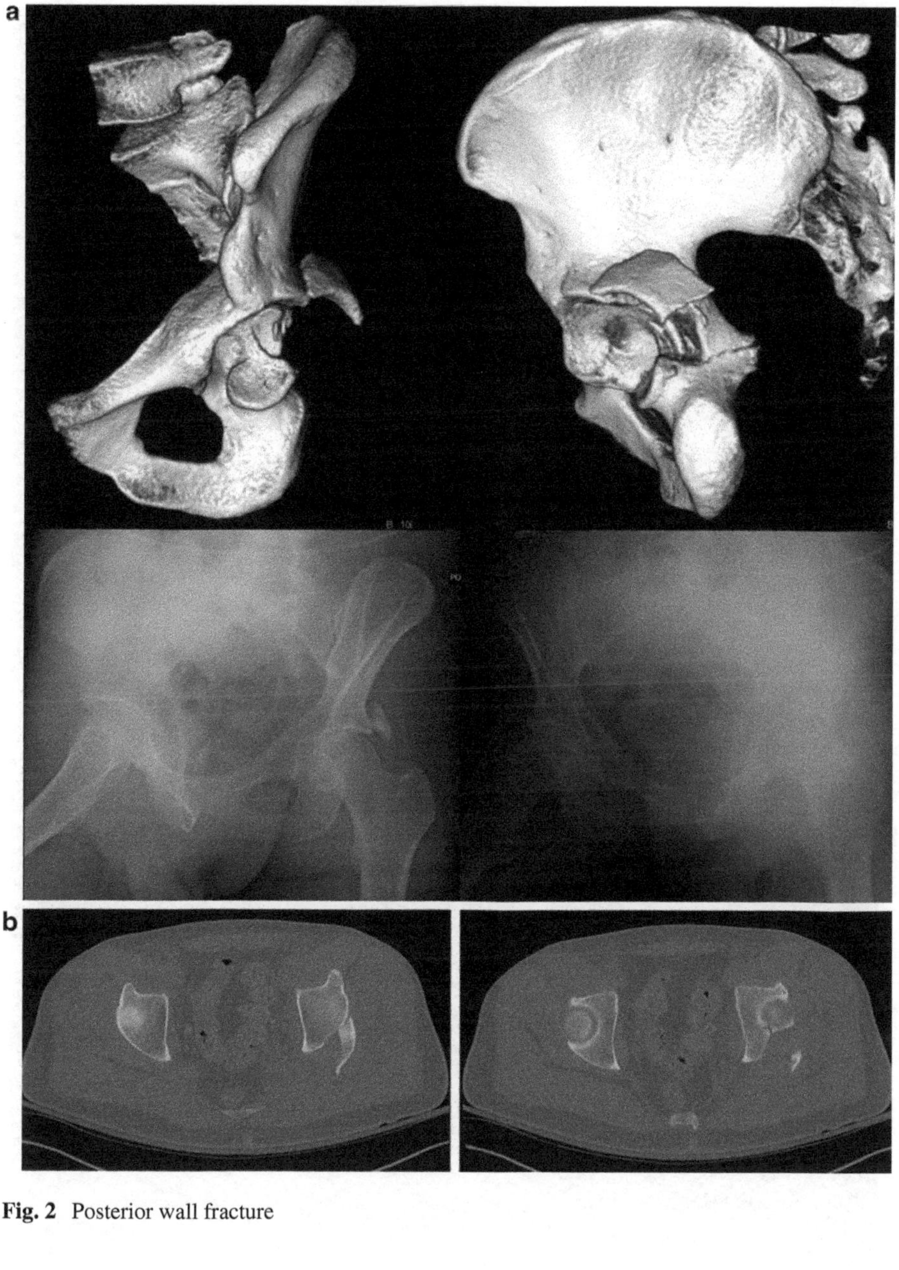

Fig. 2 Posterior wall fracture

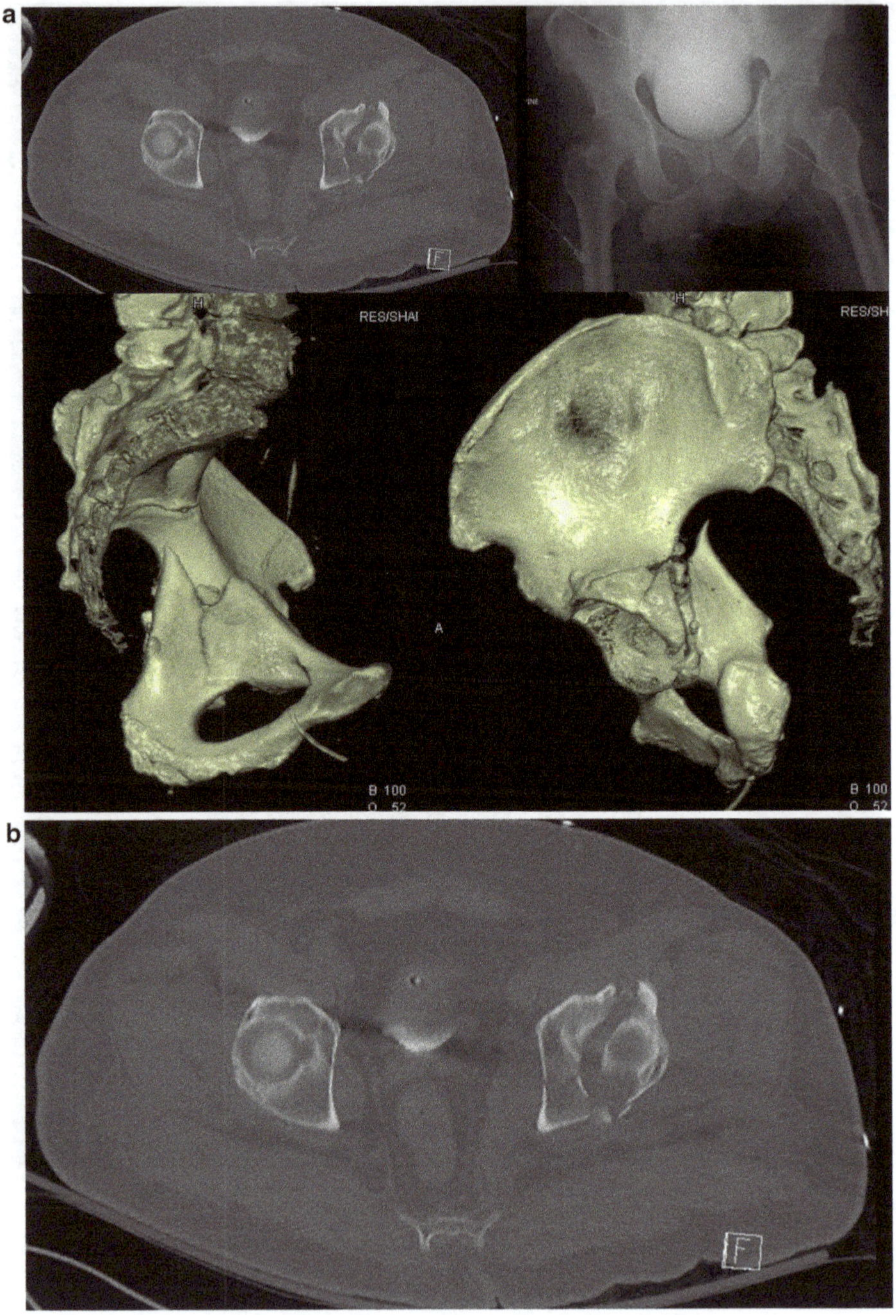

Fig. 3 Transverse + posterior wall fracture

Treatment Plan

Treatment is based on restoring a congruent acetabulum that is stable to physiologic stresses. Acetabular fractures associated with unstable hip joint may require closed hip reduction (Appendix B: Hip reduction technique), followed by skeletal traction application (Appendix B: Traction technique guide).

Nonoperative

Nonoperative treatment is protected weight bearing (usually "toe touch" or "touch-down" weight bearing) for 6–8 weeks. For minimally displaced fractures (<2 mm) or small posterior wall fractures (sometimes defined as <20 % posterior wall involvement) with a stable hip joint. May require exam under anesthesia to test joint stability. Geriatric associated both column fractures with medialization of acetabulum but a congruent joint around femoral head are also frequently treated nonoperatively.

Operative

Open reduction and internal fixation treatment of choice for displaced, unstable fracture patterns.

References

Moed BR, Carr SE, Gruson KI, Watson JT, Craig JG. Computed tomographic assessment of fractures of the posterior wall of the acetabulum after operative treatment. J Bone Joint Surg Am. 2003;85-A(3):512–22.

Plaisier BR, Meldon SW, Super DM, et al. Improved outcome after early fixation of acetabular fractures. Injury. 2000;31:81–4.

Tornetta 3rd P. Displaced acetabular fractures: indications for operative and nonoperative management. J Am Acad Orthop Surg. 2001;9(1):18–28.

ACL Rupture

Common ligamentous injury to the knee, frequently operatively reconstructed on an elective basis.

History

- Often during sports, can be a contact injury or a noncontact injury (e.g., with cutting)
- Classic history is a "pop" in the knee with severe pain, followed by a large effusion within the next hour
- Any prior knee injuries?

Physical Exam

- Acute injuries usually associated with large effusion
- Ideally would check full ligamentous knee exam (Appendix A: Ligamentous knee exam), although may be limited by pain/guarding in an acute setting
- Examine hip as well (especially in younger patients) to confirm "knee pain" not actually referred hip pain
- Confirm NVID lower extremity (Appendix A: LE neuro exam)

M.C. Makhni et al. (eds.), *Orthopedic Emergencies*,
DOI 10.1007/978-3-319-31524-9_54

Diagnosis

Imaging

- X-rays of knee should be acquired in ED to rule out fracture but usually negative
- MRI is confirmatory study but does not need to be done in initial ED visit–usually done on an elective/outpatient basis

Treatment Plan

Initial ED treatment consists of pain control and immobilization with outpatient orthopedic follow-up

Nonoperative

Pain control, knee immobilizer for comfort +/− crutches, and ice in acute period

Operative

May ultimately be surgically reconstructed but usually done on an elective basis once initial injury pain and stiffness have improved

References

Boden BP, Sheehan FT, Torg JS, Hewett TE. Noncontact anterior cruciate ligament injuries: mechanisms and risk factors. J Am Acad Orthop Surg. 2010;18(9):520–7.

Carey JL, Shea KG. AAOS Clinical Practice Guideline: management of anterior cruciate ligament injuries: evidence-based guideline. J Am Acad Orthop Surg. 2015;23(5):e6–8. doi:10.5435/JAAOS-D-15-00095. Epub 2015 Mar 20.

Distal Femur Fracture

Metaphyseal fractures with management based on displacement and articular involvement.

History

- Typical bimodal distribution (young high energy vs. elderly fragility fractures)
- Check for associated injuries, other complaints

Physical Exam

- Full trauma exam (Appendix A: Trauma exam)
- Skin intact?
- If laceration or punctate wound, consider saline load to assess communication with joint (Appendix B: Saline load of knee technique)
- Distal neurovascular exam before and after skeletal traction (Appendix A: LE neuro exam)

Diagnosis

Imaging

- XR should visualize entire length of femur, including the joint above and below the injury
- AP, lateral, and two 45° oblique views of the distal femur

M.C. Makhni et al. (eds.), *Orthopedic Emergencies*,
DOI 10.1007/978-3-319-31524-9_55

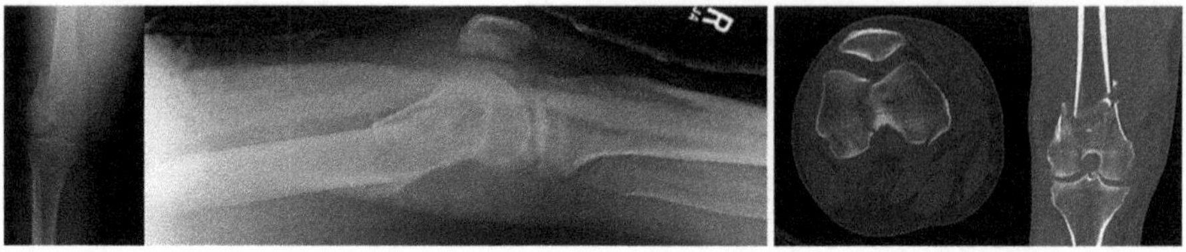

Fig. 1 Distal femur fracture with simple intra-articular extension

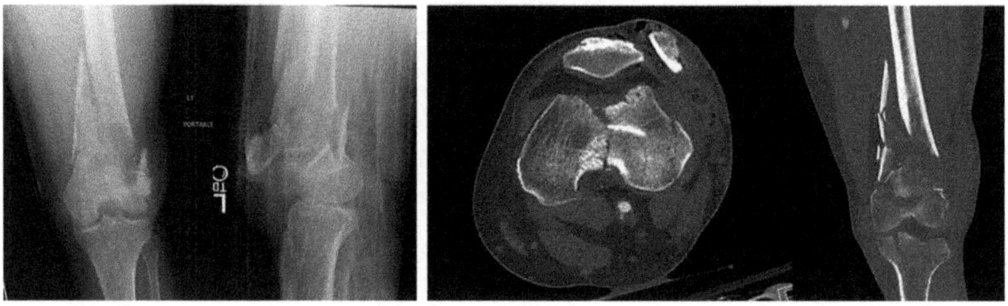

Fig. 2 Distal femur fracture with complex intra-articular extension

- Tunnel view of the notch may help evaluate displacement of vertical fractures into the joint
- Consider traction views and contralateral films for preoperative planning
- CT if concern for traumatic arthrotomy (look for free air in joint), coronal fracture (Hoffa fragment), or for preoperative planning in complex intra-articular fractures (Figs. 1 and 2)

Classification

Descriptive based on:

Skin integrity (open, closed)
Location and articular involvement (extra- vs. intra-articular, supracondylar, condylar)
Pattern (spiral, oblique, transverse, comminution/butterfly)
Displacement (shortening, translation)

AO classification

Treatment Plan

Treatment based on articular involvement and displacement.

Nonoperative

Nondisplaced fractures or patient with significant underlying medical comorbidities
All temporized with bulky Jones dressing to allow for swelling, knee immobilizer, and NWB
May consider tibial traction pin if significantly shortened (Appendix: Traction technique guide)
If stable, transition to hinged knee brace with PWB to allow knee ROM.
If unstable, transition to long leg casting for 2–3 months with goal of restoring mechanical axis of LE

Operative

Most displaced fractures are treated with open reduction internal fixation during patient hospitalization
AO pillars are respected: anatomic joint reconstruction, stable fixation to allow early ROM, and preservation of blood supply.
Fixation of articular fragments to shaft may be done using bridging technique and percutaneous instrumentation.

Reference

Gwathmey Jr FW, Jones-Quaidoo SM, Kahler D, Hurwitz S, Cui Q. Distal femoral fractures: current concepts. J Am Acad Orthop Surg. 2010;18(10):597–607.

Femoral Head Fracture

Rare high energy fracture, frequently associated with hip dislocation. Frequently (although not universally) require operative treatment

History

- Classically high energy injury, similar to native hip dislocation

Physical Exam

- Full trauma exam (Appendix A: Trauma exam)
- Leg length discrepancy
- **Good detailed distal neurologic exam of affected limb**, as traction injuries to sciatic nerve frequently occur (Appendix A: LE neuro exam).

Diagnosis

Imaging

- AP pelvis, AP and lateral hip XRs
- CT usually indicated to better assess fracture morphology. If associated with dislocation, obtain after closed reduction of hip.

M.C. Makhni et al. (eds.), *Orthopedic Emergencies*,
DOI 10.1007/978-3-319-31524-9_56

Classification

Pipkin classification:

- Type 1: Below fovea
- Type 2: Above fovea
- Type 3: With associated femoral neck fracture
- Type 4: With associated posterior wall fracture

Treatment Plan

Immediate treatment includes closed reduction of hip dislocation (if present) (Appendix B: Hip reduction technique). Treatment principles involve restoring a congruent, stable hip joint and minimizing risk of avascular necrosis of the head.

Nonoperative

TTWB for 4–6 weeks with restricted adduction and internal rotation. Indicated in most Pipkin 1 fractures and Pipkin 2 fractures with <1 mm step-off, and Pipkin 4 fractures with a stable hip joint (based on acetabular fracture) pattern.

Operative

Open reduction and internal fixation. Indicated for displaced Pipkin 2, most Pipkin 3 fractures, and Pipkin 4 fractures with an unstable hip joint based on the acetabular fracture pattern.

References

Droll KP, Broekhuyse H, O'Brien P. Fracture of the femoral head. J Am Acad Orthop Surg. 2007;15(12):716–27.

Henle P, Kloen P, Siebenrock KA. Femoral head injuries: which treatment strategy can be recommended? Injury. 2007;38(4):478–88.

Femoral Shaft Fracture

High-energy injury of the femur. Almost always operative.

History

- Almost always high energy trauma when in the adult population
- If mechanism inconsistent with level of trauma, suspect pathologic cause
- Check for associated injuries, other complaints

Physical Exam (Fig. 1)

- Full trauma exam (Appendix A: Trauma exam)
- Skin intact? Internal degloving?
- Distal neurovascular exam before and after skeletal traction (Appendix A: LE neuro exam)

Diagnosis

Imaging

- AP and lateral of entire femur
- AP pelvis and dedicated hip views to rule out ipsilateral femoral neck fracture
- Dedicated ipsilateral knee films

M.C. Makhni et al. (eds.), *Orthopedic Emergencies*,
DOI 10.1007/978-3-319-31524-9_57

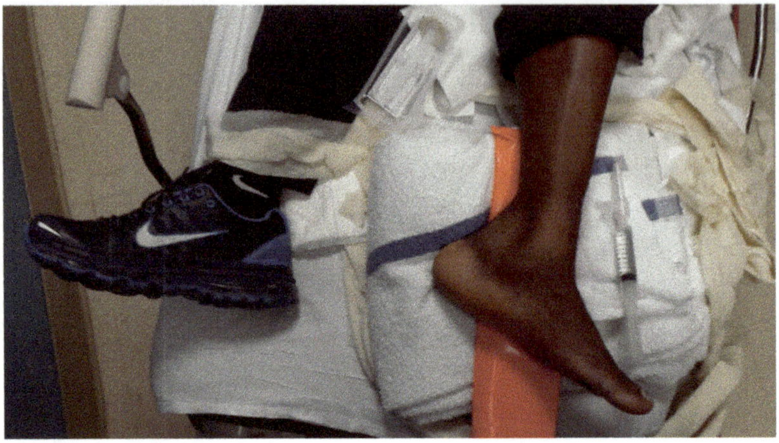

Fig. 1 Limb shortening in a patient with a femoral shaft fracture

- MUST EVALUATE FOR CONCOMITTANT FEMORAL NECK FRACTURE. This can be done with:
  - Fine-cut CT through the femoral neck (often included in trauma series CT scans)
  - Dedicated hip imaging pre-op
  - Intraoperative fluoroscopy

Other Workup

- Pulmonary status is critical, as it can help determine whether definitive care (IM nail) or temporizing "damage control orthopedics" (e.g. external fixator) is appropriate:
  - Lactate level? Trending up or down?
  - Base deficit?
  - Intubated? If so, vent settings/PEEP?
  - Known pulmonary contusions?

Classification

Descriptive based on:

Skin integrity (open, closed)
Location (proximal, middle, distal third)

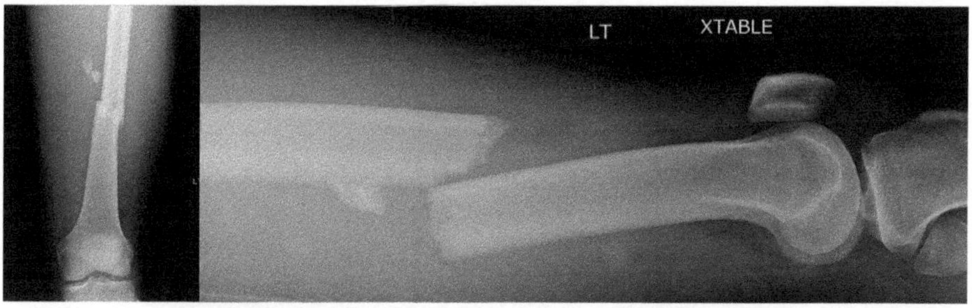

Fig. 2 Transverse femoral shaft fracture

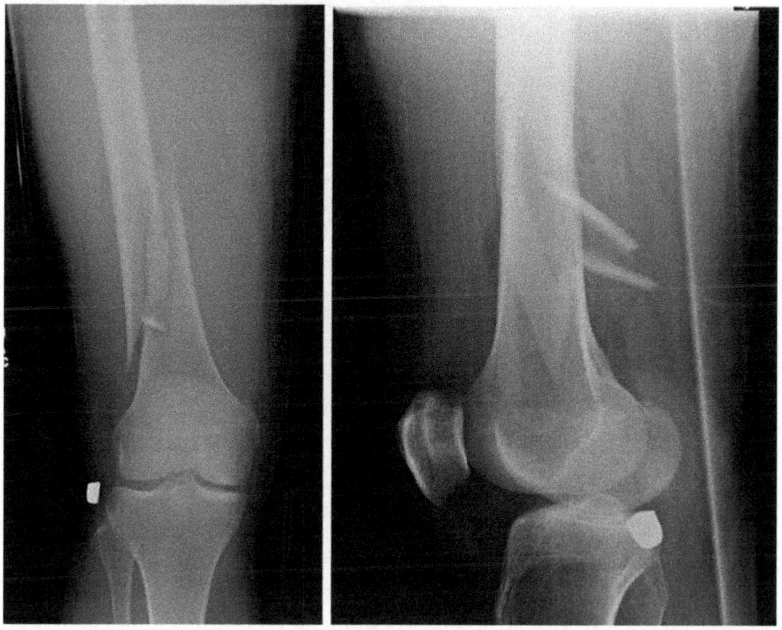

Fig. 3 Oblique femoral shaft fracture

Pattern (spiral, oblique, transverse, comminution/butterfly) (Figs. 2 and 3)
Displacement (shortening, translation)

AO classification

Treatment Plan

Operative stabilization is standard of care for nearly all femoral shaft fractures.

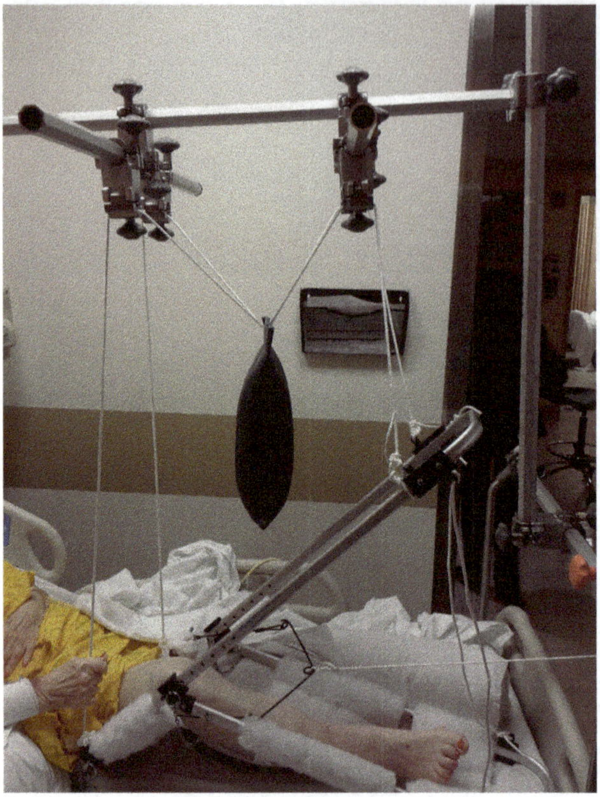

Fig. 4 Balanced skeletal traction

Nonoperative

Skeletal traction to restore length, improve pain, and minimize blood loss into thigh (Fig. 4).

Often temporizing until surgical stabilization, unless patient not safe for surgical management

Tibial traction standard unless ipsilateral acetabular fracture when femoral traction employed (Appendix B: Traction technique guide)

Operative

Surgical stabilization should be performed within 48 h if possible.

Typically intramedullary implant, unless patient unstable where external fixation may be preferable

References

Nahm NJ, Como JJ, Wilber JH, Vallier HA. Early appropriate care: definitive stabilization of femoral fractures within 24 hours of injury is safe in most patients with multiple injuries. J Trauma. 2011;71(1):175–85.

Tornetta 3rd P, Kain MS, Creevy WR. Diagnosis of femoral neck fractures in patients with a femoral shaft fracture. Improvement with a standard protocol. J Bone Joint Surg Am. 2007;89(1):39–43.

Hip Dislocation (Native)

Relatively uncommon injuries, usually high energy. Require emergent reduction, followed by evaluation for associated injuries.

History

- Classic mechanism is "dashboard injury" in MVC where knee is driven into dashboard of car and femoral head dislocates postero-superiorly out of acetabulum.
- Ask about tingling/numbness/paresthesia

Physical Exam

- Full trauma exam (Appendix A: Trauma exam)
- Leg length discrepancy
- **Good detailed distal neurologic exam of affected limb**, as traction injuries to sciatic nerve frequently occur (Appendix A: LE neuro exam)

Diagnosis

Imaging

- AP pelvis, dedicated AP and cross table lateral of hip (Fig. 1) to confirm (a) direction of dislocation, and (b) no femoral neck fracture (contraindication to closed reduction)

M.C. Makhni et al. (eds.), *Orthopedic Emergencies*,
DOI 10.1007/978-3-319-31524-9_58

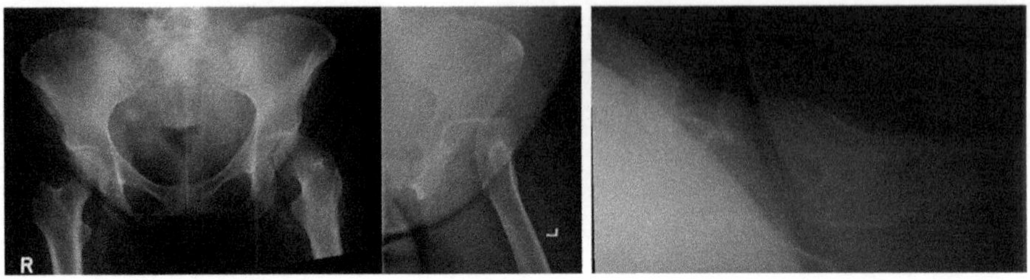

Fig. 1 Anterior hip dislocation

- Consider Judet views of pelvis to evaluate for posterior wall fracture
- CT always indicated post-reduction to check for associated femur or acetabular fracture and intra-articular loose bodies.
- CT can be considered pre-reduction if reduction attempts are unsuccessful to evaluate for other barriers to reduction.
- Role of acute MRI controversial, currently not supported.

Classification

Classified as simple versus complex (associated with acetabulum or femur fracture), and by direction of dislocation (posterior vs. anterior).

Treatment Plan

Immediate (emergent) closed reduction is critical (Appendix B: Hip reduction technique). Post-reduction, CT is performed which determines treatment plan (treatment of any associated injuries). If associated with acetabular and the joint is unstable may require skeletal traction application after reduction (Appendix B: Skeletal traction technique).

Nonoperative

If hip is stable after reduction without associated fractures or intra-articular loose bodies, can treat nonoperatively with protected weight bearing for 6–8 weeks.

Operative

Operative treatment is directed by associated injuries, and may include open reduction of associated acetabular or femoral fractures, or removal of loose bodies.

References

Foulk DM, Mullis BH. Hip dislocation: evaluation and management. J Am Acad Orthop Surg. 2010;18(4):199–209.
Moed BR, Ajibade DA, Israel H. Computed tomography as a predictor of hip stability status in posterior wall fractures of the acetabulum. J Orthop Trauma. 2009;23(1):7–15.

Hip Dislocation (Total Hip Arthroplasty)

Relatively common complication following total hip replacement. Requires urgent reduction, further treatment based on multifactorial algorithm.

History

- Usually based on accidental provocative maneuver
  - Posterior: flexion, internal rotation, adduction, like getting up from a low seat (e.g., bed, toilet)
  - Anterior: extension, external rotation
- Surgical history/date/surgeon/approach used.
- History of prior dislocations?

Physical Exam

- Leg length discrepancy (Fig. 1)
- **Good detailed distal neurologic exam of affected limb**, as traction injuries to sciatic nerve frequently occur (Appendix A: LE neuro exam) .

M.C. Makhni et al. (eds.), *Orthopedic Emergencies*,
DOI 10.1007/978-3-319-31524-9_59

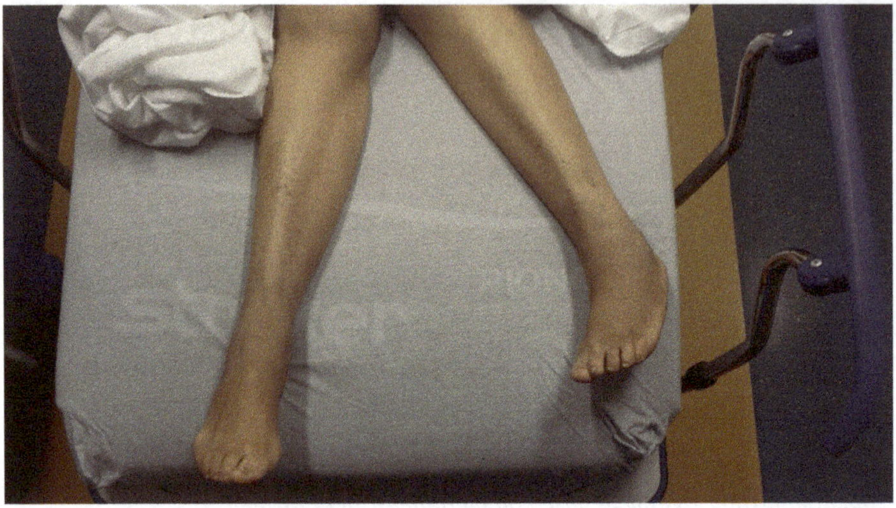

Fig. 1 Clinical appearance of dislocated THA

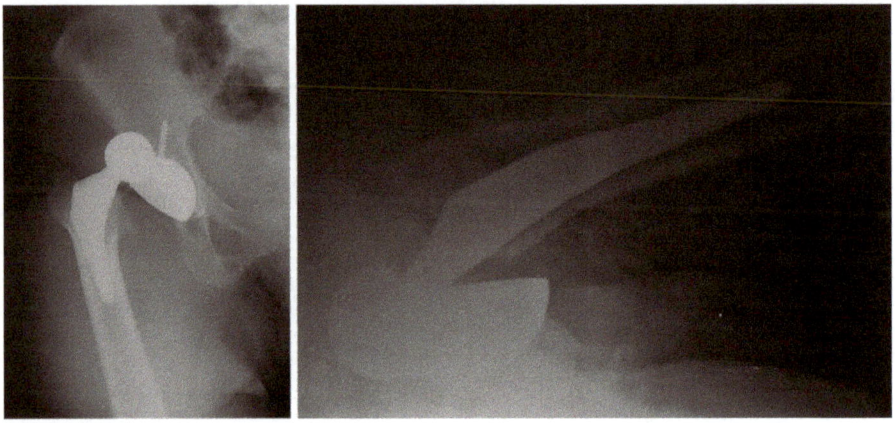

Fig. 2 Posterior THA dislocation (pre-reduction)

Diagnosis

Imaging

- AP pelvis, dedicated AP and cross table lateral of hip to confirm direction of dislocation (Figs. 2 and 3).
- Usually no acute role in CT/MRI. CT may be helpful to assess component position for long-term decision-making, but unlikely to alter emergency management unless hip is irreducible.

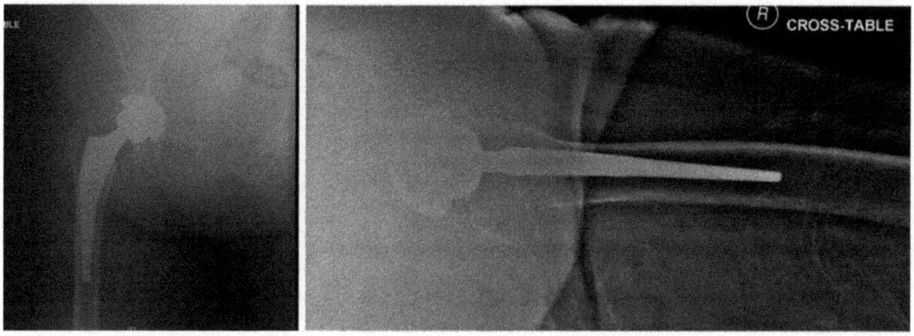

Fig. 3 Posterior THA dislocation (post-reduction)

Treatment Plan

Emergency department treatment consists of immediate closed reduction in ED (Appendix B: Hip reduction technique).

Nonoperative

Nonoperative treatment usually for first time dislocations with stable exam after reduction. Usually protected weight-bearing with early orthopedic follow-up to confirm stability. May include hip brace as well.

Operative

Revision arthroplasty for hips with multiple dislocations or for certain types of primary dislocations (constrained liner).

References

Alberton GM, High WA, Morrey BF. Dislocation after revision total hip arthroplasty: an analysis of risk factors and treatment options. J Bone Joint Surg Am. 2002;84-A(10):1788–92.

Soong M, Rubash HE, Macaulay W. Dislocation after total hip arthroplasty. J Am Acad Orthop Surg. 2004;12(5):314–21.

Impending Fractures

Impending or insufficiency fractures are often prophylactically stabilized to prevent catastrophic fracture.

History

- Atraumatic
- Osteoporosis and history of bisphosphonate use
- Family and personal history of cancer
- Pain with ambulation, night pain, weight loss, constitutional symptoms
- Remember myeloma presentation of hypercalcemia, renal failure, back pain, anemia

Physical Exam

- Examination of entire skeletal system, often multiple bones affected
- Examination of gait and station
- Distal neurovascular exam

Diagnosis

Imaging

- XR of entire bone affected and any areas of tenderness on exam
- Impending bisphosphonate fractures often in subtrochanteric or diaphyseal region with circumferential cortical thickening and stress reaction
- If no known primary neoplasm, consider MRI to determine skip lesions in the bone

M.C. Makhni et al. (eds.), *Orthopedic Emergencies*,
DOI 10.1007/978-3-319-31524-9_60

Table 1 Mirel scoring system determines the need for prophylactic fixation of long bones due to lesions

	1	2	3
Site	Upper extremity	Lower extremity	Petitrochanteric
Pain	Mild	Moderate	Functional
X-ray appearance	Blastic	Mixed	Lytic
Size	<1/3 bone diameter	1/3–2/3 bone diameter	>2/3 bone diameter

Classification (Table 1)

A score >8 suggests that prophylactic fixation may be beneficial
Harrington Criteria
Based on amount of bone destruction, region of involvement, and pain after radiotherapy

Treatment Plan

Immediate alteration of weight-bearing status to NWB or TDWB
Typically stabilized surgically

Non-operative

Almost all operative, unless known primary neoplasm and Mirel <8 may be treated with radiation alone.

Primary tumor work-up: CT chest, abdomen, pelvis. SPEP/UPEP. CBC with differential. BMP, ESR, LFTs, LDH, Ca, Phos, AlkPhos.

Operative

If no known primary, treating surgeon must obtain tissue with biopsy prior to surgical stabilization.

If primary bone neoplasm, neoadjuvant chemotherapy or radiation may be helpful.

Type of fixation depends on location of lesion and disease type; however, our goals of stabilization are the same: allow early weight bearing and mobilization, internally splint entire bone, and prevent catastrophic fracture.

References

Harrington KD. Orthopaedic management of extremity and pelvic lesions. Clin Orthop Relat Res. 1995;312:136–47.

Mirels H. Metastatic disease in long bones. A proposed scoring system for diagnosing impending pathologic fractures. Clin Orthop Relat Res. 1989;249:256–64.

Intertrochanteric/Subtrochanteric Fracture

Fractures more common in elderly, osteoporotic patients. Almost universally require operative treatment following preoperative medial optimization.

History

- Usually low-energy mechanisms (e.g., fall from standing)
- Important to determine preoperative ambulatory status/independence

Physical Exam

- Full trauma exam (Appendix A: Trauma exam)
- Log roll, heel strike (Appendix A: Hip fracture exam) (Fig. 1)
- Confirm NVID lower extremity (Appendix A: LE neuro exam)

Diagnosis

Imaging

- AP pelvis, AP, and cross-table lateral of hip
- Traction/internal rotation view may be helpful to better evaluate if fracture is in femoral neck, or lateral wall integrity (Fig. 2)
- CT usually not necessary for preoperative planning
- Full femur films needed if plans to place long cephalomedullary nail

M.C. Makhni et al. (eds.), *Orthopedic Emergencies*,
DOI 10.1007/978-3-319-31524-9_61

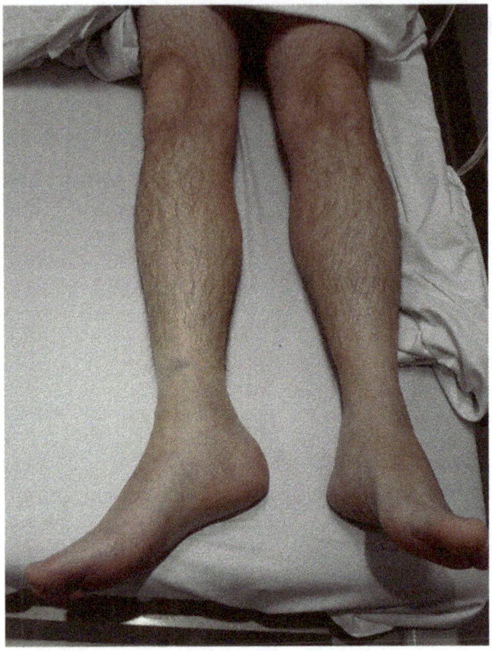

Fig. 1 Shortened, externally rotated leg after intertrochanteric fracture

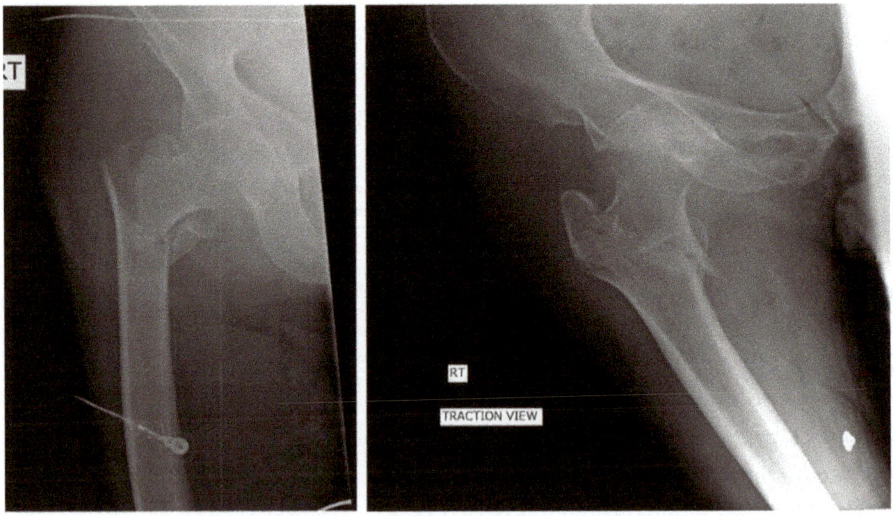

Fig. 2 Traction view can clarify fracture pattern

Classification

Multiple classification systems exist. OTA classification is commonly used:

- 31-A1: Regular obliquity, simple fracture (Fig. 3)
- 31-A2: Regular obliquity with some medial comminution (Fig. 4)
- 31-A3: Reverse obliquity (Fig. 5)

Alternate classifications include Evans, and simplified "stable" vs. "unstable."

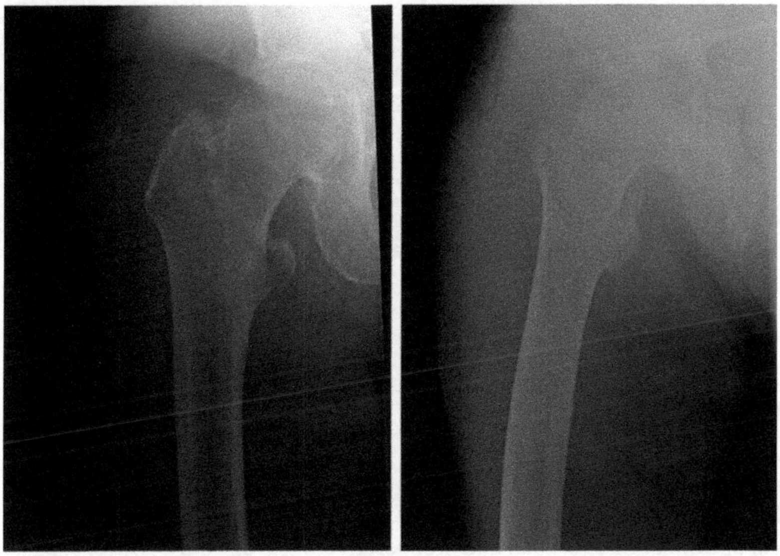

Fig. 3 A1 intertrochanteric fracture

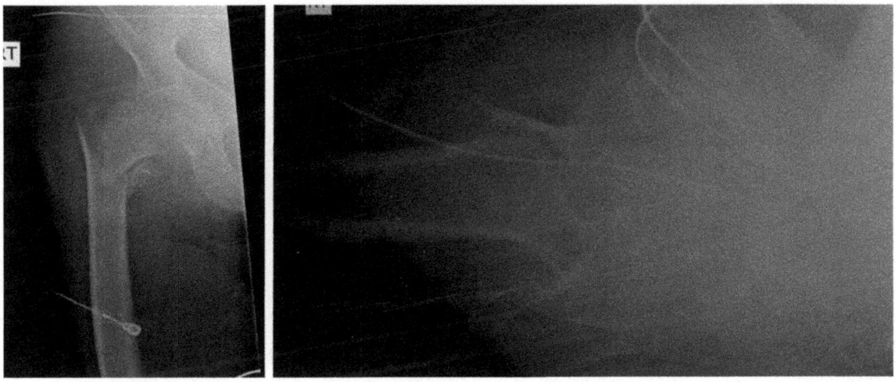

Fig. 4 A2 intertrochanteric fracture

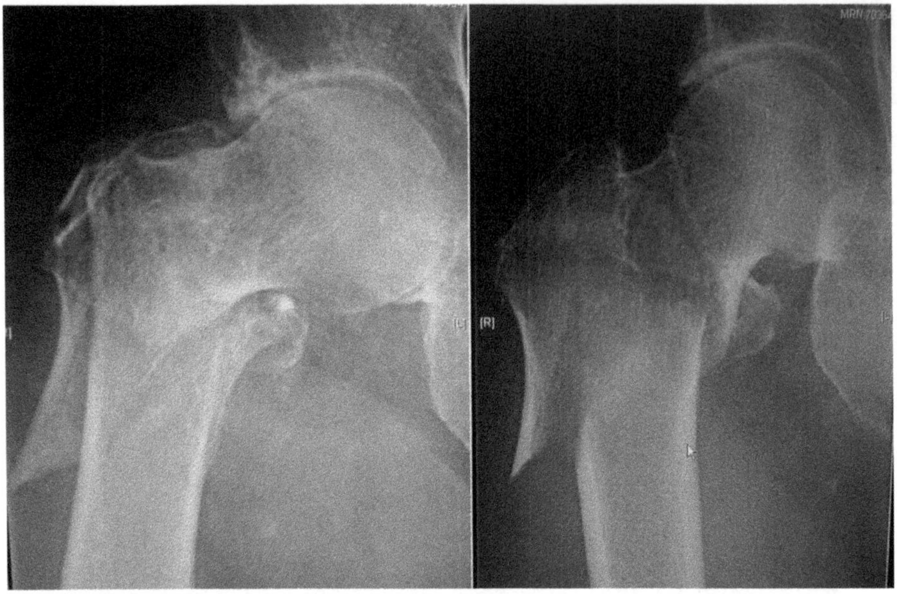

Fig. 5 A3 intertrochanteric fracture

Treatment Plan

Treatment for these fractures is almost always operative, with the goal of early mobilization and maximizing chance of return to preoperative functional levels. Medical optimization is crucial and preoperative work-up (CBC, BMP, coags, EKG, CXR, ± troponins) should be initiated as quickly as possible to facilitate clearance. The goal is operative fixation within 48 h of fracture if possible.

Non-operative

Usually reserved for patients too sick or unstable for surgery. Includes WBAT and mobilization as permitted by pain, with high-intensity nursing care while the patient is in bed.

Operative

Operative treatment is usually either cephalomedullary nail or sliding hip screw, based on fracture pattern and surgeon's preference.

References

Barton TM, Gleeson R, Topliss C, Greenwood R, Harries WJ, Chesser TJ. A comparison of the long gamma nail with the sliding hip screw for the treatment of AO/OTA 31-A2 fractures of the proximal part of the femur: a prospective randomized trial. J Bone Joint Surg Am. 2010;92(4):792–8.

Kaplan K, Miyamoto R, Levine BR, Egol KA, Zuckerman JD. Surgical management of hip fractures: an evidence-based review of the literature. II: intertrochanteric fractures. J Am Acad Orthop Surg. 2008;16(11):665–73.

Roberts KC, Brox WT, Jevsevar DS, Sevarino K. Management of hip fractures in the elderly. J Am Acad Orthop Surg. 2015;23(2):131–7. doi:10.5435/JAAOS-D-14-00432.

Femoral Neck Fractures

Can be high-energy injuries in young patients or low-energy fragility fractures in osteoporotic patients. Almost always fixed operatively. ***Considered a surgical urgency/emergency for younger patients.***

History

- Young patients: usually high-energy injury
- Older patients: frequently fall from standing
- For elderly patients:
  - Preoperative ambulatory status/independence
  - Any hip pain before injury?

Physical Exam

- Full trauma exam (Appendix A: Trauma exam)
- Leg length discrepancy
- Log roll, heel strike (Appendix A: Hip fracture exam)
- Confirm NVID lower extremity (Appendix A: LE neuro exam)

M.C. Makhni et al. (eds.), *Orthopedic Emergencies*,
DOI 10.1007/978-3-319-31524-9_62

Diagnosis

Imaging

- AP pelvis, AP and cross-table lateral of hip
- CT usually not necessary for preoperative planning

Classification

For younger patients, Pauwels classification is most helpful (Pauwels F. Stuttgart: Ferdinand Enke Verlag; 1935), based on vertical orientation of fracture line

- Pauwels type 1: Less than 30° from horizontal (Fig. 1)
- Pauwels type 2: 30–50° from horizontal
- Pauwels type 3: More than 50° from horizontal

For younger, high-energy patients, this is considered by some to be a surgical urgency/emergency, due to loss of blood supply to the femoral head. Operative treatment should be performed quickly, but whether this means emergently/overnight vs. urgently/early next day is controversial (Garden RS. J Bone Joint Surg Br. 1964;46:630–47):

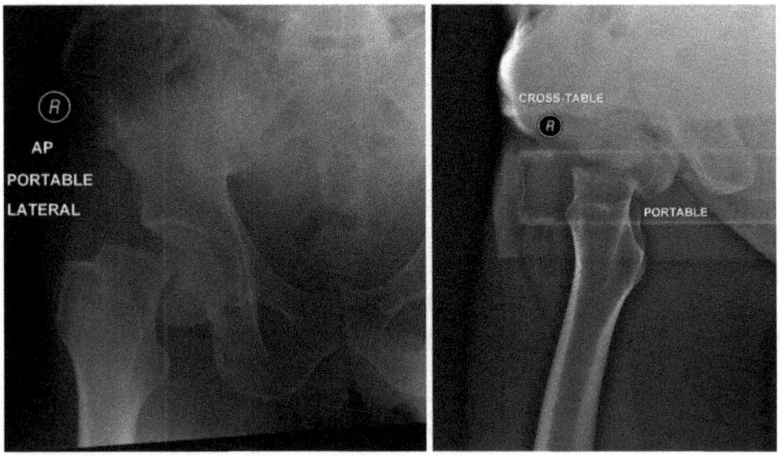

Fig. 1 Pauwels 1 fracture

- Garden type 1: Valgus impacted (Fig. 2)
- Garden type 2: Nondisplaced
- Garden type 3: Displaced less than 50 %
- Garden type 4: Displaced more than 50 % (Fig. 3)

"Simplified Garden" classification often used, which divides fractures into nondisplaced (Garden 1 and 2) and displaced (Garden 3 and 4)

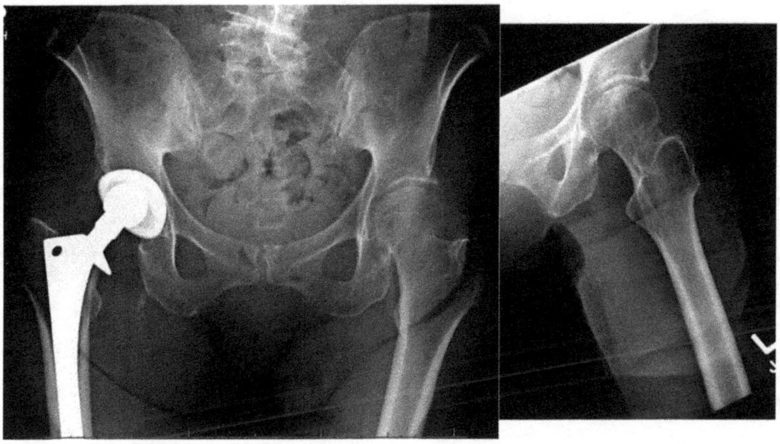

Fig. 2 Garden 1 fracture

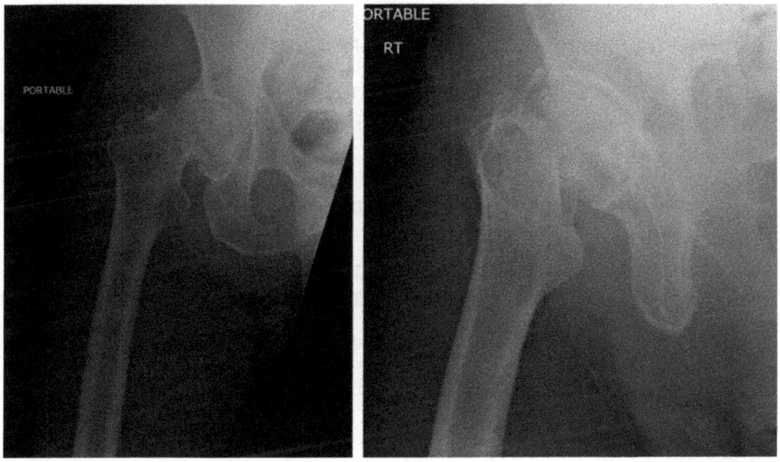

Fig. 3 Garden 4 fracture

Treatment Plan

Most fractures are treated operatively for both young and elderly patients.

- For younger, high-energy patients, this is a **surgical urgency/emergency**.
- For elderly patients medical optimization is crucial and preoperative work-up (CBC, BMP, coags, EKG, CXR, +/− troponins) should be initiated as quickly as possible to facilitate clearance. The goal is operative fixation within 48 h of fracture if possible.

Nonoperative

- Nonoperative treatment usually involves observation and mobilization as tolerated by symptoms.
- Usually reserved for patients too sick or unstable for surgery.
- Even those with extremely low demand (nonambulatory) often felt to benefit from pain control of surgery.

Operative

- For younger patients, urgent open reduction and internal fixation is the treatment of choice.
  - This is done urgently to decrease the risk of AVN and damage of blood supply to femoral head.
  - Major determinant of outcome is quality of reduction in OR.
- For elderly patients, three major operative treatment choices. Goal is early mobility and to optimize the change of return to preoperative function while minimizing the risk of requiring future operations.
  - Closed reduction and percutaneous pinning: for nondisplaced or valgus-impacted fractures (Garden 1 or 2)
  - Hemiarthroplasty: For elderly, low-demand patients
  - Total hip arthroplasty: For the "fit elderly" or higher demand elderly patients

References

Keating JF, Grant A, Masson M, Scott NW, Forbes JF. Randomized comparison of reduction and fixation, bipolar hemiarthroplasty, and total hip arthroplasty. Treatment of displaced intracapsular hip fractures in healthy older patients. J Bone Joint Surg Am. 2006;88(2):249–60.

Probe R, Ward R. Internal fixation of femoral neck fractures. J Am Acad Orthop Surg. 2006;14(9):565–71.

Roberts KC, Brox WT. AAOS Clinical Practice Guideline: Management of Hip Fractures in the Elderly. J Am Acad Orthop Surg. 2015;23(2):138–40.

Roberts KC, Brox WT, Jevsevar DS, Sevarino K. Management of hip fractures in the elderly. J Am Acad Orthop Surg. 2015;23(2):131–7. doi:10.5435/JAAOS-D-14-00432.

Knee Dislocation

High-energy injury with multiple ligament ruptures, frequently associated with vascular compromise. Almost always require operative repair vs reconstruction, although timing may vary

History

- High-energy injury frequently from MVCs or falls from height. Can also be associated with athletic collisions.

Physical Exam

- Full trauma exams
- Ligamentous knee exam
- **Distal neurovascular exam is crucial** as 5–15 % of dislocations are associated with vascular injuries
  - **Must check ABI**. If ABI is < 0.9, requires further arterial studies (ultrasound vs. CT angiography)

Diagnosis

Imaging

- Full knee X-rays needed (Fig. 1)
- Arterial ultrasound of CT angio when concern for arterial injury (ABI < 0.9)

M.C. Makhni et al. (eds.), *Orthopedic Emergencies*,
DOI 10.1007/978-3-319-31524-9_63

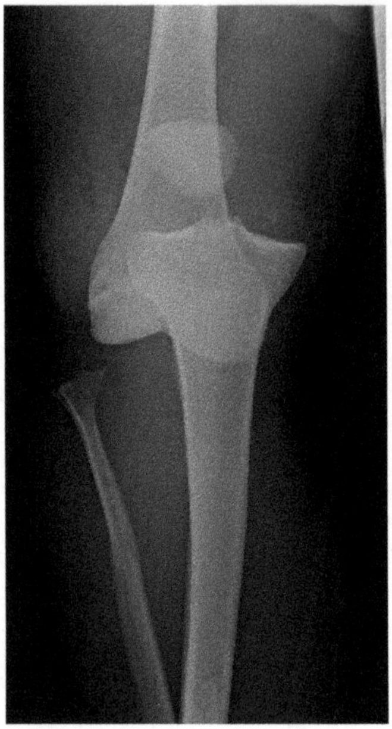

Fig. 1 High-energy knee dislocation

- MRI usually needed as part of preoperative evaluation but not part of emergent initial evaluation

Classification

Can be descriptive based on direction of injury

Also used is Schenck Classification, based on the number of torn ligaments:

- KD1—1 ligament torn: ACL or PCL
- KD2—2 ligaments torn: ACL AND PCL
- KD3—3 ligaments torn: ACL+PCL and PMC OR PLC
- KD4—4 ligaments town: ACL+PCL and PMC+PLC
- KD5—Dislocation + multiligamentous injury associated with peri-articular fracture

Treatment Plan

Immediate treatment is emergent closed reduction (may require sedation) and reevaluation of vascular status.

Nonoperative

Virtually always treated operatively except in patients too medically unstable to tolerate surgery

Operative

- If knee is grossly unstable after initial reduction, may require immediate external fixation to temporarily restore stability before definitive repair/reconstruction.
    - Can be done in conjunction with vascular surgery if emergent arterial injury
- Ultimately, almost all of these require elective repair/reconstruction although this is done on a nonurgent basis once the initial soft tissue swelling has resolved.

References

Mills WJ, Barei DP, McNair P. The value of the ankle-brachial index for diagnosing arterial injury after knee dislocation: a prospective study. J Trauma. 2004;56(6):1261–5.

Rihn JA, Groff YJ, Harner CD, Cha PS. The acutely dislocated knee: evaluation and management. J Am Acad Orthop Surg. 2004;12(5):334–46.

Stannard JP, Sheils TM, Lopez-Ben RR, McGwin Jr G, Robinson JT, Volgas DA. Vascular injuries in knee dislocations: the role of physical examination in determining the need for arteriography. J Bone Joint Surg Am. 2004;86-A(5):910–5.

Meniscus Tear

Acute or chronic injuries of the meniscus in the knee, initially treated with symptomatic relief

History

- Classically occurs during a twisting episode to the knee
- May be associated with clicking or mechanical symptoms
- In severe cases (bucket handle tears), the knee may become "stuck" in flexion or extension intermittently

Physical Exam

- Acute injuries may be associated with small or moderate effusion
- Inability to fully passively extend knee should be concerning for a bucket handle tear
- Ideally would check full ligamentous knee exam (Appendix A: Full ligamentous knee exam), although may be limited by pain/guarding in an acute setting
- Examine hip as well (especially in younger patients) to confirm "knee pain" not actually referred hip pain
- Confirm NVID lower extremity (Appendix A: LE neuro exam)

M.C. Makhni et al. (eds.), *Orthopedic Emergencies*,
DOI 10.1007/978-3-319-31524-9_64

Diagnosis

Imaging

- X-rays of knee should be acquired in ED to rule out fracture but usually negative
- MRI is confirmatory study but does not need to be done in initial ED visit—usually done on an elective/outpatient basis
  - Exception: If strong clinical concern for a bucket handle tear, may need more urgent referral with earlier follow-up

Classification

Generally descriptive, location of tear (inner third, middle third, or outer third), and morphology of tear (e.g. radial, horizontal, parrot beak, complex). Does not usually effect acute ED management with the exception of bucket handle tears.

Treatment Plan

Initial ED treatment consists of pain control and immobilization with outpatient orthopedic follow-up

Nonoperative

Pain control, ± knee immobilizer for comfort, ± crutches, and ice in acute period

Operative

May ultimately be surgically repaired or debrided but usually done on an elective basis only if patient has failed nonoperative treatment

References

Belzer JP, Cannon Jr WD. Meniscus tears: treatment in the stable and unstable knee. J Am Acad Orthop Surg. 1993;1(1):41–7. PMID: 10675855.

Kramer DE, Micheli LJ. Meniscal tears and discoid meniscus in children: diagnosis and treatment. J Am Acad Orthop Surg. 2009;17(11):698–707. Review.

Quadriceps or Patellar Tendon Rupture

Common injuries to the knee extensor mechanism, usually managed with acute surgical repair on a non-emergent basis

History

- Did you hear a "pop?"
- Do you have knee pain?
- Are you able to keep your knee straight when you try to walk on it?

Physical Exam

- Palpable defect in tendon above or below patella
- Unable to perform active straight leg raise (if pain is limiting exam, could consider intra-articular lidocaine)
- Full ligamentous knee exam to rule out other injury (Appendix A: Ligamentous knee exam)

M.C. Makhni et al. (eds.), *Orthopedic Emergencies*,
DOI 10.1007/978-3-319-31524-9_65

Diagnosis:

Imaging

- XR knee—to distinguish from patellar fracture
  - Lateral XR can be used to measure patella baja or alta to show quadriceps or patellar tendon injuries, respectively
- Ultrasound—when physical exam is equivocal can detect both complete and partial tears

Classification

- Partial or Complete

Treatment Plan

Usually treated with operative repair, although this can be done on an urgent outpatient basis

Initial treatment is a knee immobilizer with early orthopedic follow-up.

Nonoperative

Reserved for partial injuries with intact extensor mechanism (able to actively extend knee and perform straight leg raise), or those too medically unstable for surgery. Consists of prolonged immobilization in extension with a knee immobilizer or brace.

Operative

Treatment: Tendon repair

Indications: acute, complete injuries

References

Ilan DI, Tejwani N, Keschner M, Leibman M. Quadriceps tendon rupture. J Am Acad Orthop Surg. 2003;11(3):192–200.
Matava MJ. Patellar tendon ruptures. J Am Acad Orthop Surg. 1996;4(6):287–96.

Patella Fracture

Common fracture, sometimes requiring operative treatment but frequently able to be successfully treated without surgery

History

- Classic mechanism is a fall directly onto the knee

Physical Exam

- Full knee exam and distal neurovascular exam
- **Integrity of extensor mechanism is critical**—evaluate by checking for ability to actively extend the knee or perform a straight leg raise.
  - In the acute post-injury period, this exam is frequently limited by pain. If the exam is unclear, some patients may require an intra-articular lidocaine injection to get a better examination of the extensor mechanism
- **Skin check is critical** to look for abrasions over front of knee—can affect surgical planning if the injury is operative

M.C. Makhni et al. (eds.), *Orthopedic Emergencies*,
DOI 10.1007/978-3-319-31524-9_66

Diagnosis

Imaging

- AP and lateral X-rays of the knee plus patellar sunrise view (if possible)
  - *Beware bipartite patella which can frequently be confused for a fracture!*
- CT or MRI usually not required

Classification

Usually based on fracture pattern (transverse, nondisplaced, stellate, vertical, sleeve avulsion, etc.) (Figs. 1 and 2)

Treatment Plan

Treatment is generally based on integrity of extensor mechanism; if intact and fracture relatively non-displaced, usually can treat non-operatively. If disrupted, treated operatively.

Nonoperative

WBAT with knee immobilized in extension (brace vs. cylinder cast) for 4–6 weeks. Can usually start motion at 2–3 weeks with a brace.

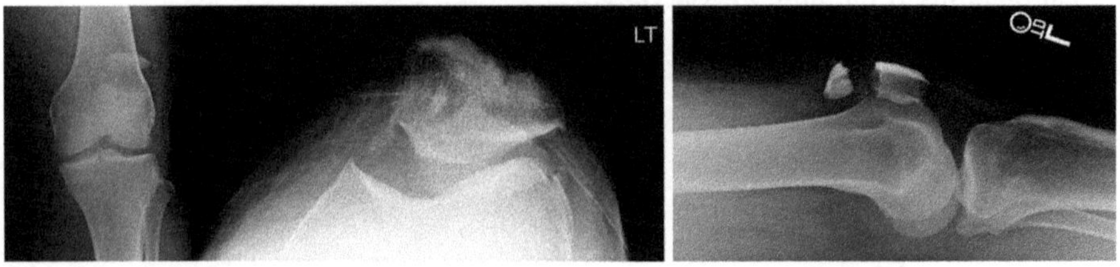

Fig. 1 Transverse patella

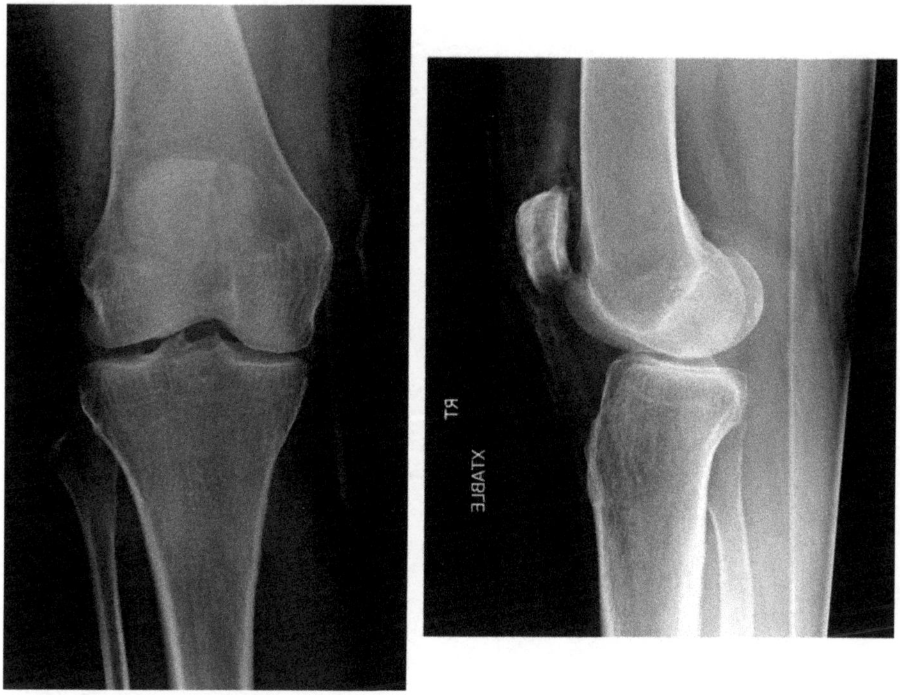

Fig. 2 Vertical patella fracture

Operative

Operative treatment is based on restoring the extensor mechanism integrity and anatomically aligning joint surface. Can usually be done electively (on a non-emergent basis) if patient can be safely discharged with knee immobilized in extension. Operative treatment may include ORIF with tension band construct, partial patellectomy, extensor mechanism repair, and/or total patellectomy based on fracture pattern and injury characteristics.

Reference

Melvin JS, Mehta S. Patellar fractures in adults. J Am Acad Orthop Surg. 2011;19(4):198–207.

Patella Dislocation

Most commonly a recurring problem that is the result of chronic ligamentous laxity, patella dislocation can also be the result of acute trauma.

Overview

- Most commonly lateral dislocation: quadriceps pulls patella laterally over femoral condyle, tearing medial retinaculum and occasionally causing osteochondral fracture.
- Recurrent dislocations more common in women, ligamentous laxity (e.g., Ehlers–Danlos), underlying patellar malalignment.

History

- Did you hear a "pop?"
- Did you see or feel your kneecap slide out to the side?
- Has this happened before?
- Do you have difficulty/weakness extending your knee?

Physical Exam

- Full ligamentous knee exam (Appendix A: Ligamentous knee exam), although can be difficult to perform in the acute setting.
- Knee pain, inability to flex knee, large palpable deformity on lateral knee, hemarthrosis (if unreduced).

M.C. Makhni et al. (eds.), *Orthopedic Emergencies*,
DOI 10.1007/978-3-319-31524-9_67

- Often maximally tender to palpation over the medial facet (where the medial patellofemoral ligament has torn off).
- Lateral patellar subluxation with knee in extension (graded by number of quadrants of patella able to sublux laterally compared to contralateral side).
- Moving patellar apprehension test: With knee extended, pressure is placed over medial patella to sublux it laterally, and the knee is slowly flexed. If positive, just before the patella engages in the trochlea the patient will describe pain/apprehension.

Diagnosis

Imaging

- XR knee: routine knee AP/lateral, Sunrise view.
  - Visualize avulsion injuries off patella or rule out concurrent injuries; usually not diagnostic.
- MRI—Rarely indicated in an acute setting. Sometimes obtained on outpatient basis when physical exam is equivocal, or in chronic/multiple dislocations for preoperative planning. Also can be used to check for intra-articular osteochondral defects or loose bodies.

Classification

Described by direction of dislocated patella: lateral, medial, superior (rare), or intra-articular (rare).

Treatment Plan

Almost all acute injuries initially managed nonoperatively with orthopaedic follow-up as an outpatient.

Attempt to reduce dislocation during initial evaluation to reduce pain.

Usually easily reduced by bringing the knee into full extension (to disengage from trochlea), then applying gentle medial pressure on patella.

For tense effusions, consider arthrocentesis. Presence of fat globules in aspirate indicates that a fracture is present.

Non-operative

Reduce Dislocation.
Hinged knee brace locked in extension or cylindrical cast with the knee in extension for 3 weeks with WBAT followed by gradually increasing flexion as patient comfort permits over the next 3 weeks
Followed by physical therapy with a focus on quadriceps strengthening.

Operative

Treatment: arthroscopy, reconstruction of the medial patellofemoral ligament, fragment excision or repair.
Indications: suspicion for osteochondral fragment, or chronic dislocators with patellar instability.

References

Archdeacon M., et al. Patella fractures and extensor mechanism injuries. Skeletal Trauma, 4th edn. Chapter 54; 2162-3.
Boden BP, Pearsall AW, Garrett Jr WE, Feagin Jr JA. Patellofemoral Instability: evaluation and management. J Am Acad Orthop Surg. 1997;5(1):47–57.
Fithian DC, Paxton EW, Stone ML, Silva P, Davis DK, Elias DA, et al. Epidemiology and natural history of acute patellar dislocation. AJSM. 2004;32:1114–21.

Pelvic Ring Injuries

High-energy injuries where the mechanical integrity of pelvic ring is disrupted. Treatment can range from nonoperative to true surgical emergency (in the case of hemodynamically unstable patient)

History

- Typically blunt trauma
- Frequently associated with other injuries

Physical Exam

- Full trauma exam (Appendix A: Trauma exam)
    - **Critical to evaluate hemodynamic status**, as **a hemodynamically unstable pelvic fracture is a true life-threatening emergency**.
- Skin intact? Amount of soft tissue swelling?
- Can test stability by gently stressing pelvis with a hand on each iliac crest
- Check for leg length discrepancy, abnormal external rotation of one or both legs

M.C. Makhni et al. (eds.), *Orthopedic Emergencies*,
DOI 10.1007/978-3-319-31524-9_68

Diagnosis

Imaging

- AP pelvis should be part of initial trauma series
- Inlet/outlet views of pelvis
- CT can help characterize injury to posterior components of the ring

Classification

Young–Burgess system (Young JWR. Baltimore, Munich, Urban & Schwarzenberg, 1987) classifies by mechanism and degree of injury:

Anterior posterior compression (APC):

- APC1: Abnormal symphysis widening, but less than 2.5 cm
- APC2: Symphysis widening > 2.5 cm, anterior SI ligaments disrupted but intact posterior SI ligaments intact as a "hinge" (Fig. 1)
- APC3: Symphysis widening > 2.5 cm with both anterior and posterior SI ligaments disrupted

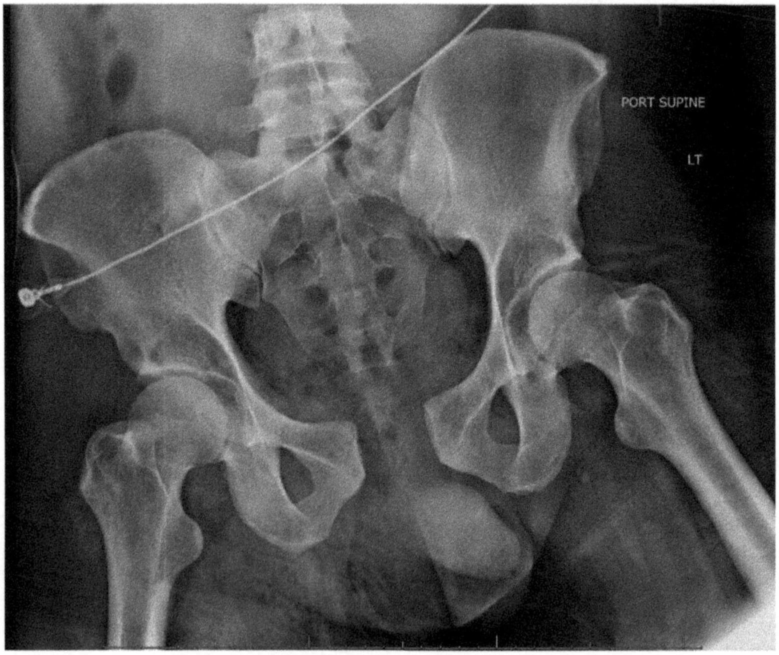

Fig. 1 APC2 injury

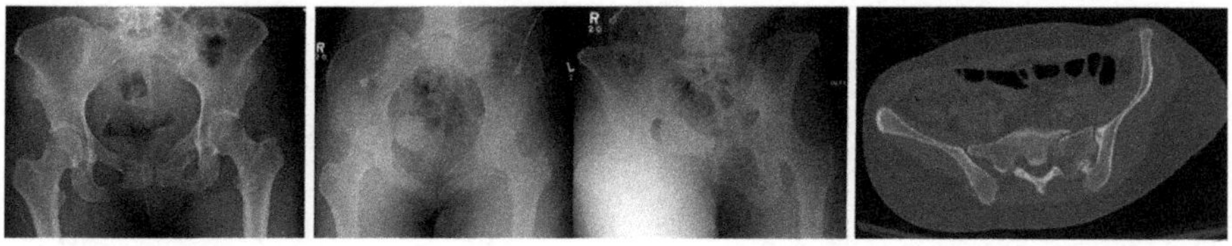

Fig. 2 LC1 injury

Lateral Compression (LC)

- LC1: Ramus fracture along with sacral ala compression fracture (Fig. 2)
- LC2: Ramus fracture along with SI fracture-dislocation (crescent fracture)
- LC3: LC type 1 or 2 on one side of pelvis combined with APC type injury to SI joint on contralateral side ("windswept pelvis")

Vertical Shear (VS)

- Superior displacement of affected hemipelvis

Alternate classifications include Tile (Tile M. J Am Assoc Orthop Surg. 1996 4:143)

Treatment Plan

Initial treatment is thorough ED workup with trauma exam. Critical differentiation is between hemodynamically stable and unstable patients

Hemodynamically Unstable

- Immediate placement of pelvic binder or wrapping with pelvic sheet (Appendix B: Pelvic binder application).
    - Once placed, frequent skin checks around binder/sheet necessary due to risk of skin necrosis.
    - Note: a pelvic binder will only stabilize an anterior component of a pelvic ring injury. A pelvic "C-clamp" is available in some institutions to treat posterior ring injuries as well.
- If continued HD instability, treatment algorithm is institutionally specific but may include:
    - Angiography/embolization by interventional radiology
    - Open pelvic packing by general surgery
    - Emergent stabilization (external fixation ± posterior SI fixation).

Nonoperative

- Appropriate for lower energy, minimally displaced injuries (usually APC1 or LC1 mechanisms)
- Treatment is WBAT or protected weightbearing with radiographic follow-up to evaluate for secondary displacement
- Risk factors for secondary displacement
  - Bilateral rami fractures
  - Complete sacral fracture (vs. impacted sacral ala)
  - Vertical sacral fracture

Operative

- Operative treatment for patients with unstable pelvic rings either shown radiographically or clinically (by inability to WBAT with pain/instability one exam despite nonoperative treatment)
- Posterior ring fixation can include:
  - Percutaneous SI screws
  - Anterior SI plating
  - Posterior SI tension band
- Anterior ring fixation can include
  - Symphyseal or anterior rami plating
  - Percutaneous anterior column screws
  - External fixation

References

Krieg JC, Mohr M, Ellis TJ, Simpson TS, Madey SM, Bottlang M. Emergent stabilization of pelvic ring injuries by controlled circumferential compression: a clinical trial. J Trauma. 2005;59(3):659–64. PMID: 16361909 (Link to Abstract).

Langford JR, Burgess AR, Liporace FA, Haidukewych GJ. Pelvic fractures: part 2. Contemporary indications and techniques for definitive surgical management. J Am Acad Orthop Surg. 2013;21(8):458–68.

Tile M. Acute pelvic fractures: I. Causation and classification. J Am Acad Orthop Surg. 1996;4(3):143–51.

Periprosthetic Hip Fracture

Proximal femur fractures around a total hip prosthesis with management depending on implant stability.

History

- Result of low-energy traumatic event after joint replacement
- Date of index procedure and previous revision surgeries
- Cemented versus cementless prosthesis
  - Cemented less likely to fracture and occur late (>5 years)
  - Cementless more likely to fracture and occur early (within first year)
- Metabolic bone disorder
- Steroid use
- Start up pain signifies prior loose component
  - Pain with first few steps that improves with prolonged ambulation

Physical Exam

- Full trauma exam (Appendix A: trauma exam)
- Skin intact?
- Distal neurovascular exam (Appendix A: LE neuro exam)

M.C. Makhni et al. (eds.), *Orthopedic Emergencies*,
DOI 10.1007/978-3-319-31524-9_69

Diagnosis

Imaging

- Imaging must include the entire length of femur
- AP pelvis
- AP and cross-table lateral femur
- Often advanced imaging is not required
- CT scan may be considered to help determine implant stability

Classification

Vancouver classification based on:

Location of fracture
Stability of implant
Bone quality

Vancouver Classification
Type A: Fracture in trochanteric region
Type B: Fracture around stem or tip

B1: well-fixed implant (Fig. 1)
B2: loose implant (Fig. 2)
B3: loose implant and poor bone quality

Type C: Fracture well below prosthesis

Treatment Plan

Excluding nondisplaced greater trochanter fractures, most are treated operatively.

Nonoperative

Vancouver A fractures that are nondisplaced and involving greater/lesser trochanter can be managed with protected weight bearing and limiting abduction.

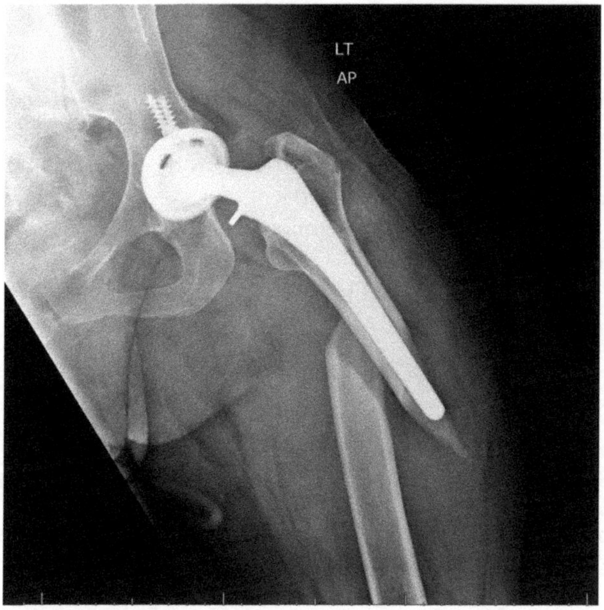

Fig. 1 Vancouver B1 periprosthetic fracture

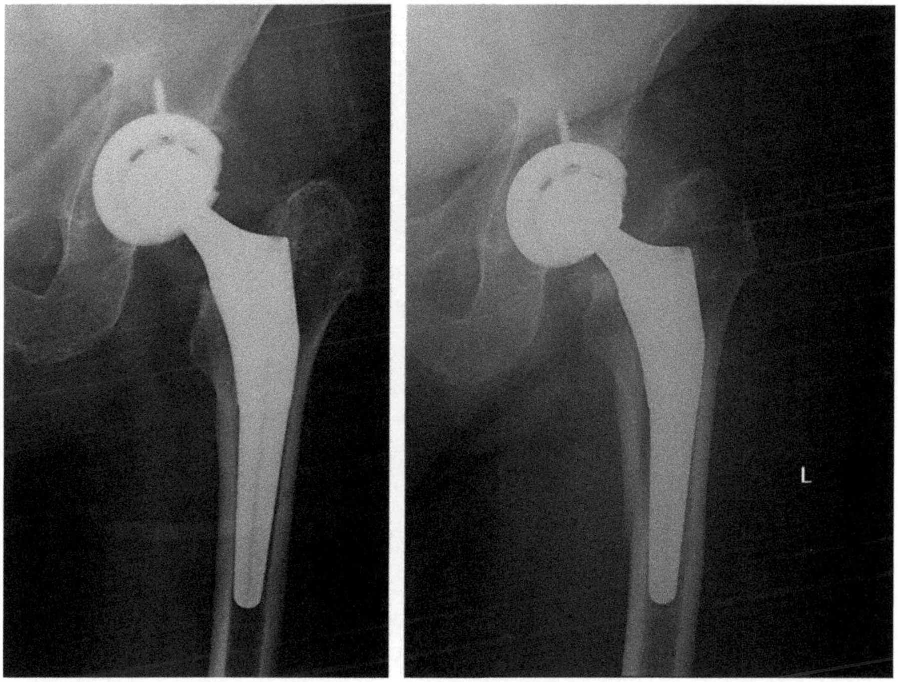

Fig. 2 Vancouver B2 periprosthetic fracture. X-rays immediately after initial surgery show stable implant. After a fall with a fracture, the implant has subsided

Operative

Displaced Vancouver A fractures are treated with ORIF.

Vancouver B1 treated with ORIF (cerclage cables and locked plates)

Vancouver B2 treated with revision to long, fully-coated femoral stem that bypasses fracture by two cortical diameters

Vancouver B3 treated with femoral component revision as in B2 fractures along with structural allograft

Vancouver C fractures are treated with ORIF.

References

Brady OH, Garbuz DS, Masri BA, Duncan CP. Classification of the hip. Orthop Clin North Am. 1999;30(2):215–20.

Parvizi J, Rapuri VR, Purtill JJ, Sharkey PF, Rothman RH, Hozack WJ. Treatment protocol for proximal femoral periprosthetic fractures. J Bone Joint Surg Am. 2004;86-A Suppl 2:8–16.

Periprosthetic Knee Femur Fracture

A complicated distal femur fracture due to the presence of prosthesis. Often surgically managed.

History

- Result of traumatic event after joint replacement
- Date of index procedure
- Any knee pain/symptoms concerning for loosening prior to fracture?
- Steroid use
- Inflammatory arthropathy
- Metabolic bone disorder
- Neurologic disorders

Physical Exam

- Full trauma exam (Appendix A: trauma exam)
- Skin intact?
- Distal neurovascular exam (Appendix A: LE neuro exam)

Diagnosis

Imaging

- XR should visualize entire length of femur
- AP, lateral, and two 45° oblique views of the distal femur

M.C. Makhni et al. (eds.), *Orthopedic Emergencies*,
DOI 10.1007/978-3-319-31524-9_70

- Consider traction views and contralateral films for preoperative planning
- May consider CT scan to help determine stability of prosthesis or if concern for coronal fracture

Classification

Many classification systems in the literature based on:

Location of fracture
Displacement of fracture
Stability of implant

Lewis and Rorabeck Classification
Type I: nondisplaced; component well-fixed
Type II: displaced; component well-fixed
Type III: displaced; component loose or failing

Treatment Plan

Treatment in emergency department setting is similar to distal femur fracture management with temporization in bulky Jones dressing, knee immobilizer, (Appendix B: Bulky Jones) and NWB.

Nonoperative

Nondisplaced fractures with well-fixed prosthesis may be managed with immobilization (casting or hinged knee bracing).

Goal is early ROM of knee to prevent stiffness.

Operative

All displaced fractures and fractures with loose components.

Displaced fractures are managed with intramedullary fixation or bridging fixed angle devices.

Loose femoral component requires revision to long stem prosthesis.

References

Aldrian S, Schuster R, Haas N, Erhart J, Strickner M, Blutsch B, et al. Fixation of supracondylar femoral fractures following total knee arthroplasty: is there any difference comparing angular stable plate fixation versus rigid interlocking nail fixation? Arch Orthop Trauma Surg. 2013;133(7):921–7.

Parvizi J, Jain N, Schmidt AH. Periprosthetic knee fractures. J Orthop Trauma. 2008;22(9):663–71.

Tibia/Fibula Shaft Fracture

Most common long bone fracture. Management predominantly based on displacement.

History

- Low-energy and high-energy fracture patterns
  - Indirect mechanism with torsion vs direct trauma
- Stress fractures can be seen in military recruits and ballet dancers
- Check for associated injuries, other complaints

Physical Exam (Fig. 1)

- Full trauma exam (Appendix A: trauma exam)
- Evaluate soft tissues and skin integrity
- Assess compartments for fullness, pain with passive stretch, and pain out of proportion to exam
- Knee ligamentous exam given concurrent injuries, although may be difficult acutely due to pain
- Distal neurovascular exam before and after reduction (Appendix A: LE neuro exam)

M.C. Makhni et al. (eds.), *Orthopedic Emergencies*,
DOI 10.1007/978-3-319-31524-9_71

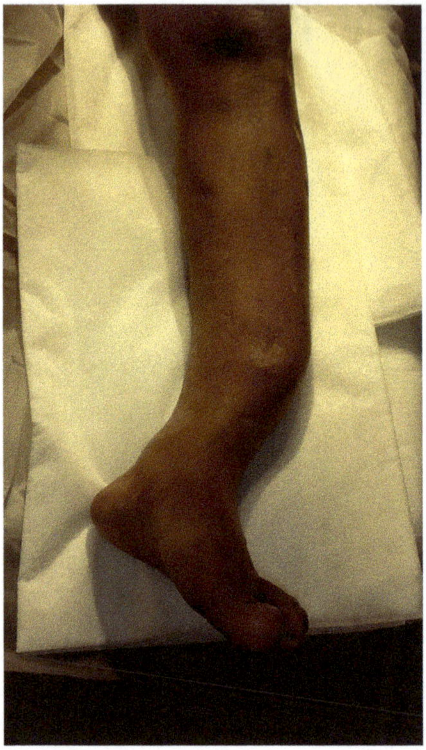

Fig. 1 Clinical appearance of tibial shaft fracture

Diagnosis

Imaging

- AP and lateral views of entire tibia with visualization of knee and ankle joints
- For distal third tibia fractures, consider CT scan of ankle to evaluate for articular extension of spiral fracture or posterior malleolus fracture
- Bone scan or MRI useful in diagnosing stress fractures not apparent on plain radiography

Classification

Descriptive based on:

Skin integrity (open, closed)
Location (proximal, middle, distal third)

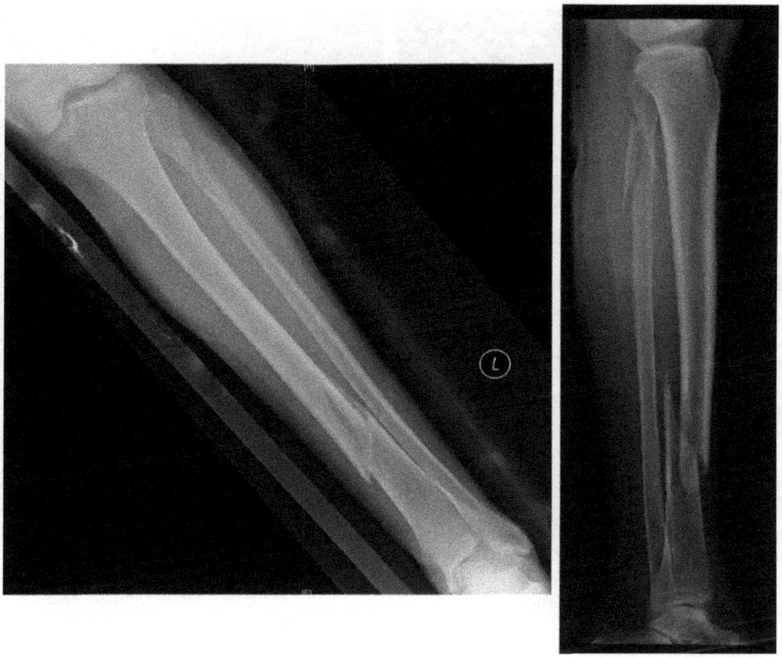

Fig. 2 Spiral tibial shaft fracture

Pattern (spiral, oblique, transverse, comminution/butterfly) (Figs. 2, 3, and 4)
Displacement (shortening, translation, angulation, rotation)

Tscherne Classification of Closed Fractures, Gustilo and Anderson Classification of Open Fractures

Treatment Plan

Treatment depends on skin integrity and fracture displacement.
Most can be temporized with padded long leg splint or cast in the emergency department. (Appendix B: long leg splint)

Nonoperative

Closed fractures with acceptable alignment after closed reduction.

Displaced fractures should be closed reduced under conscious sedation in the emergency department setting.

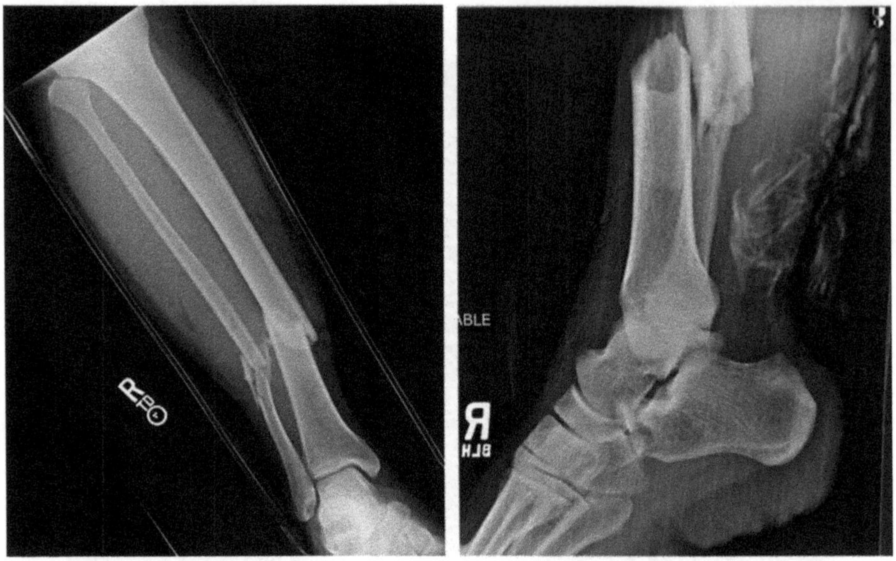

Fig. 3 Transverse tibial shaft fracture

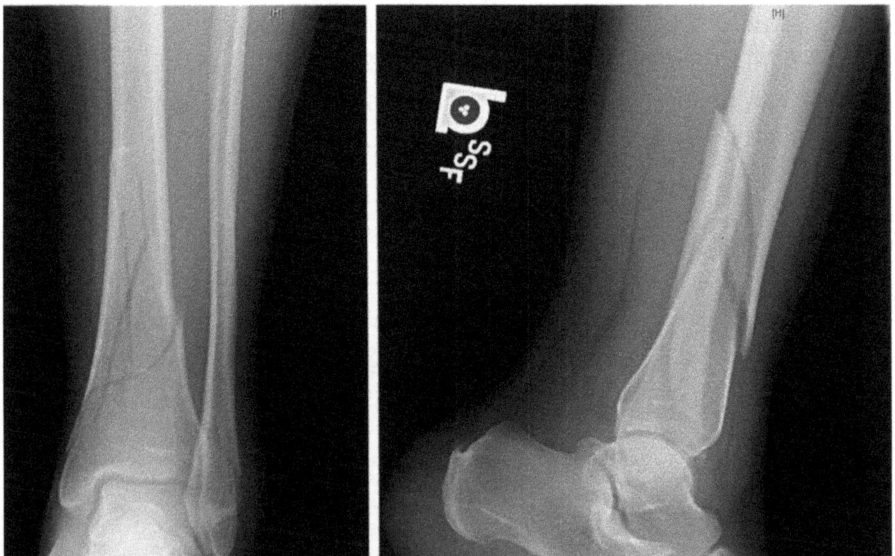

Fig. 4 Complex tibial shaft fracture

Acceptable alignment for nonoperative treatment:

<10° AP angulation
<5° varus/valgus angulation
<1 cm shortening
<10° rotational deformity
>50 % cortical apposition

Application of long leg cast with knee in 5° of flexion to allow progression of weight bearing (Appendix B: long leg casting)

Protected weight bearing in long leg cast for 3–4 weeks.

Transition to patella-bearing cast at 4–6 weeks and progress to full weight bearing.

Union is typically achieved between 14 and 18 weeks for closed fractures.

Operative

Displaced fractures outside of acceptable criteria, open fractures, associated vascular injuries, and associated compartment syndrome.

Often treated with intramedullary implant to allow for immediate weight bearing.

References

Bhandari M, Guyatt G, Tornetta III P, Schemitsch EH, Swiontkowski M, Sanders D, et al. Randomized trial of reamed and unreamed intramedullary nailing of tibial shaft fractures. J Bone Joint Surg Am. 2008;90(12):2567–78.

Sarmiento A, Gersten LM, Sobol PA, Shankwiler JA, Vangsness CT. Tibial shaft fractures treated with functional braces. Experience with 780 fractures. J Bone Joint Surg Br. 1989;71(4):602–9.

Tibial Plateau Fracture

Periarticular fractures of the proximal tibia where the soft tissues determine surgical timing.

History

- Typical bimodal distribution (high-energy trauma in young patients and low energy in older patients).
- Occurs due to varus or valgus load causing driving the femoral condyle into the plateau.
- Check for associated injuries, other complaints.

Physical Exam

- Full trauma exam (Appendix A: trauma exam).
- Skin intact? If laceration or punctate wound, consider saline load to assess communication with joint (Appendix B: saline load of knee technique).
- Assess compartments for fullness, pain with passive stretch, and pain out of proportion to exam.
- Assess varus/valgus stability, may be difficult acutely secondary to pain (Appendix A: varus/valgus knee stability).
- Dstal neurovascular exam (Appendix A: LE neuro exam).
- Any decreased pulses should be followed by immediate Ankle-Brachial Index (Appendix B: ABI technique).
- ABI <0.9 indicates arterial injury and will require vascular surgery consultation and angiography.

M.C. Makhni et al. (eds.), *Orthopedic Emergencies*,
DOI 10.1007/978-3-319-31524-9_72

Diagnosis

Imaging

- AP, lateral, and 40° IR and ER views of the knee.
- AP and lateral of the joint above and below the injury.
- Consider traction views and contralateral films for preoperative planning.
- Consider plateau view to better visualize articular depression.
- CT scan is indicated for any displaced plateau fracture to assess depression and comminution.

Classification

Schatzker Classification.
Type I: Lateral plateau, split fracture.
Type II: Lateral plateau, split depression fracture.
Type III: Lateral plateau, depression fracture.
Type IV: Medial plateau fracture.
Type V: Bicondylar fracture.
Type VI: Metaphyseal-diaphyseal dissociation (Figs. 1 and 2).

Moore Classification.
Type I: Coronal split fracture.
Type II: Entire condylar fracture.
Type III: Rim avulsion fracture of lateral plateau.
Type IV: Rim compression fracture.
Type V: Four-part fracture.

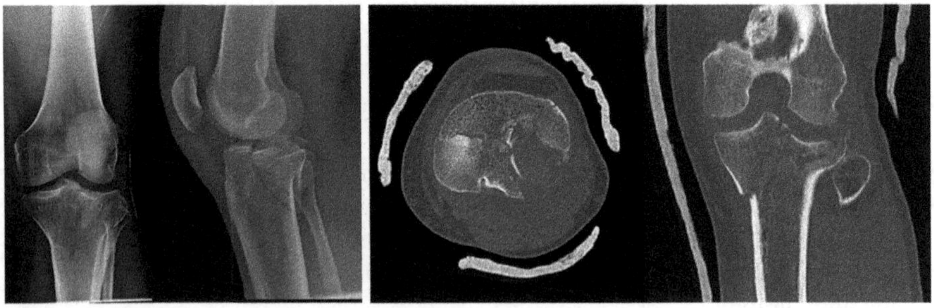

Fig. 1 "Simple" bicondylar plateau fracture

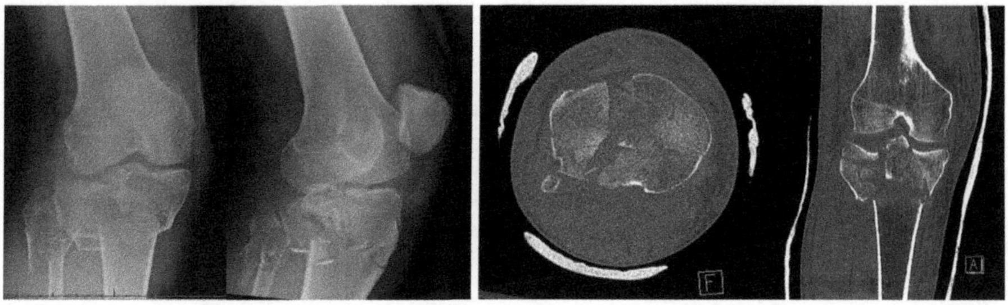

Fig. 2 Complex bicondylar plateau fracture

Treatment Plan

Early ROM is essential to optimal patient outcome.

Non-operative

Stable, minimally displaced fractures.

Nonambulatory patients or patients with extensive comorbidities precluding safe surgical intervention.

Initial temporization in ED with bulky Jones dressing, knee immobilizer, and NWB.

Transition to hinged knee brace with early ROM but prolonged period of protected weight bearing.

NWB × 6 weeks with goal ROM of 90° by 4 weeks.

PWB 6–12 weeks progressed to FWB at 12 weeks.

Operative

Displaced fractures with varus/valgus instability >10°, condylar widening >5 mm, bicondylar fractures, medial fractures, open fractures, associated vascular injuries, and associated compartment syndrome.

There is no definitive amount of articular depression that mandates surgery (ranges from 2 mm to 1 cm).

Temporizing bridging external fixation with reduction by ligamentotaxis in polytrauma and patients with significant soft-tissue compromise.

Definitive internal fixation 7–14 days later after soft-tissue rest and strict elevation.

Definitive internal fixation can be a combination of percutaneous inserted screws and plates along with formal buttress and locked plating to respect soft-tissue integrity.

Soft-tissue reconstruction (collateral ligaments and meniscal repair) is essential for optimal surgical outcome.

References

Koval KJ, Helfet DL. Tibial plateau fractures: evaluation and treatment. J Am Acad Orthop Surg. 1995;3(2):86–94.

Schatzker J, McBroom R, Bruce D. The tibial plateau fracture. The Toronto experience 1968–1975. Clin Orthop Relat Res. 1979;138:94–104.

Part VII
Foot and Ankle

Thomas Hickernell and Jon-Michael Caldwell

Achilles Tendon Rupture 331
Ankle Fracture 335
Calcaneus Fracture 347
Jones Fracture (Proximal Fifth Metatarsal) 351
Lisfranc Injury 355
Metatarsal Fractures 359
Tarsal Navicular Fracture 361
Tibial Plafond (Pilon) Fracture 365
Talar Neck Fracture 371
Lateral Process of Talus Fracture 375
Phalanx Fractures of the Foot 379

Achilles Tendon Rupture

Most common traumatically ruptured tendon in the body. Commonly associated with sports injuries involving either sudden plantarflexion of the foot or violent dorsiflexion of a plantarflexed foot. May be treated nonoperatively with bracing/splinting and early functional rehabilitation, or surgically.

History

- Did you hear a "pop?"
- Do you have heel pain?
- Do you have difficulty/weakness with walking, or are you unable to bear weight?

Physical Exam

- Palpable defect in Achilles tendon.
- Increased dorsiflexion of affected ankle to gravity in prone position (Fig. 1).
- Inability to plantar flex the ankle/weakness with plantarflexion.
- Calf atrophy (suggestive of chronic injury).
- Thompson test: Lack of plantar flexion with compression of the calf muscle. Compare to contralateral side.

M.C. Makhni et al. (eds.), *Orthopedic Emergencies*,
DOI 10.1007/978-3-319-31524-9_73

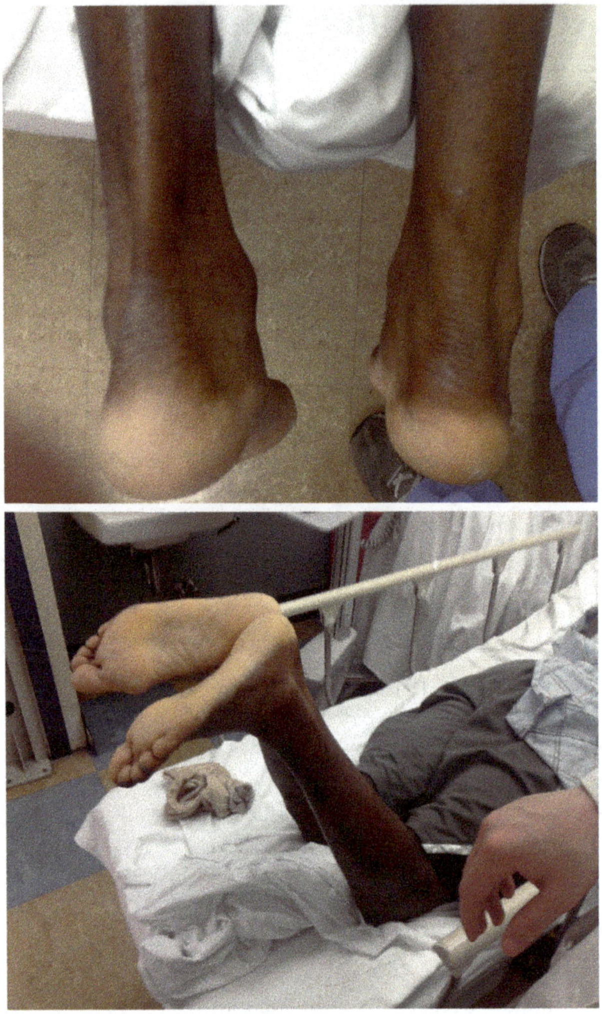

Fig. 1 Clinical appearance of Achilles tendon rupture

Diagnosis

Imaging

- XR ankle and foot—to visualize avulsion injuries off calcaneus, rule out concurrent injuries; usually not diagnostic.
- Ultrasound—when physical exam is equivocal can detect both complete and partial tears.
- MRI—when physical exam is equivocal, or in chronic ruptures.

Classification

- Partial or Complete.
- Midsubstance (most common) or avulsion off calcaneus.

Treatment Plan

Controversial: similar outcomes between surgical repair and nonoperative management, and decision for treatment plan should consider patient preferences.

Surgical repair (compared to nonoperative treatment) has demonstrated:

Quicker return to work.
Higher complication rate.
Equivalent re-rupture rates to nonoperative treatment **that includes early functional rehabilitation.** * IMPORTANT *

Nonoperative

Consider for:

- Acute injuries
- Any patient predisposed to wound complications (diabetes, neuropathy, immunocompromised states, age above 65, tobacco use, sedentary lifestyle, obesity (BMI >30), peripheral vascular disease or local/systemic dermatologic disorders)

Consists of functional bracing or immobilization in resting equinus (CAM boot with a heel lift, short leg splint in resting equinus) followed by early range of motion and functional rehabilitation.

Operative

Consider for acute or chronic injuries.

- Acute: Open or percutaneous end-to-end tendon repair. Minimally invasive techniques may offer a decreased rate of wound-related complications and improved cosmesis though with higher risk of sural nerve injury than open procedures. Early postoperative mobilization (beginning 2–4 weeks post op) recommended.
- Chronic: Tendon reconstruction with VY lengthening +/– tendon transfer

References

Chiodo CP et al. Diagnosis and treatment of acute Achilles tendon rupture. J Am Acad Orthop Surg. 2010;18(8):503–10.

Soroceanu A, Sidhwa F, Aarabi S, Kaufman A, Glazebrook M. Surgical versus nonsurgical treatment of acute Achilles tendon rupture. J Bone Joint Surg. 2012;94(23):2136–43. doi:10.2106/JBJS.K.00917.

Ankle Fracture

A variable collection of low- and high-energy injuries about the ankle—typically rotational injuries. Operative versus nonoperative based on severity/pattern of injury.

Overview

- Typically a rotational/axial load injury after taking a misstep or slipping while ambulating, versus more high energy mechanisms

History

- Can you bear weight?
- Which side(s) of your ankle hurts?
- Do you have any leg or knee pain?

Physical Exam

- Knee exam for possible ipsilateral knee injury.
- Skin exam: any openings concern for open fracture. Check for degree of swelling and any blistering as either could potentially complicate operative intervention (Fig. 1).

M.C. Makhni et al. (eds.), *Orthopedic Emergencies*,
DOI 10.1007/978-3-319-31524-9_74

Diagnosis

Imaging

- Ankle XR—Mortise view, AP, lateral.
- External rotation stress view to assess for medial clear space widening (Fig. 2).
- Talocrural angle comparison of contralateral/uninjured ankle to assess for fibular shortening.

Classification

Lauge-Hansen (debatable if fracture patterns caused predictably by these mechanisms, but widely used classification system used to describe fracture patterns) (Figs. 3–6).

- Supination-adduction (SA) (Fig. 7).
- Supination-external rotation (SER) (Figs. 8 and 9).
- Pronation-abduction (PA).
- Pronation-external rotation (PER) (Fig. 10).

Danis-Weber

- A—infrasyndesmotic.
- B—transsyndesmotic.
- C—suprasyndesmotic.

Anatomic/Descriptive

- Isolated medial or lateral malleolus fracture.
- Bimalleolar fracture.
- Trimalleolar fracture (medial, lateral, posterior malleolus).
- Fracture-dislocation (Fig. 11).

Treatment

Nonoperative

Indications

Nondisplaced, isolated distal fibula fracture without medial clear space widening or talar shift

Nondisplaced, isolated medial malleolus fracture or tip avulsions

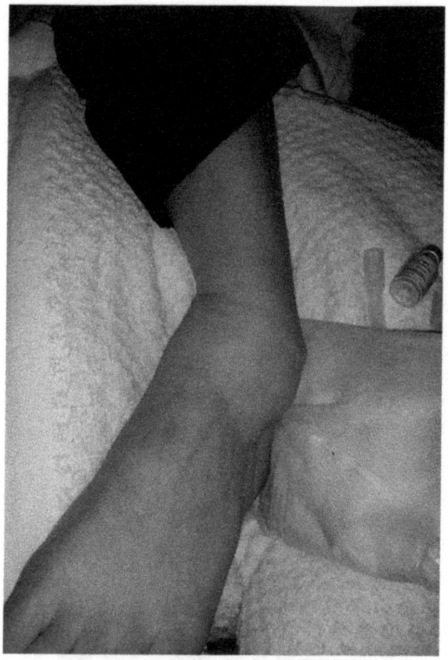

Fig. 1 Ankle fracture dislocation

Isolated posterior malleolus fracture with less than 25 % joint involvement or <2 mm intra-articular step-off

Treatment: Short leg walking cast or walking (CAM) boot

Operative

Indicated for

Displaced, isolated medial malleolus
Displaced, isolated lateral malleolus
Any talar displacement
Medial malleolus fracture with associated proximal fibula fracture (Maisonneuve fracture)

Treatment: Initial management consists of closed reduction and well-padded short leg splint in ER, followed by ORIF when the swelling subsides

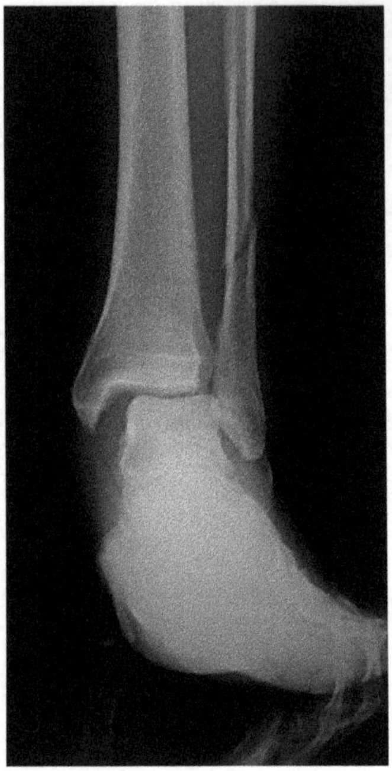

Fig. 2 Positive stress test

Treatment: Reduction and immobilization in ER followed by fixation as necessary (Appendix B: "Ankle Fracture Reduction" and "Short leg splint"). Fixation may be done acutely, but can often be done electively after discharge once swelling from the injury has subsided.

Isolated lateral malleolar fracture with increased medial clear space (bimalleolar equivalent)

Posterior malleolus fracture with greater than 25 % articular involvement or >2 mm step-off

Fracture-dislocation

Primary goal: Anatomic reduction of the joint surface and restoration of length.

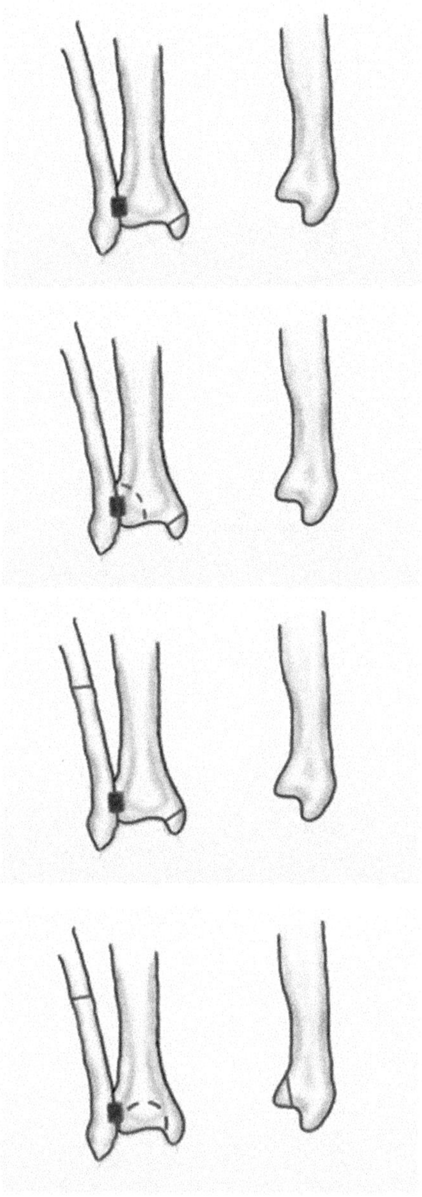

Fig. 3 Pronation External Rotation Types 1–4

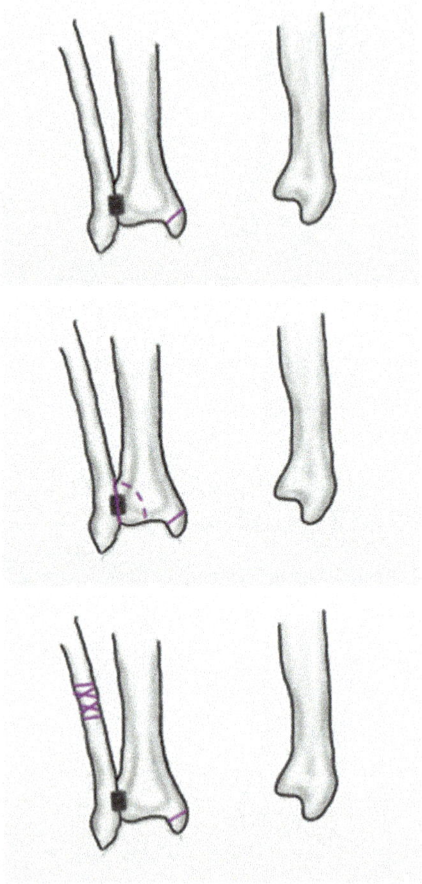

Fig. 4 Pronation Abduction Types 1–3

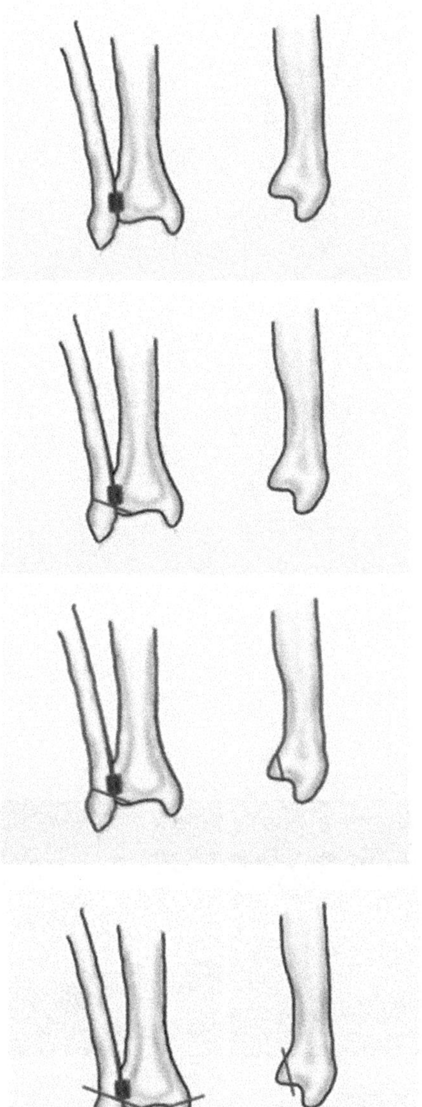

Fig. 5 Supination External Rotation Types 1–4

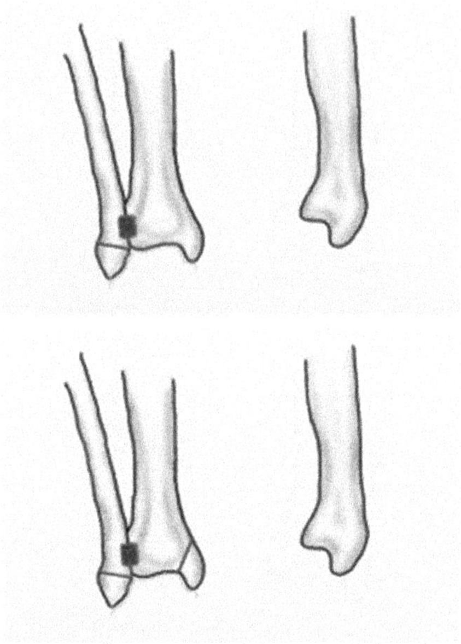

Fig. 6 Supination Adduction Types 1–2

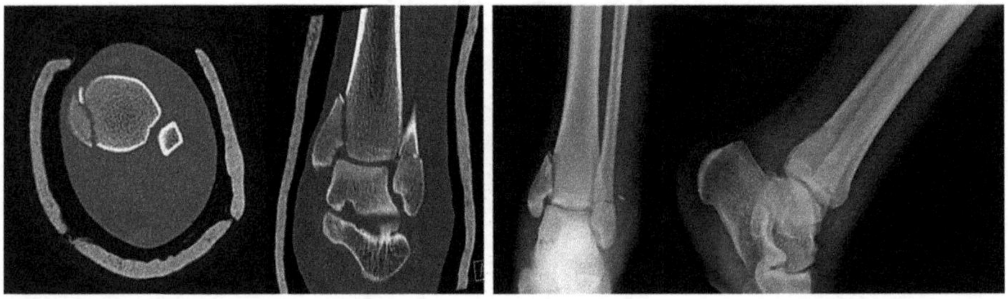

Fig. 7 Supination-adduction injury

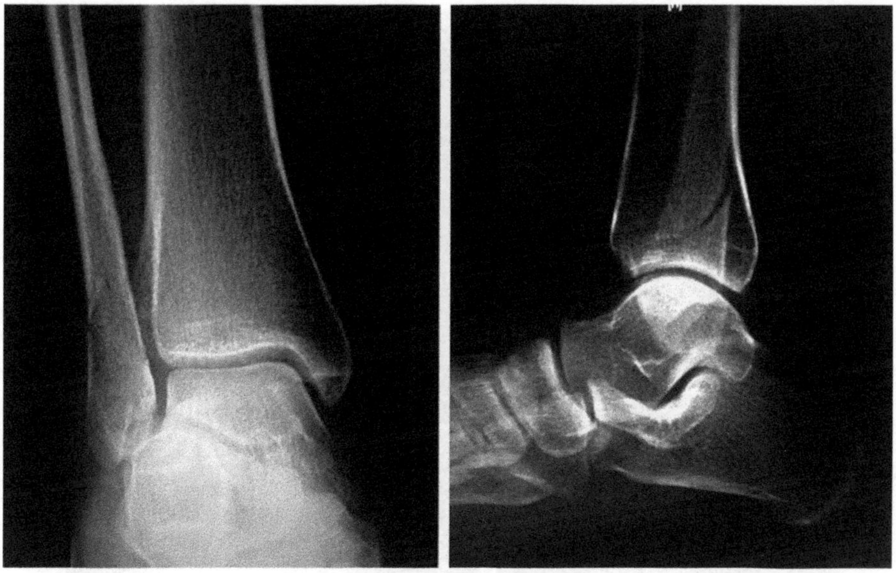

Fig. 8 SER2 injury

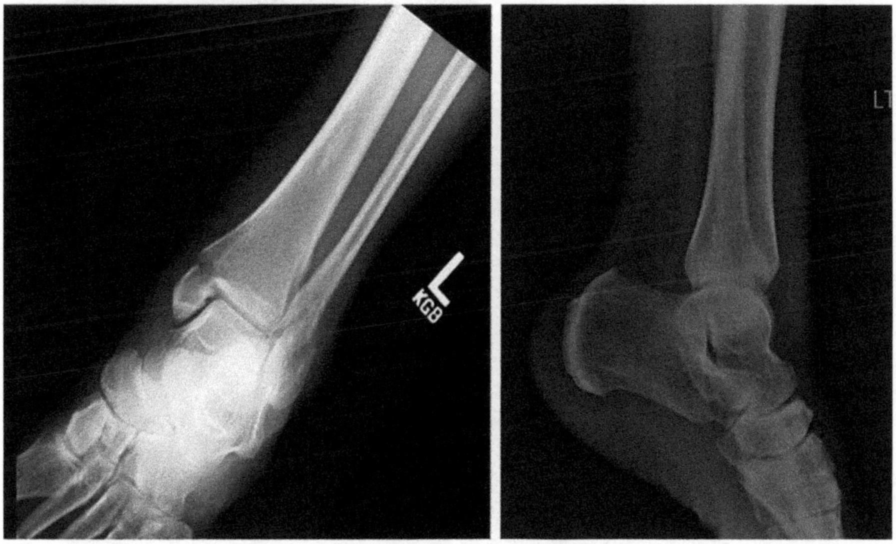

Fig. 9 SER4 injury

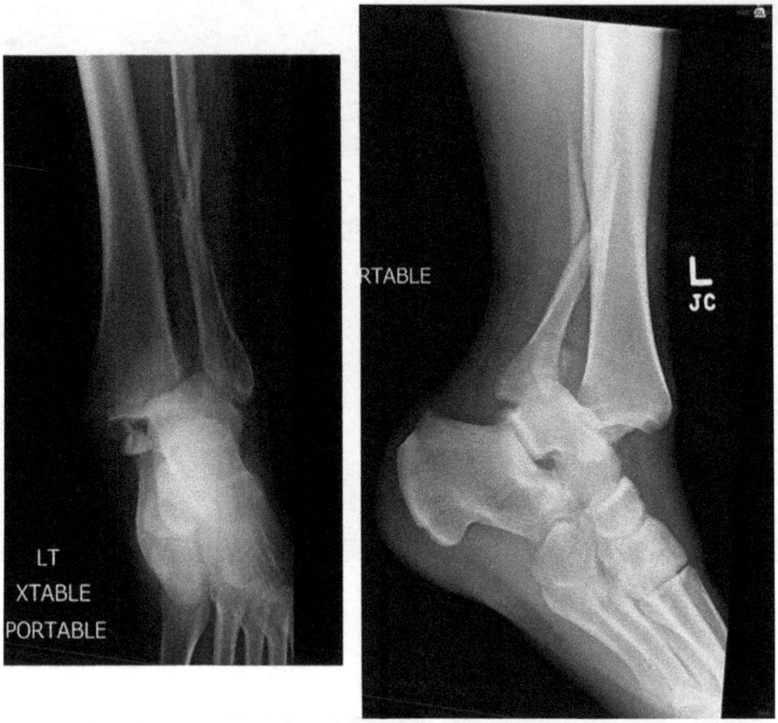

Fig. 10 PER injury

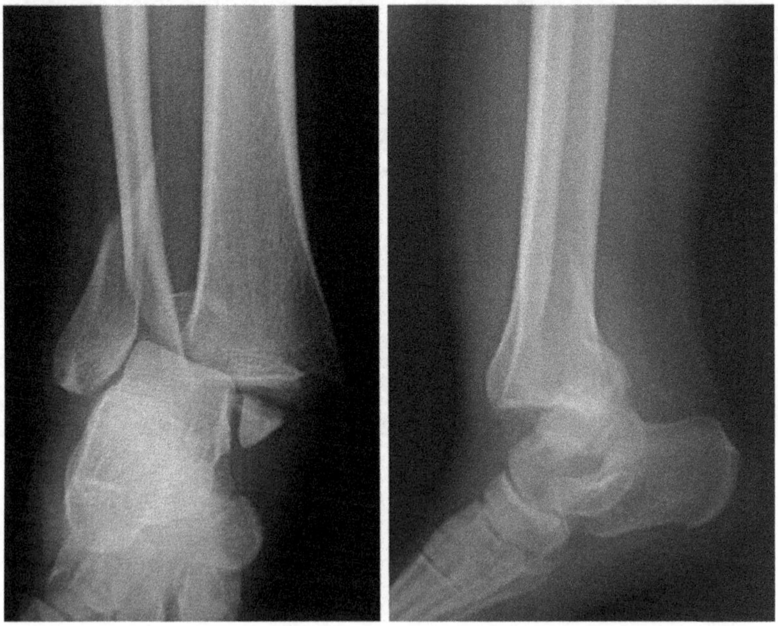

Fig. 11 SER4 fracture-dislocation

References

Egol KA, Amirtharajah M, Tejwani NC, Capla EL, Koval KJ. Ankle stress test for predicting the need for surgical fixation of isolated fibular fractures. J Bone Joint Surg Am. 2004;86-A(11):2393–8.

Kwon JY, Gitajn IL, Walton P, Miller TJ, Appleton P, Rodriguez EK. A cadaver study revisiting the original methodology of Lauge-Hansen and a commentary on modern usage. J Bone Joint Surg Am. 2015;97(7):605–9.

Michelson JD. Ankle fractures resulting from rotational injuries. J Am Acad Orthop Surg. 2003;11(6):403–12.

Zalavras C, Thordarson D. Ankle syndesmotic injury. J Am Acad Orthop Surg. 2007;15(6):330–9.

Calcaneus Fracture

High-energy injuries; debated whether benefit exists of operative over non-operative treatment.

History

- Classically due to axial load on heel—fall/jump from height common.
- Frequently associated with other injuries, e.g.: contralateral calcaneus (10 %), vertebral injuries (10 %).

Physical Exam

- Full trauma exam (Appendix A).
- Skin check is critical. Some fracture types may threaten posterior skin around heel—this is a true surgical emergency to prevent impending open fracture. * IMPORTANT *
- Distal neurovascular exam (Appendix A).

Diagnosis

Imaging

X-rays: AP, lateral, and oblique of foot required.

- Harris view of heel is optional to better visualize calcaneal tuberosity.

M.C. Makhni et al. (eds.), *Orthopedic Emergencies*,
DOI 10.1007/978-3-319-31524-9_75

CT: appropriate for evaluation of intra-articular component; integral in decision for operative vs. non-operative management.

Classification

Sanders classification—based on number of articular fragments seen on coronal CT at widest point of posterior facet.

- Type 1: nondisplaced,
- Type 2: 2 fragments of posterior facet (1 fracture line) (Fig. 1),
- Type 3: 3 fragments of posterior facet (2 fracture lines).
- Type 4: Comminuted with 4 or more fragments of posterior facet (3+ fracture lines) (Fig. 2).

Alternative classifications include Essex-Lopresti.

Treatment Plan

- Threatened skin from a posteriorly displaced tuberosity fragment ("tongue type") is the only true surgically emergent calcaneus fracture.
- Otherwise, most fractures can be temporized with immobilization in a well-padded short leg splint (Appendix B: Short leg splint).
  - Discharge home from ED if no other significant injuries and patient safe to care for self while maintaining NWB status.
- Ultimate decision between non-operative and operative treatment is controversial and a function of intra-articular displacement and calcaneal deformity (loss of height, varus deformity).

Non-operative

- Minimally displaced fractures without a loss of height are amenable to non-operative treatment.
- Treatment consists of short leg splint and NWB for 10–12 weeks

Operative

- Surgical options include ORIF and subtalar arthrodesis.
- Controversial indications. Goals of surgery to anatomically restore subtalar joint articular surface and calcaneal architecture.
- Often performed electively once soft-tissue swelling has resolved, usually 10–14 days after injury.

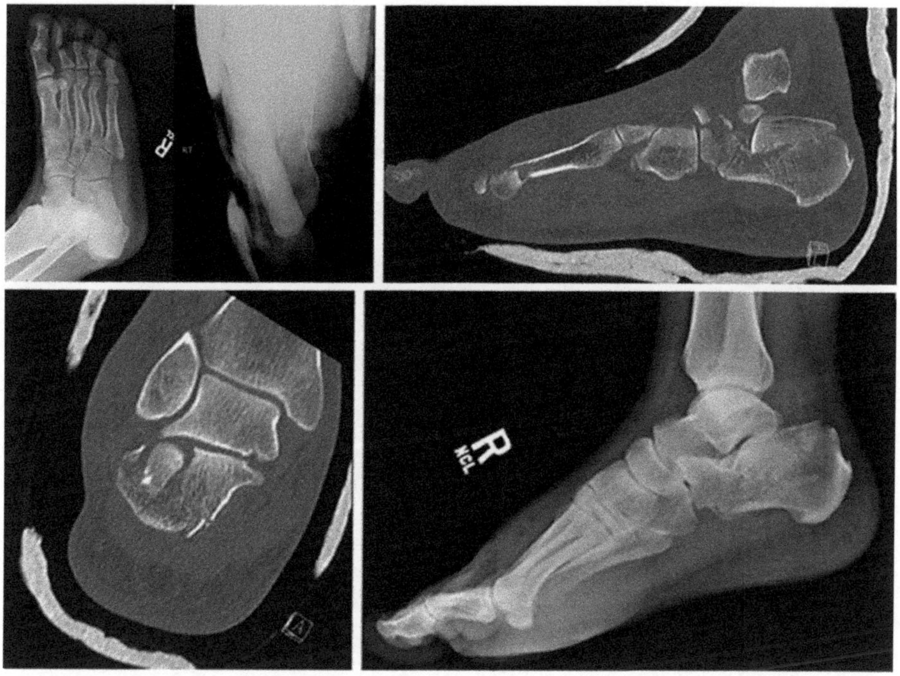

Fig. 1 Sanders 2 calcaneus fracture

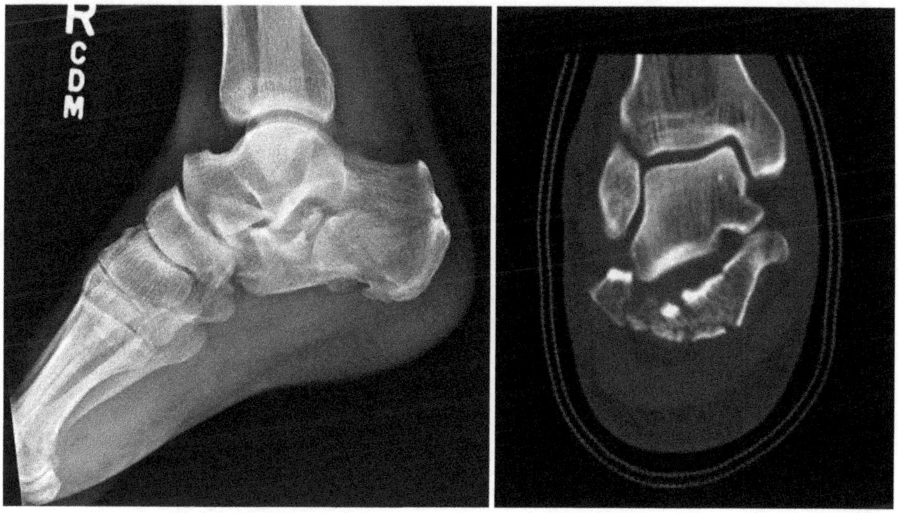

Fig. 2 Sanders 4 calcaneus fracture

References

Guerado E, Bertrand ML, Cano JR. Management of calcaneal fractures: what have we learnt over the years? Injury. 2012;43(10):1640–50.
Banerjee R, Chao JC, Taylor R, Siddiqui A. Management of calcaneal tuberosity fractures. J Am Acad Orthop Surg. 2012;20(4):253–8.
Epstein N, Chandran S, Chou L. Current concepts review: intra-articular fractures of the calcaneus. Foot Ankle Int. 2012;33(1):79–86.

Proximal Fifth Metatarsal Fracture

Common injury to the foot treated nonoperatively for proximal fractures and operatively for more distal fractures

Overview

- The mechanism of injury generally corresponds with the location of the injury (described in detail below).
    - Zone 1 injury: forced acute hindfoot inversion.
    - Zone 2 injury: strong forefoot abduction (especially in a plantarflexed foot).
    - Zone 3 injury: repetitive microtrauma (stress fracture).
- Can be associated with other injuries to the midfoot (Lisfranc fractures) or foot deformities (cavus foot, varus hindfoot).

History

- Are you an athlete/do you frequently exercise or play sports?
- Did the pain start suddenly or did it have gradual onset?
- Was there an acute injury?
- Do you have pain when weight bearing (especially over lateral aspect of foot)?

Physical Exam

- Tender to palpation over lateral aspect of foot.
- Pain with resisted eversion of foot.

M.C. Makhni et al. (eds.), *Orthopedic Emergencies*,
DOI 10.1007/978-3-319-31524-9_76

Fig. 1 Type 1 fracture

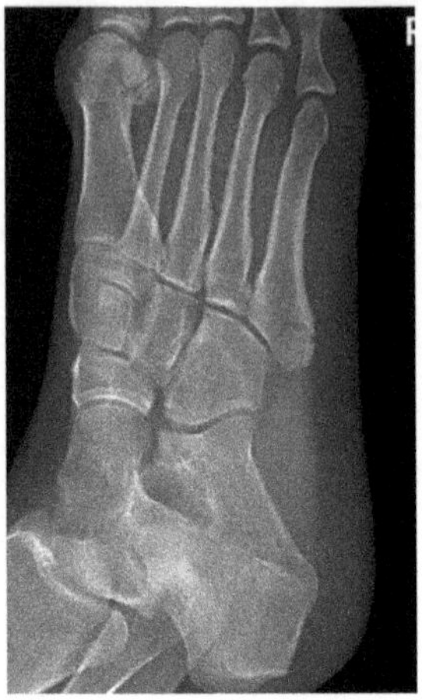

- Examine for associated conditions: cavovarus foot deformity, neuropathy, ankle ligamentous injuries.

Diagnosis

Imaging

- XR foot—AP, lateral, oblique views of the foot. Preferred imaging method (Fig. 1).
- CT/MRI foot—Not usually indicated in acute setting.

Classification

Lawrence and Botte classification (Fig. 2)

- Zone 1: Tuberosity avulsion fracture ("pseudo-Jones fracture").
- Zone 2: Metaphyseal-diaphyseal junction (true "Jones fracture").
- Zone 3: Proximal diaphysis/stress fracture.

Alternate classifications

- Recent meta-analysis shows no difference in outcome or prognosis for zone 1 and 2 injuries and suggests separating these fractures as either proximal or distal to the distal end of the 4th–5th metatarsal articulation.

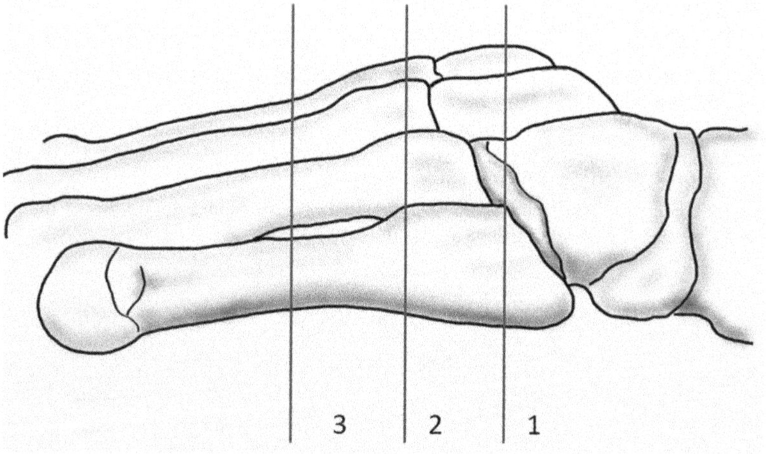

Fig. 2 Lawrence and Botte classification

Treatment Plan

Treatment plan dictated by the zone of injury.

Zone 2 is a watershed area, in and distal to which the risk of nonunion increases.

Zone 1

- Nonoperative management: indicated for nearly all zone 1 fractures regardless of number of fragments, intra-articular involvement, or displacement.
- Treatment: protected weight bearing with hard-soled shoe for comfort.

Zone 2–3

- Nonoperative: Non-weight bearing in short leg cast for 6-8 weeks pending radiographic healing. Associated with significantly longer time to return to activity and higher nonunion rate.
- Zone 2 fractures debated.
  - Traditional teaching that these have higher nonunion risk due to watershed region.
  - Recent literature suggests bony healing with weight bearing and functional treatment.
  - Consider surgery for zone 2 fracture in elite athlete.
- Operative treatment: Intermedullary screw fixation.

References

Lawrence S et al. Jones' fractures and related fractures of the proximal fifth metatarsal. Foot Ankle. 1993;14:358–65.

Polzer H et al. Acute fractures to the proximal fifth metatarsal bone: development of classification and treatment recommendations based on the current evidence. Injury. 2012;43(10):1626–32. doi:10.1016/j.injury.2012.03.010. Epub 2012 Mar 30.

Rosenberg GA, Sferra JJ. Treatment strategies for acute fractures and nonunions of the proximal fifth metatarsal. J Am Acad Orthop Surg. 2000;8(5):332–8.

Lisfranc Injury

Tarsometatarsal fracture-dislocation—usually operative.

Overview

- Lisfranc ligament complex.
  - Plantar medial cuneiform to base of second MT.
  - Plantar (stronger) and dorsal TMT ligaments.
  - Inter-MT ligaments (second to fifth MTs).
- Often due to axial load through hyperplantar-flexed foot (most commonly from MVC, fall from height, stirrup injuries (horse, motorcycle)).

History

- What was the mechanism of injury?
- Are you able to bear weight?

Physical Exam

- Medial plantar ecchymosis.
- Diffuse swelling throughout midfoot.
- Tenderness over tarsometatarsal joints.
- Dorsally subluxable forefoot (if plantar ligaments ruptured).
- Pain with pronation/abduction of forefoot.
- Inability to bear weight.

M.C. Makhni et al. (eds.), *Orthopedic Emergencies*,
DOI 10.1007/978-3-319-31524-9_77

Imaging

- XR foot—AP, lateral, and oblique.
- Bilateral weight-bearing (stress views) AP XR of foot (Figs. 1, 2, and 3).
  - Widening between the first and second ray.
  - Disruption of line (normally straight) from medial base of second MT to medial side of medial cuneiform.
  - Disruption of the medial column line (line drawn along the medial aspect of the medial cuneiform and the navicular).
  - Fleck sign—bony fragment in the space between first and second MTs from avulsion of Lisfranc ligament off base of second MT.
- Oblique XR—disruption of line between medial side of base of fourth MT and medial side of cuboid.
- Lateral XR—dorsal subluxation of the metatarsal base(s).
- CT scan—helpful for diagnosis and operative planning.
- MRI—not usually indicated. Can be used to evaluate purely ligamentous injuries.

Classification

Not commonly used and not very helpful in diagnosis/treatment.

Homo-lateral—all five MTs displaced in the same direction.
Isolated—one or two MTs displaced from the others.
Divergent—MTs displaced in sagittal and coronal planes.

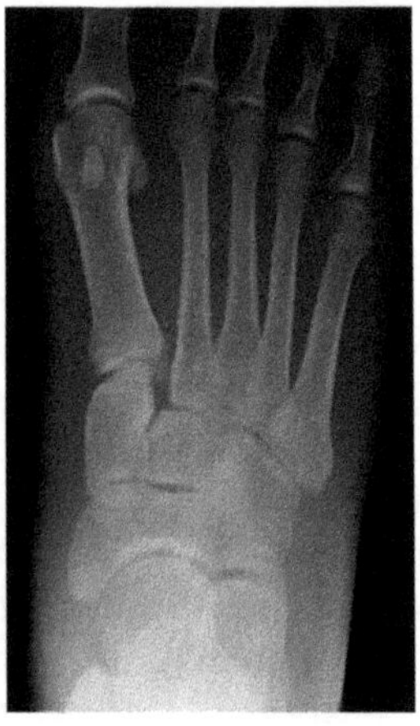

Fig. 1 Ligamentous Lisfranc injury

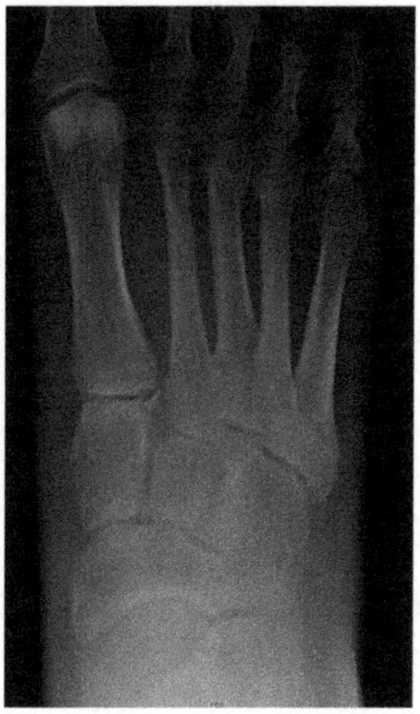

Fig. 2 Bony Lisfranc injury

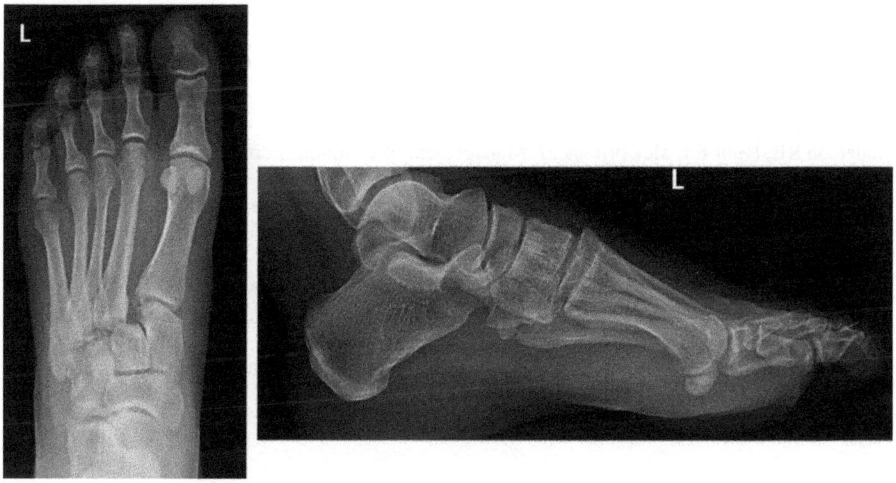

Fig. 3 Complex Lisfranc injury with multiple TMT dislocations

Treatment Plan

ED Management: immobilize (see Appendix B: Short leg splint) and restrict weight bearing.

Non-operative

Indications:

Truly non-displaced fractures.
Patients who are non-ambulatory or medically unable to tolerate surgery.

Treatment: Initial NWB in a short-leg cast.

Operative

ORIF with inter-cuneiform fixation as well as TMT transarticular screws.
Arthrodesis of TMT joints (denude of cartilage, cortical screws, ± bone graft).

Achieve better functional outcomes than ORIF.
Lower rates of hardware removal than ORIF.

Protected or non-weight bearing postoperatively.

References

Anderson RB, Hunt KJ, McCormick JJ. Management of common sports-related injuries about the foot and ankle. J Am Acad Orthop Surg. 2010;18(9):546–56.

Henning JA, Jones CB, Sietsema DL, Bohay DR, Anderson JG. Open reduction internal fixation versus primary arthrodesis for Lisfranc injuries: a prospective randomized study. Foot Ankle Int. 2009;30(10):913–22.

Ly TV, Coetzee JC. Treatment of primarily ligamentous Lisfranc joint injuries: primary arthrodesis compared with open reduction and internal fixation. A prospective, randomized study. J Bone Joint Surg Am. 2006;88(3):514–20.

Watson TS, Shurnas PS, Denker J. Treatment of Lisfranc joint injury: current concepts. J Am Acad Orthop Surg. 2010;18(12):718–28.

Metatarsal Fractures

Common foot injuries that usually heal uneventfully.

Overview

- Most frequently caused by direct trauma (e.g., a crush injury) or torque about a fixed forefoot.
- Fifth metatarsal is most frequently injured.
- Often associated with other injuries (e.g., nearly 2/3 of third metatarsal fractures are associated with fractures of second and fourth metatarsals as well).
- Insidious onset of pain may suggest a stress fracture, especially in certain athletes or dancers (ballet).

History

- Have you had pain at this site before?

Physical Exam

- Palpation along each metatarsal shaft and base, sagittal stress of the shaft and TMT joint, or axial loading of each toe will often reveal deformity or elicit pain.
- Examine soft tissue and compartments. Compartment syndrome of the foot can occur, especially in crush injuries.
- Distal neurovascular exam (Appendix A).

M.C. Makhni et al. (eds.), *Orthopedic Emergencies*,
DOI 10.1007/978-3-319-31524-9_78

Diagnosis

Imaging

- Foot XR: AP/lateral/oblique.
- Weight-bearing tangential view of metatarsal heads useful to evaluate sagittal plane alignment.
- Advanced imaging rarely indicated.

Classification

Classified by anatomic location (base, shaft, neck, or head).

Treatment Plan

Non-operative

Indicated for most nondisplaced or minimally displaced metatarsal fractures.

Treatment: WBAT in supportive shoe, CAM boot, compressive wrap, or short leg split.

Operative

Indications

- Displaced first metatarsal fracture.
- >10° angulation, >3–4 mm displacement, rotational abnormality, or shortening of central metatarsals.
- Some proximal fifth MT fractures (see Chap. "Proximal Fifth Metatarsal Fracture").

Reference

Banerjee R et al. Foot injuries. Skeletal trauma, 4th edition. Chapter 61. p. 2703–9, 2008.

Tarsal Navicular Fracture

Atraumatic stress fractures or acute and traumatic—usually nonoperative treatment trialed initially.

Overview

- Various acute mechanisms of injury:
  - Eversion of foot with simultaneous contraction of the PTT (traumatic tuberosity fracture or widening/fracture of an accessory navicular).
  - Axial loading (traumatic body fracture).
  - Plantar flexion (navicular avulsion fracture).
- Chronic from overuse (common amongst baseball players or athletes running on hard surfaces).

History

- Have you had prior pain at this site?

Physical Exam

- Midfoot pain and swelling.
- Midfoot tenderness to palpation.
- Maintained ankle and subtalar ROM.

M.C. Makhni et al. (eds.), *Orthopedic Emergencies*,
DOI 10.1007/978-3-319-31524-9_79

Diagnosis

Imaging

- Foot XR: AP/lateral/oblique.
- CT: order if suspect fracture despite negative XR.

Classification

Sangeorzan Classification

- Type 1—transverse fracture, resulting in dorsal and plantar fragments.
- Type 2—oblique fracture, associated with forefoot adduction (most common type).
- Type 3—comminuted, displaced fragments, associated with abduction.

Treatment Plan

Nonoperative

Initial treatment for most navicular fractures.
Treatment: cast immobilization, non-weight bearing.

Operative

Indications: persistent symptoms despite nonoperative treatment.

- Fragment excision: avulsion fracture that failed nonoperative treatment.
- ORIF:
  - Stress fracture in athlete.
  - Displaced type 1 and 2 fractures.
  - Fracture with >25 % articular surface involvement or >5 mm widening.
- Arthrodesis
  - Type 3 fracture.

References

Miller CM, Winter WG, Bucknell AL, Jonassen EA. Injuries to the midtarsal joint and lesser tarsal bones. J Am Acad Orthop Surg. 1998;6(4):249–58.

Shindle MK, Endo Y, Warren RF, Lane JM, Helfet DL, Schwartz EN, et al. Stress fractures about the tibia, foot, and ankle. J Am Acad Orthop Surg. 2012;20(3):167–76. doi:10.5435/JAAOS-20-03-167.

Torg JS, Moyer J, Gaughan JP, Boden BP. Management of tarsal navicular stress fractures: conservative versus surgical treatment: a meta-analysis. Am J Sports Med. 2010;38(5):1048–53.

References

Tibial Plafond (Pilon) Fracture

High energy injury of the distal tibia, with impaction of the talus caused by axial loading; almost always operative.

History

- Assess for associated injuries or other complaints

Physical Exam

- Full trauma exam (Appendix A)
- Skin intact? Amount of soft tissue swelling?
- Distal neurovascular exam (Appendix A)

Diagnosis

Imaging

- XR: tibia, ankle, and foot
- CT: usually required to determine articular displacement and proximal extent of fracture
    - If doing external fixation, CT performed afterward *IMPORTANT*

M.C. Makhni et al. (eds.), *Orthopedic Emergencies*,
DOI 10.1007/978-3-319-31524-9_80

Classification

Most common is standard AO classification

- 43-A: Extra-articular
- 43-B: Partial articular (Fig. 1)
- 43-C: Complete articular (Fig. 2)

Alternative classifications include Ruedi and Allgower

- I: nondisplaced
- II: displaced articular surface
- III: comminuted, displaced articular surface

Treatment

Almost always operative
Soft tissue management is crucial for long-term success

Nonoperative

Indications: nondisplaced fractures (rare), or medically unstable patients
Treatment: short leg splint, non-weightbearing

Operative

- Initial management:
  - Goal to re-establish joint alignment and limb length
  - Provisional immobilization with reduction and short leg splint for length-stable fractures (Appendix B): Short leg splint
  - Immediate spanning external fixation for length-unstable fractures
- Delayed ORIF once soft tissue swelling has resolved, frequently >10 days after injury

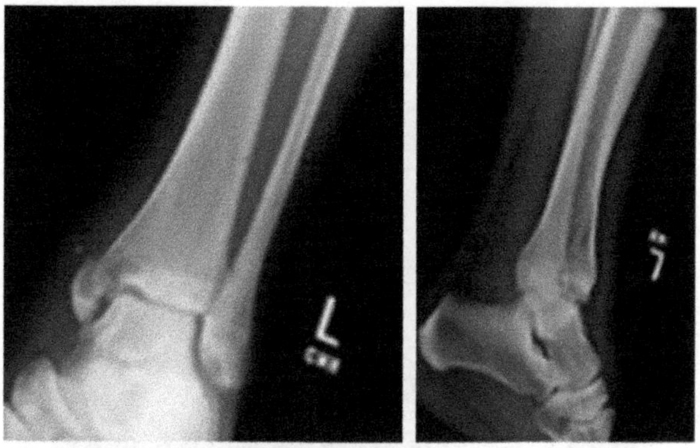

Section: Tibial Plafond (Pilon) Fracture
Image Title: Partial Articular Pilon Fracture

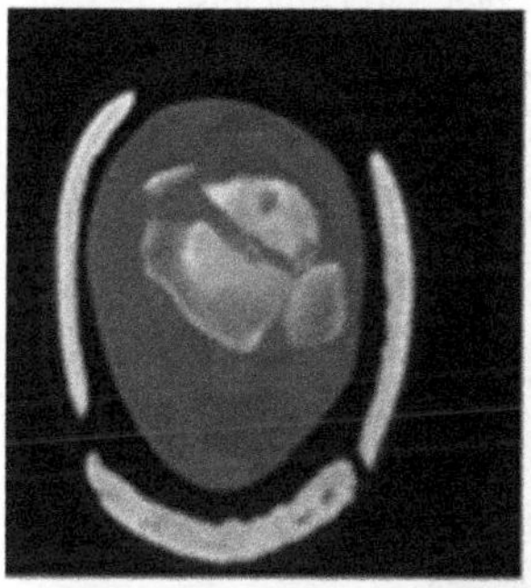

Section: Tibial Plafond (Pilon) Fracture
Image Title: Partial Articular Pilon Fracture

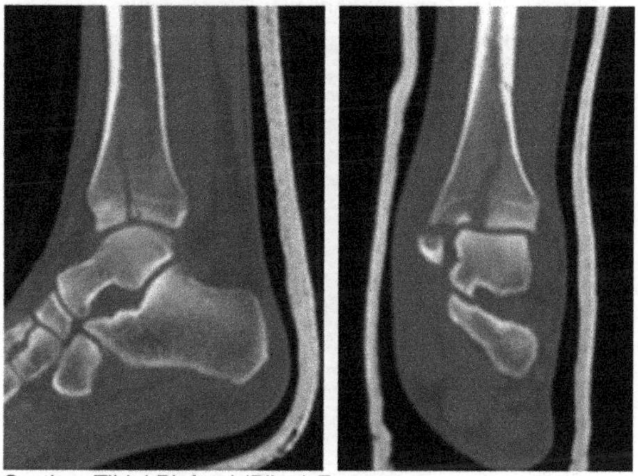

Section: Tibial Plafond (Pilon) Fracture
Image Title: Partial Articular Pilon Fracture

Fig. 1 Partial articular pilon fracture

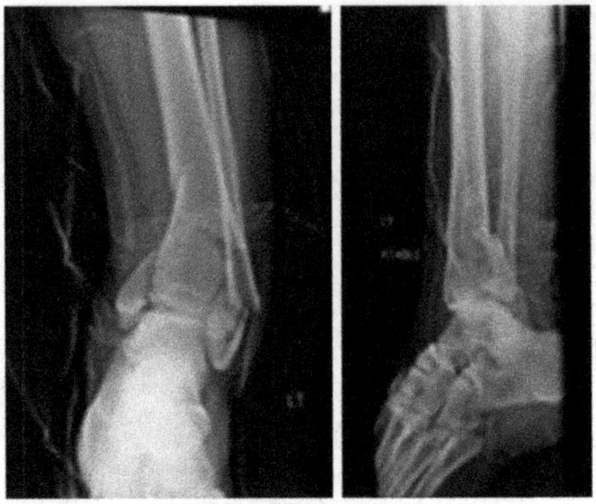

Section: Tibial Plafond (Pilon) Fracture
Image Title: Complete Articular Pilon Fracture

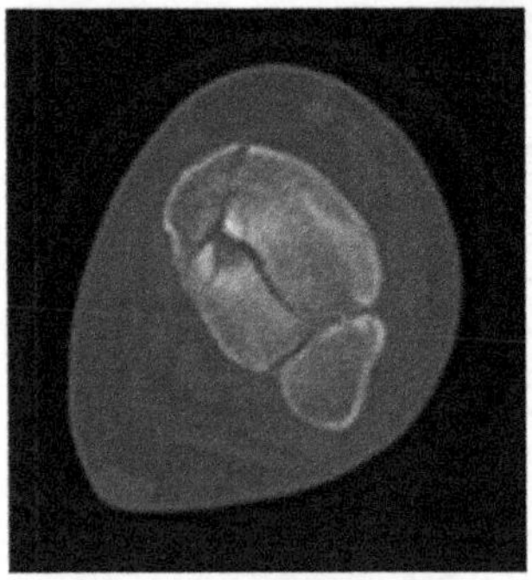

Section: Tibial Plafond (Pilon) Fracture
Image Title: Complete Articular Pilon Fracture

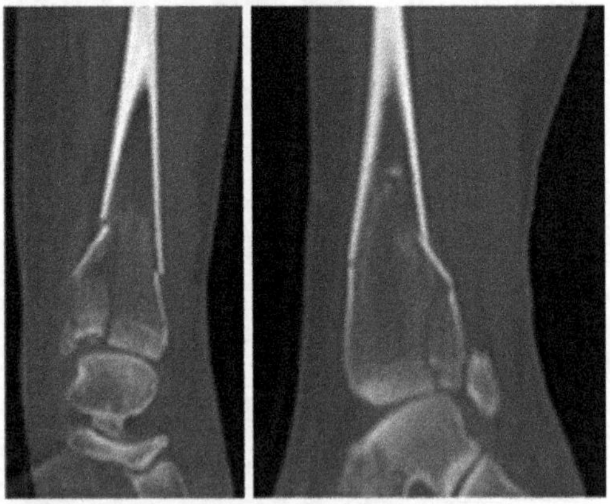

Section: Tibial Plafond (Pilon) Fracture
Image Title: Complete Articular Pilon Fracture

Fig. 2 Complete articular pilon fracture

References

Liporace FA, Yoon RS. Decisions and staging leading to definitive open management of pilon fractures: where have we come from and where are we now? J Orthop Trauma. 2012;26(8):488–98.

Crist BD, Khazzam M, Murtha YM, Della Rocca GJ. Pilon fractures: advances in surgical management. J Am Acad Orthop Surg. 2011;19(10):612–22.

Talar Neck Fractures

High energy injuries usually resulting from dorsiflexion and axial loading, often associated with other injuries and dislocations. Usually require operative fixation to minimize the risk of avascular necrosis.

History

- Do you have any other pain along your back or legs?

Physical Exam

- Skin intact? Amount of soft tissue swelling? (Fig. 1)
- Full trauma exam (Appendix A)
- Distal neurovascular exam (Appendix A)

Diagnosis

Imaging

- XR foot—AP and Lateral
- Can include Canale view to visualize talar neck
- CT scan virtually always necessary to better define fracture anatomy/displacement. Can also help identify other associated fractures (common)

M.C. Makhni et al. (eds.), *Orthopedic Emergencies*,
DOI 10.1007/978-3-319-31524-9_81

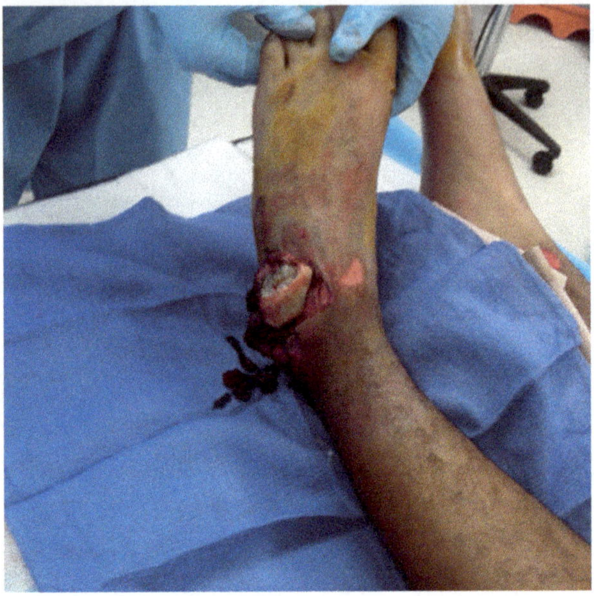

Fig. 1 Open talus fracture

Classification

Hawkins classification system, based on associated dislocations

- Type 1: Nondisplaced
- Type 2: Subtalar dislocation/subluxation (Fig. 2)
- Type 3: Subtalar, tibiotalar dislocation (Fig. 3)
- Type 4: Subtalar, tibiotalar, talonavicular dislocation

Classification predicts AVN rate up to: (Type 1: 10 %, type 2: 50 %, type 3: 75–90 %, Type 4: 100 %)

Treatment Plan

Emergent closed reduction of any associated dislocations (flex knee, plantar flex forefoot, traction, direct pressure on talar body and varus/valgus force as needed), short let splint placement (Appendix B: Short leg splint), followed by CT **AFTER** closed reduction, then ORIF of any displaced fracture.

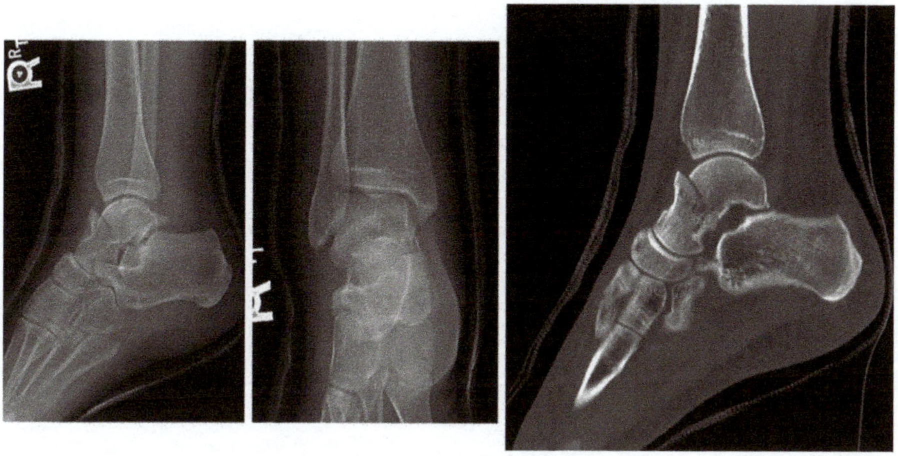

Fig. 2 Hawkins 2 talar neck fracture

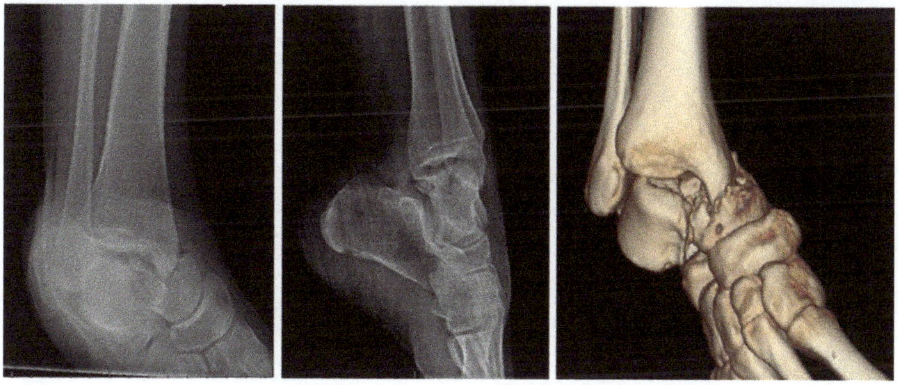

Fig. 3 Hawkins 3 talar neck fracture

Nonoperative

Indications: nondisplaced (Hawkins 1) fracture
Treatment: Non-weight-bearing short leg cast for 4–6 weeks then removable brace and early motion (may consider percutaneous screw with early motion).

Operative

Urgent open reduction and internal fixation. Had formerly been considered a true emergency, although recent literature has demonstrated that it may not be as emergent (can be done the next morning).

References

Fortin PT, Balazsy JE. Talus fractures: evaluation and treatment. J Am Acad Orthop Surg. 2001;9(2):114–27.
Hawkins LG. J Bone Joint Surg Am. 1970;53A:991–1002.
Patel R, Van Bergeyk A, Pinney S. Are displaced talar neck fractures surgical emergencies? A survey of orthopaedic trauma experts. Foot Ankle Int. 2005;26(5):378–81.
Vallier HA, Nork SE, Benirschke SK, Sangeorzan BJ. Surgical treatment of talar body fractures. J Bone Joint Surg Am. 2004;86-A Suppl 1(Pt 2):180–92.

Lateral Process of Talus Fracture

Moderate energy injury—treatment dictated by articular congruity.

Overview

- Classic mechanism is inversion with dorsiflexion and axial load ("Snowboarder's fracture")
- Frequently missed on plain radiographs so high index of suspicion for patients with severe pain and exam consistent with "ankle sprain"

Physical Exam

- Skin intact? Amount of soft tissue swelling?
- Distal neurovascular exam (Appendix B)

Diagnosis

Imaging

- AP and Lateral XR of foot (lateral process best viewed on AP image) (Fig. 1)
- CT scan can help with diagnosis when clinical concern but X-rays negative. Also helpful in determining ultimate treatment (operative vs. nonoperative) based on fracture displacement.

M.C. Makhni et al. (eds.), *Orthopedic Emergencies*,
DOI 10.1007/978-3-319-31524-9_82

Classification

Based on anatomic location

- Type 1: Tip of lateral process (doesn't involve articular surface)
- Type 2: Lateral process involves subtalar or tibiotalar joint
- Type 3: comminuted lateral process

Treatment Plan

Decision for operative vs. nonoperative treatment based on fracture displacement/comminution.

Nonoperative

Indication: minimally displaced fractures (<2 mm).

Treatment: immobilization in a short leg cast (Appendix B: Short leg cast) 4–6 weeks, initially NWB

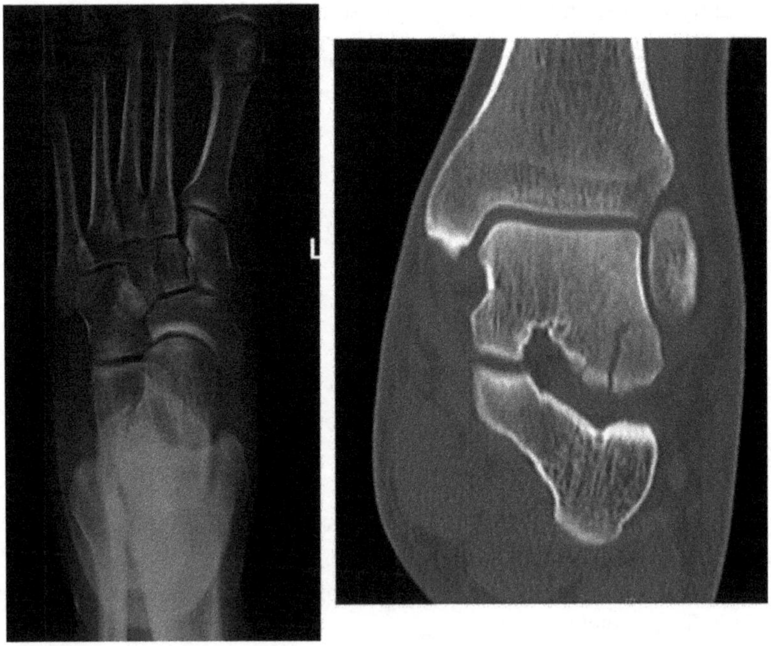

Fig. 1 Lateral process of talus fracture

Operative

Indications: fractures with >2 mm displacement or severe comminution
Treatment:

Displaced fractures—ORIF
Severely comminuted fractures—lateral process fragment excision

References

Tucker DJ, Feder JM, Boylan JP. Fractures of the lateral process of the talus: two case reports and a comprehensive literature review. Foot Ankle Int. 1998;19(9):641–6.
Vlahovich AT, Mehin R, O'Brien PJ. An unusual fracture of the talus in a snowboarder. J Orthop Trauma. 2005;19(7):498–500.

Overview

Phalanx Fractures of the Foot

Common and usually nonoperative injuries. Fractures of the hallux are treated more aggressively than fractures to the lesser toes given its biomechanical importance.

Overview

- Most commonly the result of low-energy direct trauma to an unprotected toe
- Poorly aligned lesser toe fractures can result in interdigital callus formation
- Rarely, stress fractures in the proximal phalanx of the great toe can occur in young athletes, especially with underlying hallux valgus

History

- How did the injury occur? (Crush is a common mechanism)
- Was there a cut in the skin or bleeding from the toe after anywhere
- Does it hurt anywhere in your foot other than the toe?

Physical Exam

- Tenderness to palpation, swelling, ecchymosis, are common over affected digit, usually worst 2–3 days after injury
- Distal fractures frequently associated with subungual hematoma or nailbed injury

M.C. Makhni et al. (eds.), *Orthopedic Emergencies*,
DOI 10.1007/978-3-319-31524-9_83

- Check gross stability/alignment of toes
- Confirm no other associated injuries to midfoot or forefoot

Diagnosis

Imaging

- XR Foot—AP, Lateral, Oblique views of the foot. Preferred imaging method.

Classification

- Described anatomically based on digit: (e.g. hallux vs. lesser toes), phalanx involved, and intra- or extraarticular extension

Treatment Plan

Nonoperative

- Almost always managed nonoperatively

Treatment

- Closed Reduction (if displaced)
  - Gentle traction and mobilization towards anatomic alignment
  - If dislocated, longitudinal traction is followed by hyperextension followed by rapid flexion
- No true immobilization but can buddy tape to adjacent toe for comfort
- "Hard soled shoe"—any spacious, comfortable shoe that can accommodate swelling of toe is adequate; hard sole limits stress on toe during gait
- Weight-bearing as tolerated

Indications: most nondisplaced or minimally displaced fractures, or fractures reduced into acceptable alignment

For nailbed injury, consider evacuation if >25 % of nailbed involvement

If the nail is intact and the injury is not open

Do not remove nail

Consider trephination (heated paper-clip, cautery, or an 18G needle) to carefully perforate the nail surface above the hematoma allowing blood to escape

If nailbed or matrix is disrupted, repair as would in hand (*see Nailbed Laceration Repair*)

Operative

Treatment: ORIF with crossing K-wires or lag screw fixation

Indications: Open, displaced, or unstable fractures (e.g. transverse fractures), especially in proximal phalanx of greater toe

Treatment: removal of the interposed nail bed from the physis

Indications: Seymour's fracture—open fracture of distal phalanx in child with open physis (rare)

References

Banerjee R, et al. Foot injuries. Skeletal trauma. 4th ed. Chapter 61 p. 2720–2.

Yokoe K, Kameyama Y. Relationship between stress fractures of the proximal phalanx of the great toe and hallux valgus. Am J Sports Med. 2004;32(4):1032–4.

Kensinger DR, Guille JT, Horn BD, Herman MJ. The stubbed great toe: importance of early recognition and treatment of open fractures of the distal phalanx. J Pediatr Orthop. 2001;21(1):31–4.

Part VIII
Pediatrics

Daniel Miller, Katie Rosenwasser, Anny Hsu, and Jeanne Franzone

Sedation for the Pediatric Patient 385

Casting and Immobilization in the Pediatric Patient 389

Child Abuse-Non-accidental Trauma (NAT) 393

Salter–Harris Classification 397

Clavicle Fracture 401

Proximal Humerus Fracture 405

Humeral Shaft Fracture 409

Supracondylar Humerus Fracture (SCHFx) 413

Lateral Condyle Fracture 419

Medial Epicondyle Fracture 423

Distal Humerus Physeal Separation 427

Radial Head Subluxation (Nursemaid's Elbow) 431

Radial Neck Fracture 433

Both-Bone Forearm Fracture 437

Distal Radius Fracture 443

Monteggia Fracture 447

Galeazzi Fracture 451

Pelvic Fracture 453

Avulsion Fractures of the Pelvis 457

Hip Pain: Septic Hip vs. Transient Synovitis 461

Hip Dislocation 465

Slipped Capital Femoral Epiphysis 469

Hip Fracture 473

Femur Fracture 477

Distal Femur Physeal Fracture 481

Tibial Eminence Fracture 485

Tibial Tubercle Fracture 489

Toddler's Fracture 493

Ankle Fractures 497

Sedation for the Pediatric Patient

There are many options for pain and anxiety control in the pediatric patient, and care should be taken to ensure safe and expedient treatment in the emergency department without additional emotional trauma to the child.

Principles

Generally try to use minimum amount of systemic medication to provide the following:

- Anxiolysis
- Analgesia
- Decreased consciousness

Non-pharmacologic Agents

- May be helpful to integrate games/music/television as distractions during procedures. Parental involvement with procedure to i.e.: hold child's arm during casting may ease the child's anxiety. Many pediatric EDs are equipped to offer these non-pharmacologic measures to assist in anxiolysis and minimize the need for medications.
- Consider draping in all procedures to cover patient's face and prevent direct viewing of the affected extremity in order to reduce stress.

M.C. Makhni et al. (eds.), *Orthopedic Emergencies*,
DOI 10.1007/978-3-319-31524-9_84

Local Blocks

Often used in conjunction with intranasal formulations of sedatives/anxiolytics. See chart below for specific agents (Table 1).

- Digital Block

  Injection into the base of a single digit
  Used for finger abscesses, laceration repairs, phalangeal reductions

- Hematoma Block

  Injection directly into the fracture site
  Used for distal radius fractures, both-bone fractures

- Bier Block

  Intravenous injection of local anesthetic
  Used for fractures of the forearm/wrist/hand

  (See Procedures Section for more information regarding local blocks)

Table 1 Conscious sedation

Agent	Mechanism of action	Clinical effects	Duration of effect	Appropriate use
Ketamine	*N*-Methyl-D-aspartate antagonist	Analgesia, amnesia, dissociative anesthetic state	Has dose threshold in which additional med lengthens but does not deepen state	May be used as a single agent
Fentanyl	Opioid (μ agonist)	Analgesia	Rapid onset, short duration (0.1–1.5 h)	In conjunction with sedatives. Available in intranasal formulation
Nitrous oxide	GABA agonist, NMDA antagonist	Primarily anxiolysis, minimal analgesia	Rapid onset and clearance (within minutes)	Given intranasally, does not require IV access, used in conjunction with local blocks
Midazolam (Versed)	Benzodiazepine (GABA agonist)	Anxiolysis, amnesia, spasmolyis; NO analgesia	half life of 2–4 hrs	In conjunction with analgesics

Conscious Sedation

Generally used for more complex fracture reduction (i.e., both bones, distal radius) or lengthy procedure (nail bed or laceration repair, infection I&D)

- Ensure adequate NPO time
- Obtain informed consent from parent/guardian
- May utilize local block as well for post-procedure pain control
- Choice of agent depends largely on resources and comfort level of ER physicians. It is important to discuss the anticipated length and extent of procedure to determine most appropriate combination of medications .

References

Eberson CP et al. Procedural sedation in the emergency department. Eberson CP, Hsu RY, Borenstein TR. J Am Acad Orthop Surg. 2015 Apr;23(4):233-42.

Rockwood CA, Wilkins KE, King RE. Fractures in children. Philadelphia: Lippincott; 1984.

Conscious Sedation

Casting and Immobilization in the Pediatric Patient

Proper casting and immobilization technique is crucial for the successful management of pediatric fractures. Optimal management requires close monitoring and age-appropriate techniques.

Challenges with Casting in Children

- Lower level of understanding and compliance
  - Use additional assistance with application
  - Family assistance for maintenance
- Difficulty with communication to express pain
  - Vigilant monitoring by care-giver
  - Evaluation of behavior that deviates from the norm to indicate increased pain (e.g., compartment syndrome)
- Age and size
  - Due to shorter limb length and conical limb shapes in young children, cast/splint may become loose and may easily be removed by patients
    - Extend cast (e.g., long arm cast for younger patients)
    - More frequent checks (may need to change cast after swelling from acute injury subsides)
- Children may require higher level of analgesia/sedation during reduction and casting due to anxiety and limited pain tolerance

M.C. Makhni et al. (eds.), *Orthopedic Emergencies*,
DOI 10.1007/978-3-319-31524-9_85

Casting Guidelines

- Beware of exothermic reaction with plaster/fiberglass
  - Do not dip in hot water (>24 °C or 75 °F)
  - More heat from thicker cast
- Common cast removal complication is high blade temperature causing cast saw burn
  - Change blades frequently to decrease dull blade
  - Alternate firm pressure with oscillating saw to decrease cast saw burn
  - Frequent blade cooling
  - Cast tape applied along cast removal line prior to cast application
- Fiberglass:
  - Lighter and allows for better imaging
  - May be combined with waterproof liner for water-proof cast
  - Less flexible for molding
- Plaster
  - Thicker material but easier for molding
- Pad bony prominence and cast edges → minimize ulcer/pressure points
- Minimize hyperflexion or tight casting to reduce risk of compartment syndrome/Volkman's contracture

Casting Principles

- Three point immobilization
  - Each cast/splint should closely mimic limb of immobilization
  - Wrapping should not be too tight or will otherwise act like tourniquet * IMPORTANT *
  - Anticipate pattern of fracture instability and provide counter support to minimize fracture displacement in splint
- All cast/splint should be snug without undue pressure. No focal pressure spots!
- Well fitted forearm plaster splint/cast has optimal sagittal to coronal ratio of ≤0.7 (diameter of splint on lateral view/diameter of splint on AP view)
- Limb positioning
  - Maintain fracture reduction
  - Minimize contracture (ex: foot neutral position)
  - Functional positioning (ex: long arm cast with hand in neutral instead of pronation/supination)

- Plaster and fiberglass cast may be univalved or bivalved to relieve circumferential pressure and reduce risk for compartment syndrome
- West/soiled cast should be removed and replaced to minimize skin irritation, skin breakdown, and infection

References

Charnley J. The closed treatment of common fractures. 4th ed. Cambridge, UK: Cambridge University Press; 2005.

Halanski M, Noonan KJ. Cast and splint immobilization: complications. J Am Acad Orthop Surg. 2008;16(1):30–40.

Child Abuse-Non-accidental Trauma (NAT)

Recognition is a key element of helping children who are subjected to non-accidental trauma. Suspicious cases MUST be reported.

Overview

- Child abuse is maltreatment of a child by either parents or caretakers and includes physical, sexual, and emotional abuse, in addition to emotional and physical neglect * IMPORTANT *
- Mandatory reporting of suspected abuse/neglect in all states
- May need to admit and maintain in hospital if concern for safety of child
- Significant problem

  >1 million children are victims of abuse in the US annually
  NAT is the second most common cause of death in children (after accidents)
  Half of fractures in children less than 1 year old due to abuse
  Children who return home after an unrecognized episode of abuse have a 25 % risk of serious reinjury and a 5 % risk of death

- History is critical in detecting child abuse
- A quiet area for the interview is important; ask questions in a nonjudgmental way; must sort out how the child lives, which caretakers have access to the child; interview siblings as well; may be helpful to speak with child and all involved parties independently
- Careful detailed documentation is critical

M.C. Makhni et al. (eds.), *Orthopedic Emergencies*,
DOI 10.1007/978-3-319-31524-9_86

History

- Is the history of trauma adequate to explain the severity of the injury?
- Does the given history fit the patient's developmental abilities?
- Does the story make sense? Who witnessed the event?
- Who discovered the injury?
- How soon the child received medical care?
- Look for prior ER visits; ask about prior injuries and prior ER visits to other hospitals

Physical Exam

- Initial musculoskeletal evaluation for the acute fracture is performed
- Thorough examination is essential including evaluation of the skin for bruising, burns, abrasions, any other soft tissue injuries or scars, the abdomen, the central nervous system, and the genitalia (in a chaperoned setting)
- Complete neurological evaluation
- Multidisciplinary evaluation—may include collaboration with Neurosurgery, Ophthalmology, General Surgery, Gynecology, Pediatrics

Imaging

- Appropriate radiographs of the acute fracture or injury
- Skeletal survey is crucial
- Additional imaging will depend on injuries noted

Common Types of NAT

Note: This chapter is not meant to be an exhaustive list of such injuries but rather to help raise awareness of those seeing injured children in emergency room settings

- Head injury is the most common cause of death in physical abuse
- Soft tissue injuries as noted above, bruises, and burns (skin lesions most common sign of NAT)
- Abdominal trauma is the second most common reason for death from child abuse
- Genital injuries as noted above
- Multiple fractures in different stages of healing
- Femoral fractures in non-ambulatory children
- Fractures of lateral clavicle and scapula

- Torus fractures of the metacarpals or phalanges of the hand or feet
- Rib fractures; sternal fractures
- Metaphyseal and diaphyseal fractures of long bones
- Corner or bucket-handle fracture of the metaphysis
- Distal humeral physeal separation
- Rib fractures including posterior rib fractures and disruption of the anterior costochondral junction
- Remember the differential diagnosis including systemic diseases such as scurvy, osteogenesis imperfecta, tumors, rickets, obstetric trauma, etc—the presence of metabolic disease or pathologic fracture does not, however, exclude the possibility of child abuse * IMPORTANT *

Treatment

- Admission places the child in a safe, monitored environment and allows further work-up and involvement of social services
- Appropriate musculoskeletal care must be provided for the injuries
- All suspected child abuse is required to be reported to the appropriate child protective services or legal authorities

References

Campbell Jr RM, Schrader T. Child abuse. In: Beaty JH, Kasser JR, editors. Rockwood and Wilkins' fractures in children. 6th ed. Philadelphia, PA: Lippincott Williams & Wilkins; 2006.
Jayakumar P, Barry M, Ramachandran M. Orthopaedic aspects of paediatric non-accidental injury. J Bone Joint Surg Br. 2010;92(2):189–95.
Kocher MS, Kasser JR. Orthopaedic aspects of child abuse. J Am Acad Orthop Surg. 2000;8(1):10–20.

Salter–Harris Classification

"Children are not small adults. The Salter-Harris classification describes fractures in children around a growth plate, or physis. This descriptive classification system often has treatment implications as well"

Overview

- Physis, or "growth plate," is area of growing cartilage in children's bones responsible for growth throughout childhood until reaching skeletal maturity
- Epiphysis is the region at the end of long bone—forms a secondary center of ossification and determines shape of the articular surface.
- Physeal fractures account for 15–30 % of all childhood fractures

Radiographs

- XR bone/joint of interest, including full bone/adjacent joints as needed
- May obtain contralateral X-rays to evaluate for asymmetry in subtle cases
- If fracture intra-articular, may obtain CT to further evaluate articular displacement

Classification

Salter–Harris Classification: (Fig. 1)

Mnemonic for Types I–V: *SALTR*

*S*ame = through level of physis
*A*bove = exits above physis

M.C. Makhni et al. (eds.), *Orthopedic Emergencies*,
DOI 10.1007/978-3-319-31524-9_87

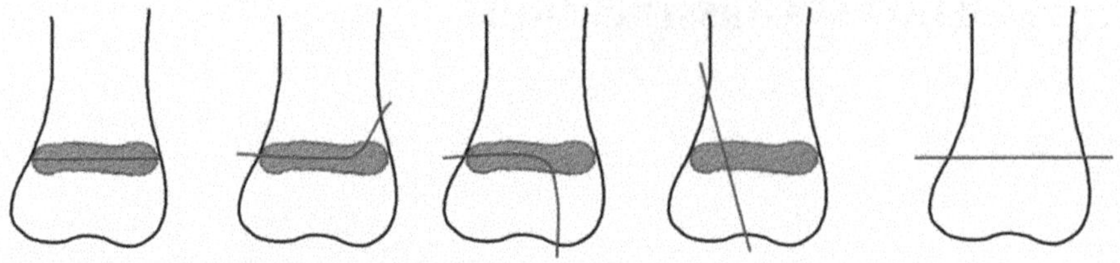

Fig. 1 Salter–Harris classification

Lower = exits below physis
Through = above and below physis
Really bad = crush injury to the physis

Type I

- Transverse fracture through the physis (i.e., transphyseal plane of injury) without metaphyseal or epiphyseal fragment
- Most commonly seen in infants and young children
- Localized swelling and point tenderness should help confirm diagnosis
- Prognosis for uninterrupted growth is quite good

Worse prognosis for rare occurrences of physeal separation of proximal or distal femur or when periosteum is trapped in the physis

Type II

- Fracture line passes through portion of growth plate and exits through a segment of the metaphysis that remains attached to the intact portion of the growth plate
- The metaphyseal fragment = Thurston Holland fragment
- Prognosis for growth resumption generally good, particularly in the distal radius

Worse prognosis in distal femur type II fractures, with growth disturbance in up to 50 % of patients.

Type III

- Fracture line traverses physis, then crosses epiphysis into articular surface
- More common in older children in whom growth arrest may be less problematic
- Often involves germinal and proliferative layers of physis
  - More guarded prognosis with respect to remaining growth
  - Intra-articular nature of these fractures necessitates anatomic reduction, which can often require surgical intervention

Type IV

- Fracture crosses all zones of the physis
- Intra-articular—traverse epiphysis, physis, and metaphysis

- High risk of growth arrest
- Intra-articular nature of these fractures necessitates anatomic reduction, which can often require surgical intervention

Type V

- Compression injury to the physis
- May not be apparent on X-rays
- Growth arrest common

Treatment

- Depends on fracture type and displacement
- Patients with non-displaced Salter–Harris Type I fractures are typically immobilized in a cast and discharged home
- As Salter–Harris Type III and IV fractures are typically intra-articular

  Advanced imaging in the form of a CT scan may be indicated
  May require anatomic reduction and fixation in the operating room

- All patients and families of patients with fractures involving the physis must be counseled regarding the possibility of growth disturbance and those with higher risk fractures must be followed through the end of their growth *IMPORTANT*

References

Price CT, Flynn JM. Management of fractures. In: Morrissy RT, Weinstein SL, editors. Lovell & winter's pediatric orthopaedics. 6th ed. Philadelphia, PA: Lippincott Williams & Wilkins; 2006.

Rang M. Children's fractures. Philadelphia, PA: J. B. Lippincott Co.; 1983.

Rathjen KE, Birch JG. Physeal injuries and growth disturbances. In: Beaty JH, Kasser JR, editors. Rockwood and Wilkins' fractures in children. 6th ed. Philadelphia, PA: Lippincott Williams & Wilkins; 2006.

Salter R, Harris WR. Injuries involving the epiphyseal plate. J Bone Joint Surg Am. 1963;45:587.

Clavicle Fracture

Clavicle fractures are common in the pediatric population and can often be treated non-operatively. Controversy exists regarding treatment of markedly displaced fractures in adolescents. Medial and distal physeal fractures are unique to the developing skeleton.

History

- Obtain birth history if associated with birth trauma.
- How did you injure your arm?
- Do you have any numbness or tingling in your arm?
- Do you have pain in your shoulder, elbow, or wrist?
- Do you have any difficulty breathing or swallowing?

Physical Exam

- Examine for deformity or evidence of soft-tissue compromise/skin tenting *IMPORTANT*
- Palpate for swelling or crepitus about the clavicle
- Percuss entire extremity to evaluate for tenderness
- Assess range of motion of extremity; limited shoulder range of motion should raise suspicion for possible glenohumeral dislocation
- In infants, eliciting a Moro reflex can help distinguish between guarding 2/2 pain and paralysis
- UE neuro exam (Appendix A), with careful attention to the vascular exam in setting of medial physeal fracture *IMPORTANT*

M.C. Makhni et al. (eds.), *Orthopedic Emergencies*,
DOI 10.1007/978-3-319-31524-9_88

Diagnosis

Imaging

- Chest and clavicle X-rays including AP, and serendipity (40° cephalic tilt) views
  - Examine for evidence of fracture comminution, shortening, or segmental injury. Comparison with the contralateral side provides better appreciation of fracture shortening
  - Medial physeal fracture is difficult to appreciate on AP view and is better visualized on the serendipity view as superior or inferior displacement
- Obtain shoulder X-rays including axillary view if concern for concomitant shoulder injury or dislocation.
- CT scan can be used to distinguish between medial physeal fracture (more common in patients <25 years) and sternoclavicular dislocation (more common in adults) (Fig. 1)

Classification

No commonly used classification exists for pediatric clavicle fractures. Fractures described by location, pattern, displacement, and presence of soft-tissue injury.

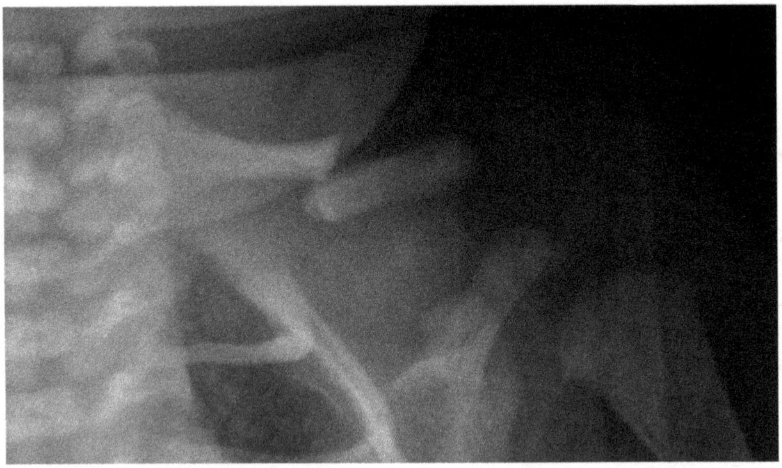

Fig. 1 Clavicle fracture

Treatment Plan

Nonoperative

- **Treatment:** Immobilization in sling or figure of eight brace
  - 2–4 weeks
  - Followed by gradual resumption of motion and strengthening
- **Indications:**
  - Nearly universal in patients <10 years old
  - Minimally to mildly displaced shaft fractures (<15–20 mm shortened and <100 % displaced) in adolescents
  - Distal physeal fractures given the tendency for the periosteum to remain intact
  - Relative indications are controversial (see below) particularly in adolescents
- **Treatment:** Closed reduction under anesthesia
- **Indications:**
  - Displaced medial physeal fractures (anterior or posterior)
- **Treatment:** Open reduction and internal fixation with plating or intramedullary nailing.
- **Indications:**
  - Open fractures (with I&D)
  - Impending open fractures 2/2 skin tenting
  - Associated scapular neck fracture (e.g., floating shoulder)
  - Significantly displaced fractures in adolescents nearing skeletal maturity (>15–20 mm shortened and/or >100 % displaced) (relative/controversial)
  - Polytrauma patients (relative)

References

Caird MS. Clavicle shaft fractures: are children little adults? J Pediatr Orthop. 2012;32 Suppl 1:S1–4.

Pandya NK, Namdari S, Hosalkar HS. Displaced clavicle fractures in adolescents: facts, controversies, and current trends. J Am Acad Orthop Surg. 2012;20(8):498–505.

Proximal Humerus Fracture

A fracture of the proximal aspect of the humerus that is often treated nonoperatively given the remarkable remodeling potential of the proximal humeral physis.

History

- Obtain birth history if associated with birth trauma
- How did you injure your shoulder?
- Do you have any numbness or tingling in your arm?
- Do you have pain in your forearm, wrist, or elbow?
- Have you ever dislocated your shoulder?
- Are you a thrower and recent throwing patterns?
- Consider NAT investigation, particularly in patients <2 years (see section on NAT) *IMPORTANT*

Physical Exam

- Examine shoulder girdle for deformity; apex anterior deformity with prominence over anterior shoulder is common
- Evaluate skin and soft tissue integrity
- Note the positioning of the arm; arm is usually held guarded in an adducted, internally rotated position
- Palpate entire extremity to evaluate for tenderness. Tenderness is usually limited to the proximal humerus; Tenderness at other areas (i.e., wrist, forearm, elbow) suggest additional injuries *IMPORTANT*

M.C. Makhni et al. (eds.), *Orthopedic Emergencies*,
DOI 10.1007/978-3-319-31524-9_89

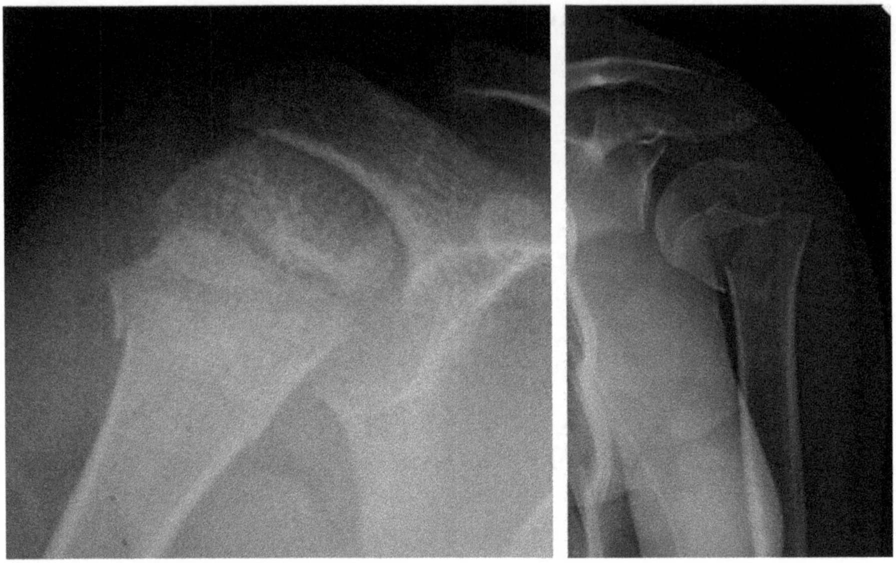

Fig. 1 Proximal humerus fractures

- Assess range of motion of extremity; pain in shoulder associated specifically with shoulder external rotation or resisted internal rotation suggests lesser tuberosity avulsion fracture
- UE neuro exam (Appendix A)
- In infants, eliciting a Moro reflex can help distinguish between guarding 2/2 pain and paralysis

Diagnosis

Imaging

- Obtain shoulder X-rays including AP, scapula Y, and axillary views (Velpeau view if patient unable to position for axillary) (Fig. 1)
  - Rule out associated glenohumeral dislocation on axillary or Velpeau view *IMPORTANT*
  - Evaluate for pathologic fracture (e.g., unicameral bone cyst)
  - Evaluate for widening of proximal humerus growth plate in overuse injury

Advanced Imaging

- Ultrasound may be used to identify fracture in a newborn if radiographs are unclear
- MRI may be obtained if there is concern for occult Salter Harris I fracture or in cases of lesser tuberosity fracture to evaluate for soft tissue pathology
- CT is rarely used but may be indicated in the setting of a lesser tuberosity avulsion fracture or in instances of fracture-dislocation.

Classification

Neer and Horowitz Classification—based on degree of displacement

Grade I—less than 5 mm displacement
Grade II—displaced <1/3 of the shaft width
Grade III—displaced >1/3, and <2/3 of the shaft width
Grade IV—displaced >2/3 of the shaft width

Treatment

Nonoperative

- Sling ± swath, hanging arm cast, or Velpeau bandages
  - Indications
    - Neer I + II fractures regardless of age
    - Neer III + IV controversial; Generally nonoperative if <10 years old or <30°–70° angulation
  - Duration of immobilization based on age; 2–3 weeks for newborns vs 3–4 for preadolescents and adolescents
- Cessation of throwing × 3 months followed by gradual rehabilitation for overuse injuries

Operative

- CRPP vs ORIF
  - Indications
    - Fractures with intra-articular displacement (including displaced SH III + IV fractures)
    - Open injuries (in conjunction with I&D)
    - Neer III + IV >10 years of age with significant displacement (>30°–70° angulation) controversial
    - Lesser tuberosity avulsion fracture ORIF (arthroscopic repair also possible)

Reference

Popkin CA, Levine WN, Ahmad CS. Evaluation and management of pediatric proximal humerus fractures. J Am Acad Orthop Surg. 2015;23(2):77–86.

Humeral Shaft Fractures

A fracture of the humeral shaft that is often treated non-operatively given the remodeling potential and propensity for healing. Recognition of concomitant injuries is critical to success.

History

- Obtain birth history if associated with birth trauma
- How did you injure your arm? (Consider pathologic fractures in fractures associated with minor trauma)
- Do you have any numbness or tingling in your arm?
- Did you have pain in your arm before this injury?
- Are you a thrower - if so, recent throwing patterns?
- Do you have pain in your elbow, forearm, or wrist? *IMPORTANT*
- Consider NAT investigation, particularly for ages 3–10 *IMPORTANT*

Physical Exam

- Examine for deformity of arm
- Evaluate skin and soft tissue integrity
- Examine for swelling or crepitus about the humeral shaft
- Percuss entire extremity to evaluate for tenderness. Tenderness is usually limited to the humeral shaft. Tenderness at other areas (i.e.: clavicle, elbow, forearm) suggest additional injuries and should be imaged appropriately *IMPORTANT*
- UE neuro exam (Appendix A), with careful attention to the radial nerve given its intimate relation to the humeral shaft
- In infants, eliciting a Moro reflex can help distinguish between guarding secondary to pain and paralysis

M.C. Makhni et al. (eds.), *Orthopedic Emergencies*,
DOI 10.1007/978-3-319-31524-9_90

Diagnosis

Imaging

- X-rays of humeral shaft (upright AP and transthoracic lateral)
  - Measure fracture displacement and angulation on AP and transthoracic views
  - Upright X-rays incorporate gravity as a reducing force
  - Transthoracic lateral is more indicative of fracture displacement compared to a standard lateral of the humerus which rotates through the fracture
  - Examine closely for any cystic or pathologic lesion, particularly in setting of minimal trauma
- Elbow X-rays (AP, lateral, and oblique views) and shoulder X-rays (AP, scapula Y, and axillary views) are recommended
  - Ensure reduction of elbow and shoulder
- Can obtain MRI or bone scan if high clinical suspicion for occult stress fracture not visualized on X-ray

Treatment Plan

Nonoperative

- **Treatment:**

Immobilization in closed methods including hanging arm cast or coaptation splint. Can convert to fracture brace when soft tissue swelling decreased.

- **Indications:**
  - Indicated in majority of closed humeral shaft fracture in absence of concomitant injury or significant soft tissue injury

Surgery

- **Treatment:**
  - Retrograde flexible intramedullary nailing most common
  - External fixator can be considered in instances of significant soft tissue injury
  - Pinning or compression plating is less commonly utilized

- **Indications:**
  - Open fractures—in conjunction with I&D
  - Pathological fractures (dependent on lesion)
  - Bilateral fractures, relative
  - Polytrauma. relative
  - Fractures with significant displacement (>25–35° angulation) despite closed reduction (relative indication)

Reference

Caviglia H, Garrido CP, Palazzi FF, Meana NV. Pediatric fractures of the humerus. Clin Orthop Relat Res. 2005;432:49–56.

Supracondylar Humerus Fracture (SCHFx)

An extra-articular fracture of the distal humerus that represents the most common elbow fracture in the pediatric population. Displaced fractures are generally treated operatively. Early identification of vascular compromise is critical to treatment success in Type IV fractures.

History

- How did you injure your arm?
- Do you have any numbness or tingling in your arm? *IMPORTANT*
- Do you have pain in your shoulder, forearm, or wrist?
- Have you ever injured your elbow before?

Physical Exam

- Examine arm for deformity and evidence of soft tissue compromise: ecchymoses, swelling, and/or skin puckering are common in type III injuries and signify significant soft tissue injury.
- Percuss entire extremity to evaluate for tenderness. Tenderness is usually limited to the elbow; Tenderness at other areas (i.e., wrist, shoulder) suggest additional injuries and should be imaged appropriately *IMPORTANT*
- UE neuro exam (Appendix A), with careful attention to radial pulse and anterior interosseous nerve *IMPORTANT*
- If a pulse is not palpable, the vascularity of the hand as judged by its color, warmth, capillary refill, and Doppler ultrasound should be assessed.

M.C. Makhni et al. (eds.), *Orthopedic Emergencies*,
DOI 10.1007/978-3-319-31524-9_91

- If there is evidence of vascular compromise, provisional reduction with gentle flexion (~30°) should be performed to decrease tenting over the brachial artery over the fracture site.

Radiographs

- XR Elbow: AP, lateral view, and internal oblique
  - Assess for posterior fat pad sign on lateral—represents effusion, and may represent occult non-displaced fracture
  - Evaluate if anterior humeral line through capitellum on lateral
  - Bauman's angle (between humeral shaft and growth plate of lateral condyle) on AP to quantify coronal displacement
- Consider XRs contralateral elbow in equivocal cases

Classification

Broadly grouped based on mechanism of injury

Extension Type—(98 %) usually caused by fall on outstretched hand with arm in full extension resulting in apex anterior angulation and anterior displacement of the proximal fracture segment.

Flexion Type—usually result from fall onto flexed elbow with resultant apex posterior angulation and posterior displacement of the proximal fracture segment (Fig. 1).

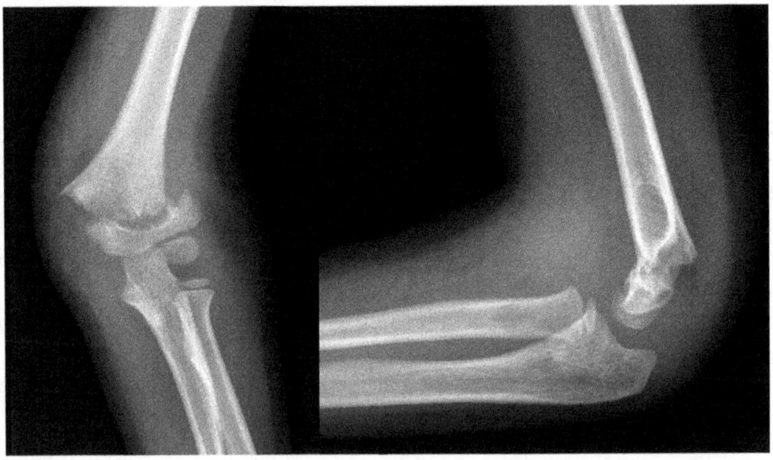

Fig. 1 Flexion Type SCHFx

Modified Gartland Classification

Of extension type fractures only
Based on degree of displacement and the integrity of posterior hinge

Type I—Non-displaced or minimally displaced (<2 mm). The anterior humeral line should extend through the central third of the capitellum when viewed on a true lateral radiograph. A discrete fracture may not be visualized but suggested by the posterior fat pad sign (Fig. 2).

Type II—Displaced by >2 mm with a hinged, but presumable intact, posterior humeral cortex. Because of the displacement, the anterior humeral line will not traverse the central third of the capitellum on a true lateral radiograph.

Type III—Displaced by >2 mm with no cortical contact. These injuries are associated with higher degree of injury to surrounding soft tissue as well as an increased risk of neurovascular injury.

Type IV—Significantly displaced fracture with circumferential soft tissue stripping and associated multidirectional instability. This is often determined at the time of surgery and as such does not have significant influence on the preoperative workup (Fig 3).

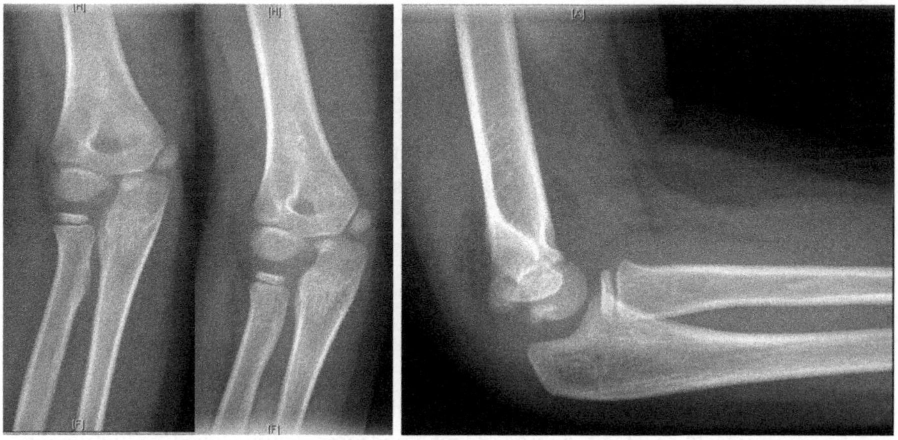

Fig. 2 Extension Type 1 SCHFx

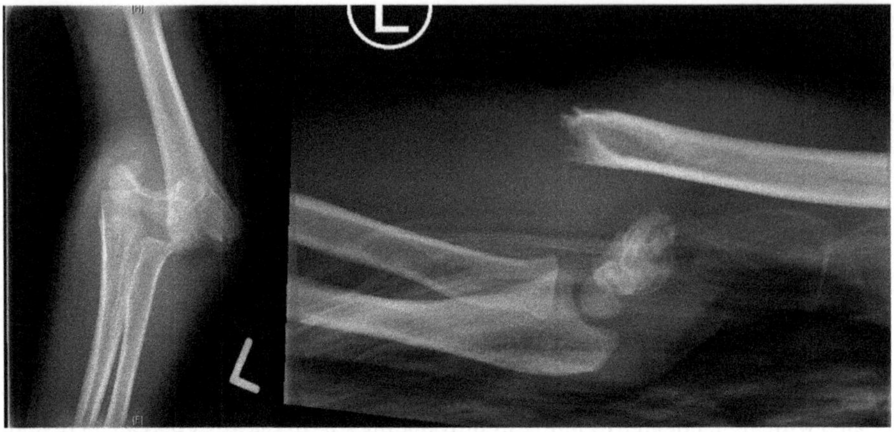

Fig. 3 Extension Type 4 SCHFx

Treatment Plan

Nonoperative

Long arm cast in ~70–90° of flexion. Generally 3–4 weeks total of immobilization.

- **Indications:**
  - Gartland Type I fractures;
  - Can consider in Gartland Type II fractures with minimal swelling, minimal displacement, and no medial comminution (controversial)

    No strong evidence indicating surgery for these; however, due to minimal risks from percutaneous pinning, consider fixation for all displaced supracondylar fractures

Surgery

Goal to prevent cubitus varus deformity (usually not associated functional deficits) and to minimize the risk of compartment syndrome from closed reduction and immobilization in flexion.

- **Treatment:** Closed reduction and percutaneous pinning
- **Indications:**
  - Displaced fractures (Types 2–4)
  - Often non-emergent unless cold, pulseless hand

References

Franklin CC, Skaggs DL. Approach to the pediatric supracondylar humeral fracture with neurovascular compromise. Instr Course Lect. 2013;62:429–33.

Mulpuri K, Hosalkar H, Howard A. AAOS clinical practice guideline: the treatment of pediatric supracondylar humerus fractures. J Am Acad Orthop Surg. 2012;20(5):328–30.

Omid R, Choi PD, Skaggs DL. Supracondylar humeral fractures in children. J Bone Joint Surg Am. 2008;90(5):1121–32.

Lateral Condyle Fracture

A fracture of the lateral condyle of the elbow that is often treated operatively given the intra-articular nature of the fracture. These injuries are frequently missed, so a high level of suspicion is important. Vigilance for fracture displacement during non-operative management is critical.

History

- Do you have pain in your forearm, wrist, or shoulder?
- Have you ever injured your elbow before?

Physical Exam

- Evaluate limb for evidence of deformity; gross deformity is usually absent.
- Evaluate skin and soft-tissue integrity; swelling and/or ecchymoses are generally limited to lateral elbow as opposed to a supracondylar fracture.
- Percuss entire extremity to evaluate for tenderness. Tenderness at other areas (i.e.: wrist, forearm, shoulder) suggests additional injuries *IMPORTANT*
- UE ROM.
- UE neuro exam (Appendix A).

M.C. Makhni et al. (eds.), *Orthopedic Emergencies*,
DOI 10.1007/978-3-319-31524-9_92

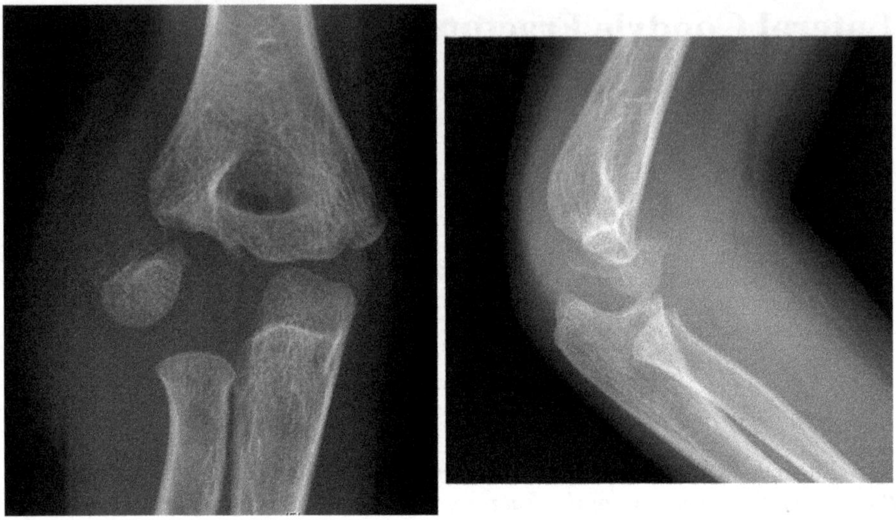

Fig. 1 Displaced lateral condyle fractures

Diagnosis

Imaging

- Obtain complete elbow X-rays including AP, lateral, and internal oblique views (Fig. 1):
  - Examine for fracture displacement (both translation or rotation), the internal oblique view is often the best radiograph for determining the maximum amount of displacement
- Contralateral views of elbow may be helpful in equivocal cases
  - MRI or ultrasound can be used to identify the presence of cartilaginous hinge but rarely is necessary
  - Arthrography can be utilized to characterize fracture displacement, intra-articular step-off, and the presence of a cartilaginous hinge. This generally is performed in the operating room

Classification

Milch classification—based on location and orientation of fracture (Fig. 2)

Type I—lateral wall of the trochlea remains attached to the main mass of the humerus (fracture through the ossific nucleus)

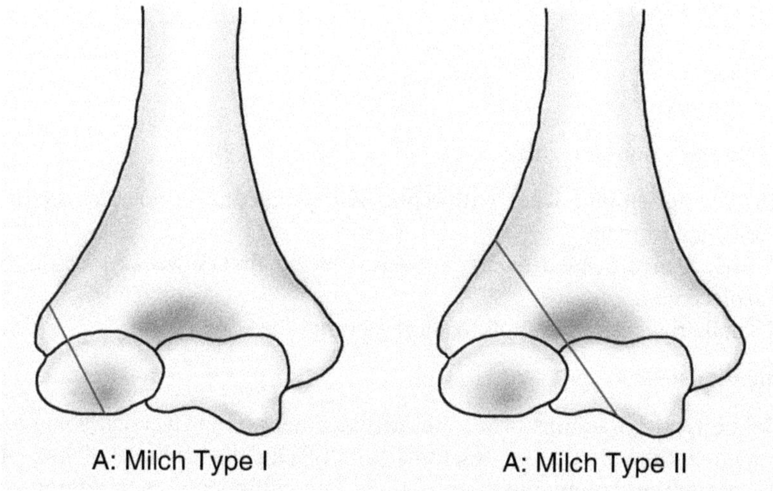

Fig. 2 Lateral condyle fractures (Milch)

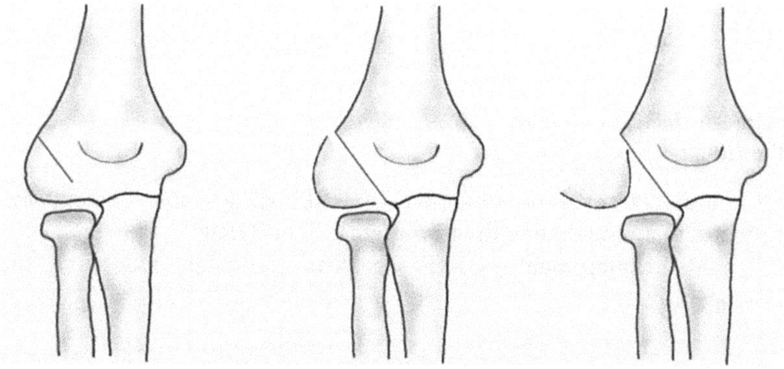

Fig. 3 Lateral condyle fractures (Jakob)

Type II—lateral wall of the trochlea remains attached to the fractured condylar fragment (fracture line is lateral to the ossific nucleus)

Jakob et al. classification—based on fracture displacement and integrity of cartilaginous hinge (Fig. 3)

Type I—non-displaced fracture with intact articular surface
Type II—moderately displaced fracture with extension to the articular surface
Type III—completely displaced fracture with intra-articular extension and a high frequency of rotational displacement

Treatment Plan

Nonoperative

- **Treatment:** Long-arm cast
  - Follow-up within a week with repeat X-rays to confirm no evidence of fracture displacement
  - Serial X-rays needed every 3–7 days during first 3 weeks to monitor for displacement
  - Usually 6 weeks of immobilization required for bony healing
- **Indications:**
  - Jakob type 1 fractures or <2 mm displacement (controversial, some recommend stabilization of all fractures prophylactically because of risk of displacement and nonunion, and to avoid late complications of cubitus valgus and tardy ulnar nerve palsy)

Surgery

- **Treatment:** CRPP vs. ORIF
- **Indications:**
  - <2 mm displacement (controversial) → CRPP (if articular hinge intact, confirm articular reduction with arthrogram) versus ORIF
  - >2 mm displacement → ORIF (confirm articular reduction directly intraoperatively)

References

Sullivan JA. Fractures of the lateral condyle of the humerus. J Am Acad Orthop Surg. 2006;14(1):58–62.

Song KS, Kang CH, Min BW, Bae KC, Cho CH. Internal oblique radiographs for diagnosis of nondisplaced or minimally displaced lateral condylar fractures of the humerus in children. J Bone Joint Surg Am. 2007;89(1):58–63.

Medial Epicondyle Fracture

A fracture of the medial epicondyle is frequently associated with an elbow dislocation. Treatment is controversial and is influenced by the amount of displacement and patient's athletic pursuits.

History

- How did you injure your arm?
- Do you have any numbness or tingling in your hand? *IMPORTANT*
- Do you have pain in your shoulder, forearm, or wrist?
- Did you feel your elbow pop out or dislocate?
- Have you ever injured your elbow before?
- Are you an athlete and/or have goals of high-level competitive athletics?

Physical Exam

- Examine for deformity of elbow that may suggest dislocation. Dislocation is most commonly posterolateral.
- Evaluate skin and soft-tissue integrity including evidence of open fracture.
- Examine for swelling or crepitus about the medial aspect of the elbow.
- Assess elbow range of motion with careful attention to any blocks to motion.
- Assess stability to varus/valgus stress at various degrees of flexion/extension.
- Percuss entire extremity to evaluate for tenderness. Tenderness is usually limited to the medial elbow. Tenderness at other areas (i.e.: wrist, shoulder) suggests additional injuries and should be imaged appropriately. *IMPORTANT*
- UE neuro exam (Appendix A), with careful attention to the ulnar nerve given its proximity to the medial epicondyle.

M.C. Makhni et al. (eds.), *Orthopedic Emergencies*,
DOI 10.1007/978-3-319-31524-9_93

Diagnosis

Imaging

- Elbow X-rays including AP, lateral, and internal oblique views (Fig. 1)
  - Ensure complete reduction of elbow on all views.
  - Examine closely for evidence of incarcerated intra-artciular fragments, particularly if there is evidence of joint subluxation or a donor site at the medial epicondyle.
  - Check for loss of parallelism along the smooth margins of the medial physis which is present in minimally displaced fractures.
  - Measure fracture displacement. Internal oblique views often provide the best view to measure displacement.
  - A posterior fat pad is often absent because these injuries are extra-articular.
- X-rays of contralateral elbow can be helpful in equivocal cases or for preoperative planning.
- CT scan can be used to more accurately determine the degree of displacement but is infrequently utilized.

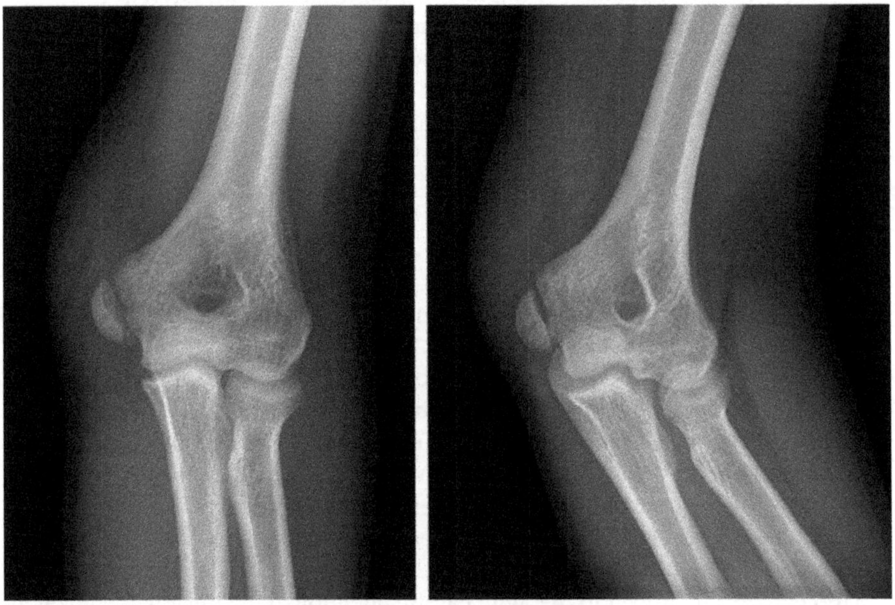

Fig. 1 Displaced medial epicondyle fracture

Classification

Though multiple classification systems have been described in the literature, fractures are more commonly described based on chronicity, degree of displacement, and the presence of an associated elbow dislocation (reduced or unreduced).

Treatment Plan

Nonoperative

- **Treatment:**
  - Immobilization in long-arm cast in ~90° of flexion
  - Total duration of treatment is ~4 weeks
- **Indications:**
  - Minimally to mildly displaced fractures (2–15 mm), relative indications are controversial (see below)

Surgery

- **Treatment:**
  - Open reduction and internal fixation with screw, pin, or suture fixation
- **Indications:**
  - Fracture fragments incarcerated in the joint unable to be extricated via closed means
  - Moderate-severe displacement (>2–15 mm, controversial)
  - Ulnar nerve dysfunction (relative)
  - Valgus instability of the elbow (relative)
  - Displaced fractures in patients with high-demand upper extremity function such as pitchers or throwing athletes (controversial)

Reference

Gottschalk HP, Eisner E, Hosalkar HS. Medial epicondyle fractures in the pediatric population. J Am Acad Orthop Surg. 2012;20(4):223–32.

Distal Humerus Physeal Separation

A transphyseal fracture of the distal humerus which occurs in children < 3 years of age. Given the lack of ossification in young children, the injuries are frequently missed or misdiagnosed. A high index of suspicion for non-accidental trauma (NAT) is required.

History

- How did this injury occur?
- How long has the child had pain?
- Has the child ever hurt that elbow before?
- Consider NAT investigation, particularly in patients <3 years *IMPORTANT*

Physical Exam

- Examine arm for deformity and of swelling
- Check for crepitus with elbow range of motion
- UE Neuro exam (Appendix A)
- Percuss entire extremity to evaluate for tenderness and fully evaluate all areas of tenderness *IMPORTANT*
- Evaluation for NAT *IMPORTANT*

M.C. Makhni et al. (eds.), *Orthopedic Emergencies*,
DOI 10.1007/978-3-319-31524-9_94

Classification

Imaging

- Elbow X-rays including AP, lateral, and oblique views
    - Check radiocapitellar line on all views
        - Capitellum should remain aligned with radial head (in contrast to an elbow dislocation or lateral condyle fracture where this relation is disrupted). Here the capitellum will be displaced in relation to the humeral shaft and metaphysis
        - The distal humeral epiphysis and radius/ulna are frequently displaced medially in relation to the humeral shaft as opposed to a an elbow dislocation where the radius and ulna are displaced laterally
- X-rays of contralateral elbow may be helpful in equivocal cases or for preoperative planning
- Consider skeletal survey if concern for NAT *IMPORTANT*
- MRI, arthrography, or ultrasound may be utilized if diagnosis is unclear. MRI and arthrography generally require sedation whereas ultrasound is operator dependent

Classification

Based on age of child, presence or absence of ossification of capitellum

Type A—Patient 0–9 months of age. Capitellum not ossified; Transphyseal injury with no metaphyseal bony fragment attached to the distal fragment/epiphysis.
Type B—Patient 7 months—3 years of age. Center of capitellum is ossified; a fragment of the metaphysis (Thurston–Holland fragment) may be displaced with the epiphysis.
Type C—Patient 3–7 years of age. Capitellum is fully ossified; a large Thurston–Holland fragment is displaced with the epiphysis.

Treatment Plan

Nonoperative

- **Treatment:** Immobilization of arm in long arm cast
    - Total duration of treatment is ~4 weeks.
- **Indications:** Subacute presentations with radiographic evidence of healing

Operative

- **Treatment:** CRPP vs. ORIF
- **Indications:** Acute fractures (high incidence of cubitus varus if untreated)

References

DeLee JC, Wilkins KE, Rogers LF, Rockwood CA. Fracture-separation of the distal humeral epiphysis. J Bone Joint Surg Am. 1980;62(1):46–51.

Oh CW, Park BC, Ihn JC, Kyung HS. Fracture separation of the distal humeral epiphysis in children younger than three years old. J Pediatr Orthop. 2000;20(2):173–6.

Radial Head Subluxation (Nursemaid's Elbow)

A subluxation of the radiocapitellar joint is frequently seen in toddlers. When recognized acutely, nonoperative management is universally successful. Operative management may be indicated in subacute presentations.

History

- How did this injury occur?
- Have you ever injured your elbow before?
- How long has the child been guarding the arm?

Physical Exam

- Examine for deformity or swelling of the elbow
- Examine how the arm is held (typically arm is held adducted with slight elbow flexion and pronation)
- Careful observation of range of motion
- Percuss entire extremity to evaluate for tenderness. Tenderness is localized to the lateral elbow
- UE neuro exam (Appendix A)

M.C. Makhni et al. (eds.), *Orthopedic Emergencies*,
DOI 10.1007/978-3-319-31524-9_95

Diagnosis

Imaging

- Usually not necessary in acute presentations
- XR Elbow: AP, lateral, and oblique views in chronic presentations or if diagnosis is uncertain
- XR Contralateral Elbow—can be helpful in equivocal cases

Treatment

Nonoperative

- **Treatment:** Closed reduction without immobilization.
  - Most common method involves full supination of forearm with arm in extension with subsequent hyperflexion and pressure applied to the radial head.
- **Indications:**
  - Acute presentations; numerous techniques of closed reduction have been described.

Operative

- **Treatment:** Open reduction
- **Indications:** Subacute presentations where closed reduction fails.

Reference

Browner EA. Nursemaid's elbow (annular ligament displacement). Pediatr Rev. 2013;34(8):366–7.

Radial Neck Fracture

More common in adolescents, this fracture is frequently treated nonoperatively unless displacement is severe or motion is limited.

History

- How did this injury occur?
- Have you ever injured your elbow before?
- Do you have numbness or tingling in your arm?

Physical Exam

- Percuss entire extremity to evaluate for skin changes, deformity, or tenderness. Tenderness is usually limited to the lateral elbow; Pain at the wrist should alert for possible DRUJ injury.
- Perform careful assessment of elbow/forearm range of motion particularly pronation/supination. Pain is often present with supination/pronation. This pain may radiate down the arm.
- UE neuro exam (Appendix A)

Diagnosis

Imaging

- Elbow XR: AP, lateral, and radiocapitellar (oblique) views
  - Measure fracture displacement and angulation

M.C. Makhni et al. (eds.), *Orthopedic Emergencies*,
DOI 10.1007/978-3-319-31524-9_96

- XR contralateral elbow if equivocal/for preoperative planning
- XR Wrist/Forearm: AP/Lateral if concern for injury to DRUJ
- Consider skeletal survey if concern for non-accidental trauma *IMPORTANT*

Classification

Based on degree of displacement

Type I: angulated <30°
Type II: angulated 30–60°
Type III: angulated >60°

Treatment

Nonoperative

- **Treatment:** immobilization in long arm cast without attempt at reduction
  - Total duration of treatment is ~3–4 weeks.
- **Indications:**
  - <30° angulation, <3 mm of translation, and >45° of pronation and supination
- **Treatment:** closed reduction with immobilization in long arm cast
  - Elbow in extension and forearm in supination, can apply traction and manual force over radial head
  - Elbow in 90° flexion and forearm in supination, can pronate forearm while applying manual force over radial head
- Total duration of treatment is ~3–4 weeks.
- **Indications:**
  - >30° angulation, 3 mm of translation, or <45° of pronation or supination

Surgery

- **Treatment:** percutaneous reduction vs retrograde ("Metaizeau") nailing
- **Indications:**
  - >30° angulation, 3 mm of translation, or < 45° of pronation or supination despite closed reduction attempts

Reference

Pring ME. Pediatric radial neck fractures: when and how to fix. J Pediatr Orthop. 2012;32 Suppl 1:S14–21.

Both-Bone Forearm Fracture

A fracture of the radius and ulna shaft. Unlike adults, the periosteum allows for successful closed management in the majority of cases.

History

- How did this injury occur?
- Have you ever injured your arm before?
- Do you have any numbness or tingling in your arm?

Physical Exam

- Examine arm for deformity and evidence of soft-tissue compromise; ecchymosis, swelling, and/or open wound (Fig. 1)
- Percuss entire extremity to evaluate for tenderness. Tenderness at other areas should be imaged appropriately
- Complete a thorough neurovascular exam   *IMPORTANT*

Diagnosis

Imaging

- Forearm X-rays including AP and lateral views
- Elbow X-rays including AP, lateral, and oblique
    - Check radiocapitellar alignment to exclude subluxation/dislocation

M.C. Makhni et al. (eds.), *Orthopedic Emergencies*,
DOI 10.1007/978-3-319-31524-9_97

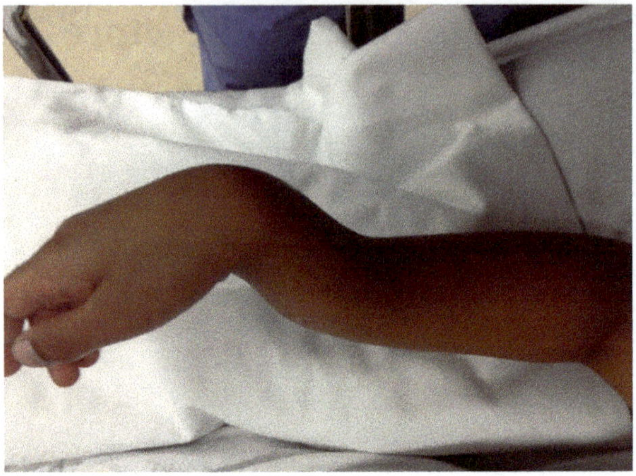

Fig. 1 Both-bone fracture clinical appearance

- Wrist X-rays including AP, lateral, and oblique
  - Examine distal radioulnar joint (Figs. 2, 3, 4, and 5)

Classification

Incomplete/Greenstick
Complete

Treatment Plan

Nonoperative

- Treatment: Closed reduction and long-arm casting
  - Total duration of treatment is ~4–8 weeks.
- Indications:
  - Greenstick injuries
  - Angulation <15–20° (controversial—the exact amount of displacement that can be tolerated is not known and is dependent on patient age and remodeling potential

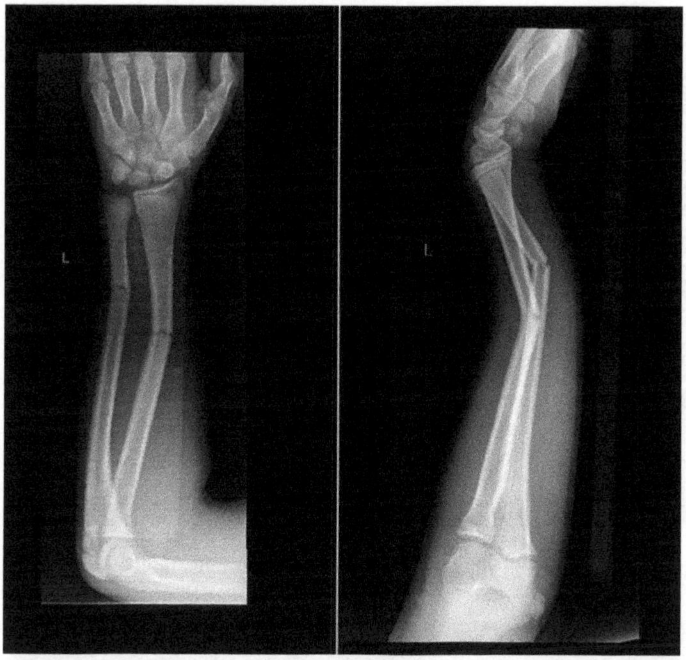

Fig. 2 Both-bone Greenstick fracture

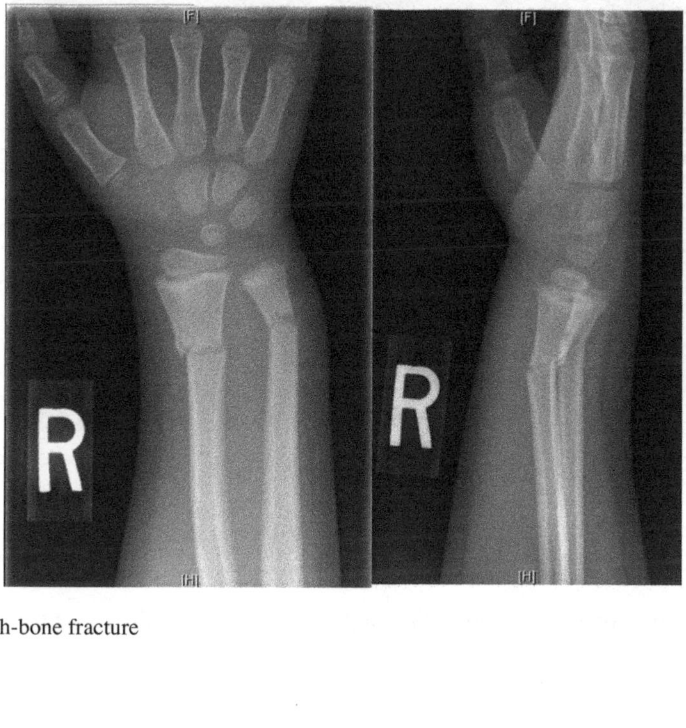

Fig. 3 Both-bone fracture

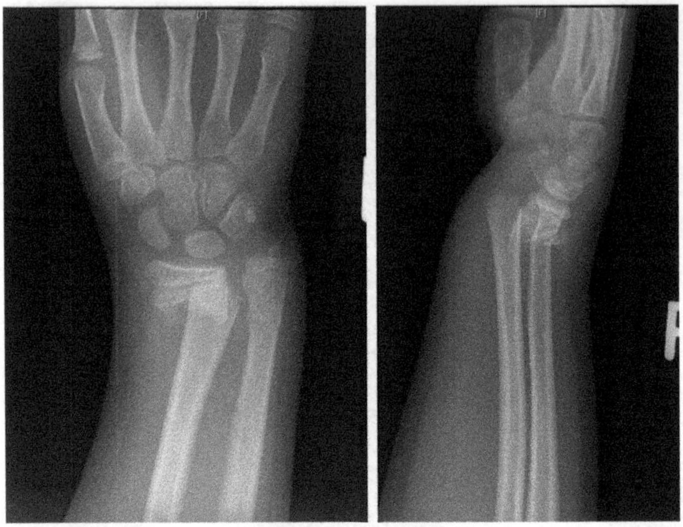

Fig. 4 Both-bone fracture with significant displacement, pre-reduction

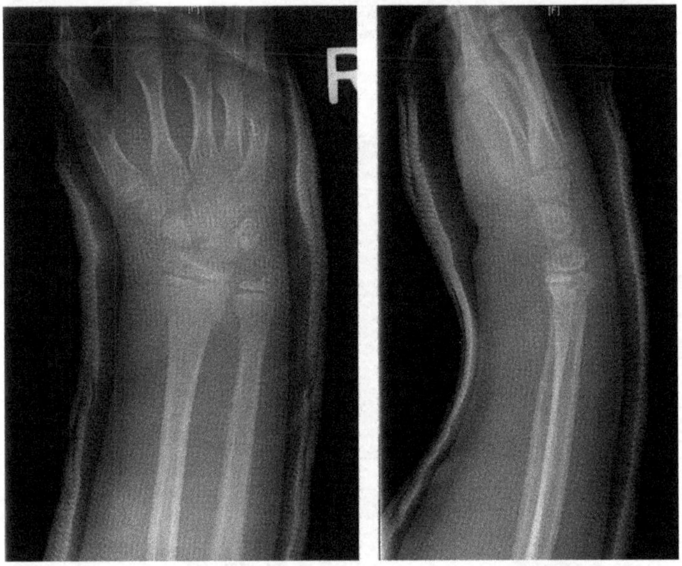

Fig. 5 Both-bone fracture with significant displacement, post-reduction

Surgery

- Treatment: Open vs. closed reduction and flexible IM nailing vs. ORIF
- Indications:
    - Open I & D—In (controversial), some literature supports the nonoperative treatment of type 1 forearm fractures.

- Angulation >15–20°
- Bayonet apposition in patients >10 years old
- Patients older than 13–15 years

References

Franklin CC, Robinson J, Noonan K, Flynn JM. Evidence-based medicine: management of pediatric forearm fractures. J Pediatr Orthop. 2012;32 Suppl 2:S131–4.
Vopat ML, Kane PM, Christino MA, Truntzer J, McClure P, Katarincic J, et al. Treatment of diaphyseal forearm fractures in children. Orthop Rev. 2014;6(2):5325.

Distal Radius Fracture

A common fracture that frequently results from a fall on an outstretched hand. These fractures are often treated non-operatively given the remodeling potential of the distal radial physis and the ability to control through closed means.

History

- How did this injury occur?
- Have you ever injured your wrist before?
- Do you have any numbness or tingling in your hand?
- Do you have pain in your shoulder, arm, or elbow?

Physical Exam

- Evaluate limb for evidence of deformity
- Evaluate skin and soft-tissue integrity including any evidence of open fracture
- Percuss entire extremity and anatomic snuffbox to evaluate for tenderness. Tenderness usually limited to wrist *IMPORTANT*
- UE neuro exam (Appendix A)

M.C. Makhni et al. (eds.), *Orthopedic Emergencies*,
DOI 10.1007/978-3-319-31524-9_98

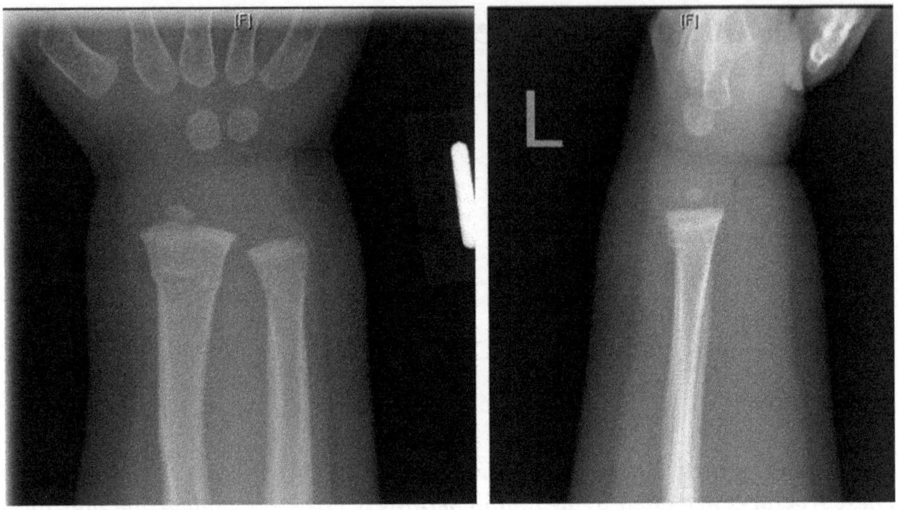

Fig. 1 Distal radius buckle fracture

Diagnosis

Imaging

- Wrist X-rays including AP, lateral, and oblique views—Examine closely to confirm reduction of the DRUJ to exclude Galeazzi fracture-dislocation.
- Advanced imaging generally not required. CT can be obtained to evaluate the pattern/extent of intra-articular displacement if present on plain films.

Classification

Physeal fractures are classified using the Salter-Harris classification system.

Torus fracture (aka Buckle fracture)—A metaphyseal compression fracture of a single cortex. The opposite cortex remains intact and no significant angulation is observed (Fig. 1).

Bicortical extraphyseal fractures are described based on their location, pattern, displacement, and presence of soft-tissue injury (Figs. 2 and 3).

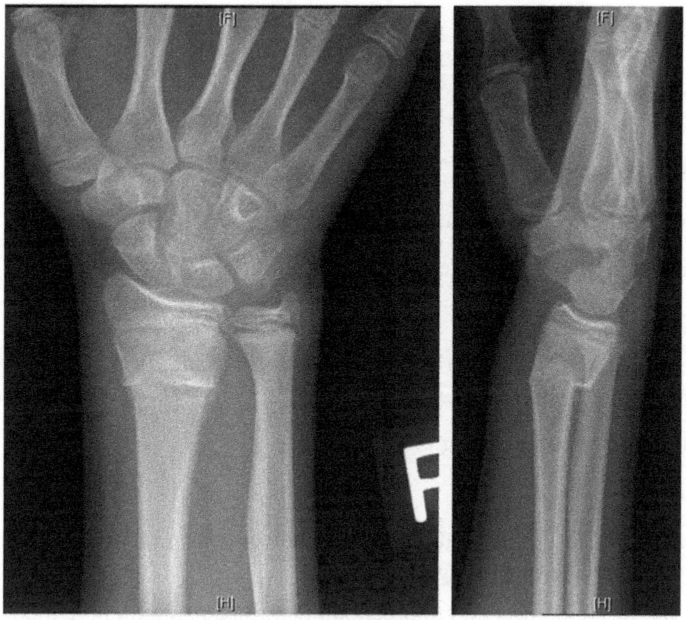

Fig. 2 Distal radius fracture with apex volar angulation

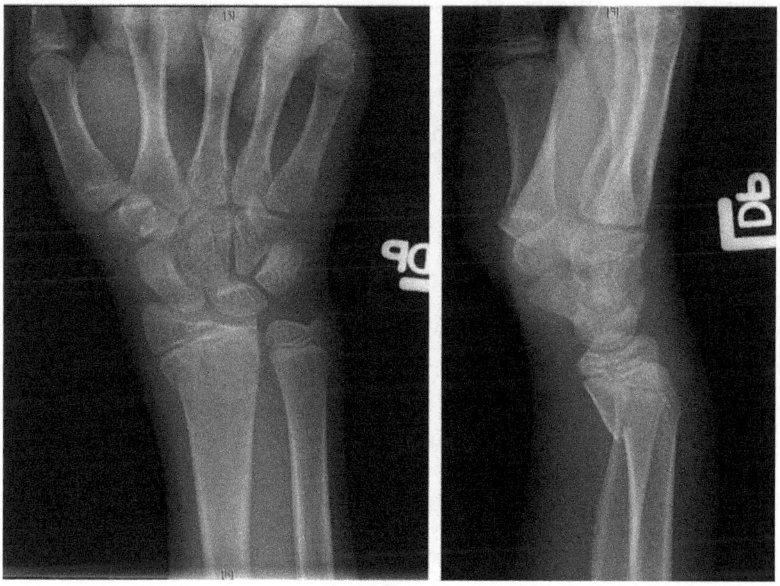

Fig. 3 Distal radius fracture with apex dorsal angulation

Treatment

Nonoperative

Torus/buckle fractures

- Treatment: Immobilization in removable wrist splint × 3–4 weeks
  - Ensure true buckle fracture (not a greenstick) *IMPORTANT*

Displaced fractures

- Treatment: Immobilization in long- vs. short-arm cast/splint (controversial) with or without closed reduction (controversial)
  - Total duration of treatment is ~4–8 weeks
- Indications:
  - "Acceptable" criteria for alignment is controversial and is dependent on fracture location and patient age
    - ~30° of angulation and bayonet apposition acceptable in patients <9 years of age
    - ~20° of angulation acceptable in patients >9
  - Avoid repeated attempts at closed reduction of physeal injuries to minimize risk of growth arrest
  - Multiple recent studies suggest that short-arm immobilization is equal to or superior to long-arm immobilization provided an adequate mold as judged by a cast index (sagittal inner width of cast at fracture/coronal inner width of cast at fracture) <0.7

Surgery

- Treatment: Closed vs. open reduction and percutaneous pinning
- Indications:
  - Open fracture—controversial, there is data supporting the non-operative treatment of type 1 open fractures
  - Inability to achieve or maintain reduction with closed means
  - SH-III and IV fractures
  - Floating elbow

References

Bae DS. Pediatric distal radius and forearm fractures. J Hand Surg Am. 2008;33(10):1911–23.

Noonan KJ, Price CT. Forearm and distal radius fractures in children. J Am Acad Orthop Surg. 1998;6(3):146–56.

Monteggia Fracture

A proximal ulna fracture with an associated radial head dislocation. Unlike in adults, nonoperative management with closed reduction and cast immobilization often yields a successful outcome.

History

- How did this injury occur?
- Have you ever injured your elbow before?
- Do you have any numbness or tingling in your arm?

Physical Exam

- Examine for deformity of elbow or arm (Fig. 2).
- UE ROM exam.
- Evaluate skin and soft-tissue integrity including any evidence of open fracture.
- Percuss entire extremity to evaluate for tenderness.
- UE neuro exam (Appendix A).

Diagnosis

Imaging

- XR elbow: AP, lateral, and oblique
    - Check for radial head subluxation/dislocation by noting alignment with capitellum—radial head should be aligned with the capitellum on all views.

M.C. Makhni et al. (eds.), *Orthopedic Emergencies*,
DOI 10.1007/978-3-319-31524-9_99

- Assess congruency of radioulnar and ulnohumeral articulations.
- Unlike in adults, ulna fracture may be plastic or minimally displaced so a high index of suspicion for ulnar fracture is needed when a radial head dislocation is present.

- XR forearm and XR wrist—AP and lateral

Classification

Bado Classification (Fig. 1)

Ulna fracture plus associated:
Type I—Anterior dislocation of radial head
Type II—Posterior dislocation of radial head
Type III—Lateral dislocation of radial head
Type IV—Proximal radial fracture and radial head dislocation

Treatment Plan

Nonoperative

- **Treatment:** closed reduction and long-arm casting in supination
- Total duration of treatment is ~4–8 weeks.
- **Indications:**
  - Ulna fracture with plastic deformation

Operative

- **Treatment:** Flexible intramedullary nail fixation vs. percutaneous pinning vs. ORIF
- **Indications:**
  - Unstable ulna fractures with complete fracture
  - Fracture dislocations that are irreducible via closed means
  - Subacute or chronic presentations (may be combined with ulnar osteotomy and/or annular ligament reconstruction)

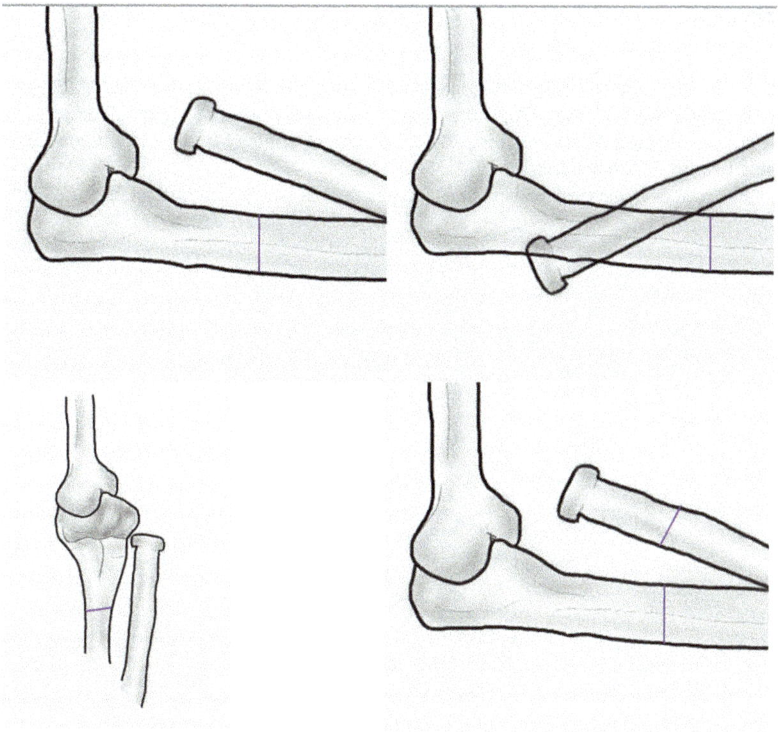

Fig. 1 Bado classification Types 1–4

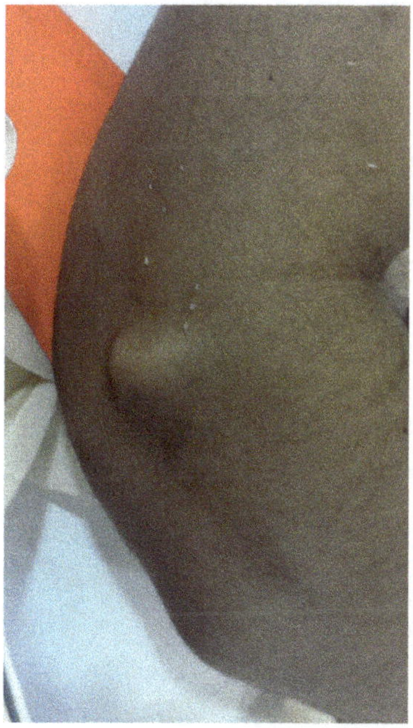

Fig. 2 Monteggia—dislocated radial head

References

Beutel BG. Monteggia fractures in pediatric and adult populations. Orthopedics. 2012;35(2):138–44.
Ramski DE, Hennrikus WP, Bae DS, Baldwin KD, Patel NM, Waters PM, et al. Pediatric monteggia fractures: a multicenter examination of treatment strategy and early clinical and radiographic results. J Pediatr Orthop. 2015;35(2):115–20.
Wilkins KE. Changes in the management of monteggia fractures. J Pediatr Orthop. 2002;22(4):548–54.

Galeazzi Fracture

A fracture of the distal radius with disruption of the distal radioulnar joint and subluxation of the ulna. Unlike in adults, closed management is often successful.

History

- Have you ever injured your wrist before?
- Do you have pain in your shoulder, arm, or elbow?
- Do you have any numbness or tingling in your hand?

Physical Exam

- Evaluate limb for evidence of deformity.
- Evaluate skin and soft-tissue integrity including any evidence of open fracture.
- Palpate entire extremity to evaluate for tenderness; tenderness usually limited to the level of the wrist.
- Prominence at the displaced ulnar head may be noted. *IMPORTANT*
- Assess the stability of the DRUJ by gentle anteroposterior stress. This can be compared to the opposite extremity.
- UE neuro exam (Appendix A).

M.C. Makhni et al. (eds.), *Orthopedic Emergencies*,
DOI 10.1007/978-3-319-31524-9_100

Diagnosis

Imaging

- Wrist X-rays including AP, lateral, and oblique views—Examine closely to assess congruity of the DRUJ. Disruption is suggested by widening on the AP view or vertical displacement on a true lateral X-ray.
- Examine for ulnar epiphyseal fracture which represents a Galeazzi equivalent.
- Contralateral wrist can be helpful in equivocal cases.
- Consider skeletal survey if concern for non-accidental trauma. *IMPORTANT*

Treatment Plan

Nonoperative

- **Treatment:** Closed reduction and immobilization in long-arm cast in supination
  - Total duration of treatment is ~4–8 weeks often successful in children.
- **Indications:** Ability to achieve stable anatomic reduction of radius and DRUJ

Surgery

- **Treatment:** Open reduction internal fixation +/− DRUJ pinning
- **Indications:** Fracture-subluxations which are irreducible by closed means

Reference

Eberl R, Singer G, Schalamon J, Petnehazy T, Hoellwarth ME. Galeazzi lesions in children and adolescents: treatment and outcome. Clin Orthop Relat Res. 2008;466(7):1705–9.

Pelvic Fracture

Uncommon injury in children (represents 1–2 % of pediatric fractures). Often treated non-operatively depending on age and displacement. Surgery mainly needed for high-energy trauma or in older patients.

Overview

- Low-energy mechanism: avulsion of apophysis
- High-energy mechanism: motor vehicle accident or peds struck
- More commonly lateral compression (vs. adults with more AP compression)
- Higher rate of single-bone fractures
- Lower rate of hemorrhage secondary to plasticity of bones, thicker cartilage
    - May be associated with: (*requires co-evaluation with trauma team*)
        - CNS or abdominal visceral injury
        - Femoral head fx/dislocation
        - GU injury

History

- Mechanism of injury?
- Other sites of pain (abdomen, back, extremities)?

M.C. Makhni et al. (eds.), *Orthopedic Emergencies*,
DOI 10.1007/978-3-319-31524-9_101

Physical Exam

- Skin intact, tenderness, ecchymosis
- Full trauma survey (often done in conjunction with trauma team) including rectal/GU survey
- Stability of pelvis to compression (AP, lateral, rotational)
- LE neuro exam (Appendix A)

Diagnosis

Imaging

- XR Pelvis: AP, inlet/outlet views
- CT pelvis without contrast—often needed as radiographs may underestimate injuries
- MRI—occasionally indicated to evaluate apophyseal injuries

Classification

Tile Classification—describing stability

Type A: stable (rotationally and vertically)
Type B: rotationally unstable; vertically stable
Type C: unstable (rotationally and vertically)

Torode/Zieg Classification—describing location

Type I: avulsion fx
Type II: iliac wing fx (usually from a direct blow)
Type III: ring fx with no segmental instability (pubic rami/symphysis fractures)
Type IV: ring fx with segmental instability (bilateral rami, straddle injuries, SI joint disruption)

- Before closure of triradiate cartilage (14 in boys, 12 in girls), iliac wing is weaker than pelvic ligaments leading to more pubic rami and iliac wing fractures.
- After closure, more likely to sustain fractures of acetabulum, diastasis of pubic symphysis, SI joint separation.

Treatment

Non-operative

- **Treatment:** Protected weight bearing → physical therapy → gradual return to activities
  - Generally less than 2 cm of displacement
- **Indications:** Generally indicated for most nondisplaced or type I/II injuries
- **Treatment:** Bedrest
- **Indications:** Type IV fracture with less than 2 cm of displacement
- **Treatment:** Consider spica casting
  - May use skeletal or Buck's traction
- **Indications:** Young patients who have trouble with weight-bearing restrictions

Surgery

- **Treatment:** Usually done in the first 24–48 h after injury
  - ORIF
  - External fixation—vertical shear patter with hemodynamic instability
- **Indications:**
  - More than 2 cm of displacement, intra-articular, triradiate cartilage displacement
  - Older children, high-energy (comminuted/displaced) fractures, open fractures, neurovascular compromise, associated injuries

References

Banerjee S et al. Paediatric pelvic fractures: 10 years experience in a trauma centre. Injury. 2009;40(4):410–3.
Holden CP et al. Pediatric pelvic fractures. J Am Acad Orthop Surg. 2007;15(3):172–7.

Avulsion Fractures of the Pelvis

Apophyseal avulsion fractures of the hip and pelvis occur most commonly in patients of age 14–25. They are usually the result of sudden forceful concentric or eccentric contraction of a muscle attached to an apophysis. These fractures are often treated nonoperatively unless significantly displaced.

Overview

Locations of apophyseal fractures:

- Ischial tuberosity (hamstrings)
- Pubic symphysis (adductors)
- Anterior superior iliac spine (ASIS) (sartorius)
- Anterior inferior iliac spine (AIIS) (rectus femoris)
- Iliac crest (abdominal muscles)
- Lesser trochanter (iliopsoas)
- Greater trochanter (hip abductors/gluteal muscles)

History

Did you feel a sudden pain during an activity or sporting event? (in contrast to an apophysitis which often presents with a more insidious onset of pain)

Is the pain worse with activity and better with rest?

M.C. Makhni et al. (eds.), *Orthopedic Emergencies*,
DOI 10.1007/978-3-319-31524-9_102

Physical Exam

- No deformity
- Swelling/ecchymosis and focal tenderness to palpation
- Evaluate gait for limp
- ROM: active/passive hip flexion, extension, abduction, adduction, IR, ER (compare to contralateral side)
- Distal neurovascular exam

Diagnosis

Imaging

- XR Pelvis: AP
- CT pelvis if clinical suspicion is high and radiographs appear normal
- MRI if ossification centers have yet to ossify
- Consider ultrasound to avoid radiation from CT scan (if have skilled technician)

Classification

- Classification is based on location and amount of displacement

Treatment

Nonoperative

Treatment

- Rest, cryotherapy, analgesics as needed for the first week after injury; crutches to assist ambulation
- After 1 week, begin gentle active and passive motion
- Once 75 % of motion is regained, progress to resistance exercises (typically 2–3 weeks post-injury)
- Usually at about 1–2 months progress to stretching and strengthening with an emphasis on sport-specific exercises
- Return to competitive sports usually takes place no earlier than 2 months post-injury

Indications:

- Acute injury with displacement <2–3 cm

Surgery

Treatment

- Fixation options include screws with or without washers or tension band techniques
- Usually non-urgent and can often follow up within 1 week with orthopedic surgeon

Indications

- Displacement >2–3 cm, particularly for avulsion fractures of ischial tuberosity or greater trochanteric apophyses
- Painful nonunion or exostosis formation
- Inability to return to competitive sports

References

Mckinney BI, Nelson C, Carrion W. Apophyseal avulsion fractures of the hip and pelvis. Orthopedics. 2009;32(1):42.

Willis BR. Sports medicine in the growing child. In: Morrissy RT, Weinstein SL, editors. Lovell & Winter's pediatric orthopaedics. 6th ed. Philadelphia, PA: Lippincott Williams & Wilkins; 2006.

Hip Pain: Septic Hip vs. Transient Synovitis

Although the most common cause of hip pain in children is transient synovitis, hip pain must be evaluated carefully for septic hip arthritis. A child with septic hip arthritis will require urgent surgical irrigation and debridement.

History

- Does your hip pain prevent you from walking?
- Have you had fever or any development of recent rash/swollen lymph node?
- Have you had any recent tick bites?
- Have you had all your vaccination?
- Did you have any recent bacterial/viral infection?
- Any history of recent trauma?

Physical Exam

- Toxic appearance
- Local groin/thigh swelling
- Effusion, erythema, tenderness in groin/thigh
- Log roll test
- Hip ROM
  - Limited due to severe pain
  - Rest in position of flexion, abduction, and external rotation. No deformity

M.C. Makhni et al. (eds.), *Orthopedic Emergencies*,
DOI 10.1007/978-3-319-31524-9_103

- ROM *(knee, ankle)*
  - Flexion/extension
  - Rotation
- LE neuro exam (Appendix A)

Diagnosis

Imaging

- XR Hip/Pelvis: AP and frog leg lateral hip, pelvis AP—widening of joint space, dislocation/subluxation
- Ultrasound—evaluation of hip joint effusion/capsule distension; (±needle aspiration if available when notable effusion)
- MRI—evaluation of joint effusion (do not delay treatment for MRI if it cannot be expeditiously obtained)

Laboratory Studies

- CBC with differential
- BMP
- Inflammatory makers: ESR and CRP
- Blood culture
- Serologic evaluation of Lyme disease

Kocher Criteria for Septic Arthritis

- WBC > 12.000 mm^3
- Non-weight bearing on affected side
- Fever > 38.5 °C
- ESR > 40 mm/h

Kocher Criteria Met	Likelihood of septic arthritis
1	3 %
2	40 %
3	93 %
4	99 %

Treatment Plan

Nonoperative

- **Treatment:**
  - IV or PO NSAID
  - Observation for 24 h
  - Allow for early weight bearing with physical therapy
- **Indications:** Kocher score <2 → likely transient synovitis
- **Treatment:**
  - Surgical I&D if ultrasound guided aspiration unavailable
  - Ultrasound guided hip aspiration
  - Can consider XR-guided hip aspiration with fluoroscopy
    - Septic arthritis suggested by any of the following:
      - WBC >50,000/mm^3 with >95 % PMN
      - Glucose 50 mg/dl less than serum level
      - High lactic acid level
- **Indications:** if concern for (or unable to r/o) septic arthritis

Surgical

- **Treatment:**
  - Urgently to OR for emergent surgical irrigation and debridement to minimize chondrolytic effect
  - IV antibiotics after surgical treatment and close monitoring
- **Indications:** Kocher score 3 = 93 % chance of having septic arthritis
  - Kocher score 2 = 40% chance of septic arthritis - surgical intervention dependent on clinical judgment as well as risks and benefits discussion between surgical team and family

References

Flynn JM, Widmann RF. The limping child: evaluation and diagnosis. J Am Acad Orthop Surg. 2001;9(2):89–95.

Sucato DJ, Schwend RM, Gillespie R. Septic arthritis of the hip in children. J Am Acad Orthop Surg. 1997;5(5):249–60.

Hip Dislocation

A rare and traumatic injury in children that requires timely management including careful closed reduction or open reduction/exploration to minimize complications such as osteonecrosis, coxa magna, osteoarthritis, and nerve injury.

History

- Mechanism/energy of injury?
- Able to bear weight?
- Ambulatory at baseline?
- Prior hip dislocations?
- Hip/groin pain?

Physical Exam

- Asymmetry of inguinal fold
- Gross deformity/palpable femoral head
- Limb length discrepancy
- Leg position
  - Abduction, ER, slight flexion suggests anterior dislocation (rare)
  - Adduction, IR, slight flexion suggests posterior dislocation
- LE neuro exam (Appendix A) *IMPORTANT*

M.C. Makhni et al. (eds.), *Orthopedic Emergencies*,
DOI 10.1007/978-3-319-31524-9_104

Diagnosis

Imaging

- XR: AP pelvis radiograph and AP and Lateral Hip radiograph:
  - Determine if anterior vs. posterior hip dislocation
  - r/o other fractures: acetabulum, femoral head, or femoral neck fractures *IMPORTANT*
- XR: Femur/knee radiograph: r/o distal fractures/injuries pre-reduction maneuver *IMPORTANT*

Classification

Thompson and Epstein Classification for Posterior Hip Dislocation

1. Posterior dislocation +/− minor fracture
2. Posterior dislocation + large posterior acetabular rim fracture
3. Posterior dislocation + comminution of acetabular ring
4. Posterior dislocation + acetabular floor fracture
5. Posterior dislocation + femoral head fracture

Treatment

Nonoperative

- For chronic hip dislocation with non-ambulatory patient, no emergent reduction warranted
  - Further evaluation of DDH warranted
- Closed Reduction
  - Urgent reduction within 6 h of injury reduce risk of osteonecrosis
  - MUST have adequate sedation or anesthesia
  - Gentle traction—special care to not displace proximal femoral epiphysis
- Post reduction
  - Check hip ROM and stability
  - Post-reduction imaging
    - Radiograph (minimum): hip AP and cross table lateral → confirm concentric reduction

- CT hip → evaluation joint congruity (+/−)
    - Labrum or capsule entrapment
    - Osteochondral fragments
    - Interposed soft tissue
- MRI (+/−): evaluation for interposed soft tissue or possible labral tear, cartilage injury, or loose body

- Post-reduction management:
  - Hip spica cast bracing with bedrest for 3–4 weeks if less than 10yo
  - Protected weight bearing for 6–12 weeks with crutches if older than 10yo

Surgical

- Treatment: Open Reduction +/− Internal Fixation
- Indications:
  - Failed closed reduction
  - Post-reduction CT reveals nonconcentric reduction or intra-articular fragment
  - Unstable acetabular fracture

References

Bressan S, Steiner IP, Shavit I. Emergency department diagnosis and treatment of traumatic hip dislocations in children under the age of 7 years: a 10 year review. Emerg Med J. 2014;31(5):425–31.

Haverstock JP, Sanders DW, Bartley DL, Lim RK. Traumatic pediatric hip dislocation in a toddler. J Emerg Med. 2013;45(1):91–4.

Herrera-Soto JA, Price CT. Traumatic hip dislocation in children and adolescents: pitfalls and complications. J Am Acad Orthop Surg. 2009;19(1):15–21.

Slipped Capital Femoral Epiphysis

Slippage of the epiphysis through the hypertrophic zone of the physis relative to femoral neck due to disorder of the proximal femoral physis. SCFE requires surgical treatment.

History

- Recent rapid growth?
- Do you have groin and thigh pain? Knee pain?
- Have you had pain for weeks or several months?
- Have you had previous radiation therapy?

Physical Exam

- Often male gender, obese
- Abnormal gait (externally rotated, Trendelenburg gait)
- Affected leg externally rotated, shortening
- Ability to ambulate
- Limb length discrepancy
- Hip ROM
  - Decrease abduction, flexion, internal rotation
  - External rotation and abduction during passive flexion of hip when supine *IMPORTANT*

M.C. Makhni et al. (eds.), *Orthopedic Emergencies*,
DOI 10.1007/978-3-319-31524-9_105

- LE neuro exam (Appendix A)
  - Thigh atrophy/weakness
  - Possible bilateral symptoms

Diagnosis

Imaging

- XR Hips: AP and frog leg lateral of both hips (Fig. 1)
  - Posteroinferior displacement of epiphysis relative to metaphysis
  - Epiphysiolysis
  - Klein's line (line drawn on AP Pelvis along superior border of femoral neck - should intersect femoral head but will be superior to head if SCFE)
  - Metaphyseal blanch sign of Steel
- MRI
  - Growth plate widening
  - Increase signal of metaphysis

Traditional SCFE Classification

1. Pre-slip: weakness, limping, exertional pain, decrease in internal rotation
2. Acute slip: symptoms <3 weeks, 1–3 months of mild symptoms, severe pain and unable to bear weight

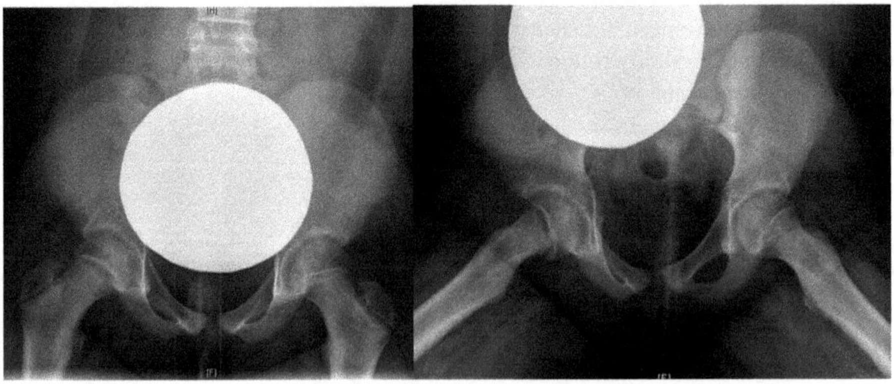

Fig. 1 Right SCFE

3. Chronic slip (most common): >3 weeks symptoms, mild form lasts for several months to years, walks with limp
4. Acute on chronic slip: sudden acute exacerbation of pain, unable to walk

Lorder Classification

1. Stable—able to bear weight without crutches
2. Unstable—unable to bear weight without crutches

Southwick Angle Classification

- Difference between both hips in femoral head shaft angle on frog lateral view
- Not accurate if bilateral SCFE present
  1. Mild <30°
  2. Moderate 30–50°
  3. Severe >50°

SCFE Severity Grading

1. Grade I 0–30 % slippage
2. Grade II 34–50 % slippages
3. Grade III >50 % slippage

Treatment

Surgical

- Stable
  - In situ percutaneous fixation with screw(s) ± arthrotomy
  - Bone graft epiphysiodesis
- Unstable (urgent)
  - In situ percutaneous fixation with screw(s) ± arthrotomy
  - Open reduction and internal fixation

- For moderate/severe slips (stable or unstable), consider cuneiform osteotomy, femoral neck osteoplasty
- For severe chronic SCFE with pain and function deficit: proximal femoral osteotomy
- Consider contralateral in situ prophylactic pinning
  - Obese boys
  - Endocrine disorder
  - Young age of SCFE (open triradiate cartilage, <10 years old)

References

Aronsson et al. Slipped capital femoral epiphysis: current concepts. J Am Acad Orthop Surg. 2006;14(12):666–70.

Aronsson et al. Stable slipped capital femoral epiphysis: evaluation and management. J Am Acad Orthop Surg. 1996;4:173–81.

Hip Fracture

Hip fractures in children are rare and account for <1 % of all pediatric fractures. They are typically associated with high complication rates and poor outcomes.

History

- Have you had recent trauma?
- Can you bear weight?
- Do you have any history of hip pain or limping?
- Any recent weight loss, night pain? Other constitutional symptoms?

Physical Exam

- Trauma evaluation (Appendix A)
- Limb deformity - affected extremity shortened and externally rotated
- Hip ROM
- Assess for other injuries → mindful for child abuse   *IMPORTANT*
- LE neuro exam (Appendix A)
- Examine ipsilateral knee and ankle for other injuries

Diagnosis

Imaging

- XR Hip: AP and lateral (cross table) (Fig. 1)
- XR Pelvis: AP

M.C. Makhni et al. (eds.), *Orthopedic Emergencies*,
DOI 10.1007/978-3-319-31524-9_106

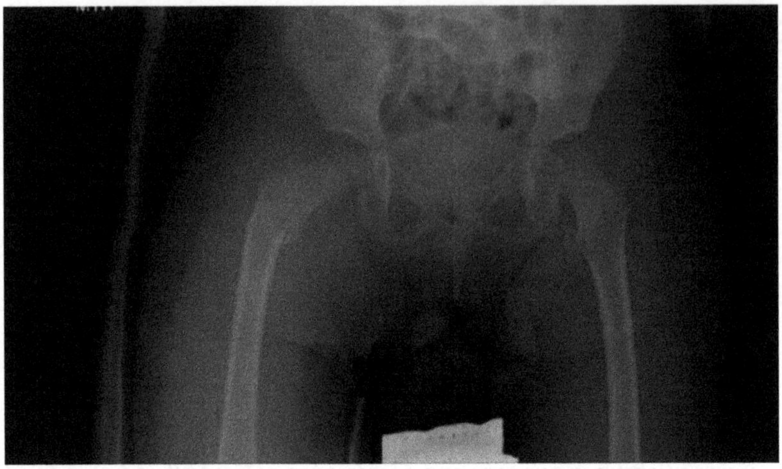

Fig. 1 Delbet IV hip fracture

- XR: Ipsilateral femur and knee radiograph to r/o other ipsilateral injuries and for preoperative planning
- MRI: primary study for high clinical fracture suspicion and equivocal radiographic finding
- CT hip: if MRI unavailable and equivocal XR finding, evaluation for occult hip fracture

Delbet Classification of Pediatric Hip Fractures

1. Type I—transphyseal fracture +/− capital femoral epiphysis dislocation
2. Type II—transcervical fracture
3. Type III—cervicotrochanteric fracture
4. Type IV—intertrochanteric fracture

Treatment

- Urgent reduction within 24 h after injury to decrease risk of osteonecrosis

Nonoperative

- **Treatment:** Hip spica casting including single leg or both legs (Fig. 2).
- **Indications:** Nondisplaced fractures
- **Treatment:** Closed reduction and hip spica casting

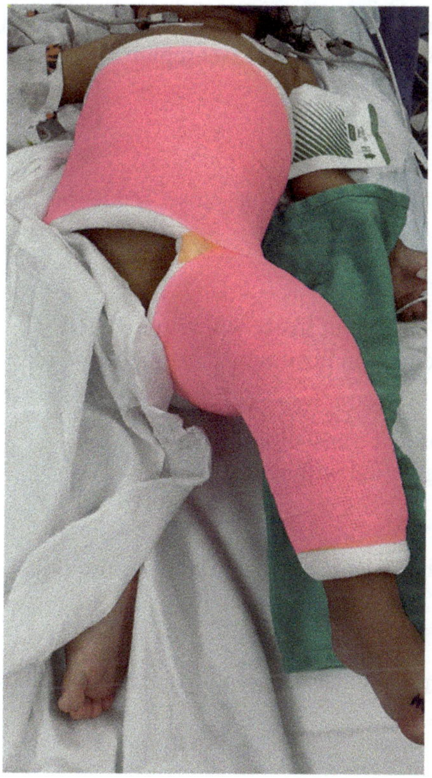

Fig. 2 Hip spica cast

- Closed reduction
  - Supine with hip in extension and slight abduction, leg internal rotation
  - Reduction maneuver consist of gentle longitudinal traction and minor adjustment of leg positioning
- **Indications:**
  - Type I, II, and III in children <4 years old
  - Type IV in children < 8 if acceptable angulation (<10°)

Surgical

- Indication for open reduction
  - Failed closed reduction
  - Displaced fracture (note below in detail)

  - Pathologic hip fracture → require culture, biopsy, grafting
  - Vascular injury → require large vessel repair
- Displaced fractures
  - Type I
    - CRPP with smooth wires or close reduction with cannulated screw fixation
  - Type II
    - May attempt CRPP but likely will require ORIF
    - Acceptable reduction position is near anatomic reduction due to high-risk AVN
      - <2 mm cortical translation
      - <5° of angulation with no malrotation
  - Type III
    - May attempt CRPP but will likely require ORIF, acceptable reduction consist of less than 10° angulation
  - Type IV
    - If children >8 years old, plan for open reduction internal fixation

References

Boardman MJ, Herman MJ, Buck B, Pizzutillo PD. Hip fractures in children. J Am Acad Orthop Surg. 2009;17(3):162–73.

Beaty JH. Fractures of the hip in children. Orthop Clin North Am. 2006;37(2):223–32 vii.

Canale ST. Fractures of the hip in children and adolescents. Orthop Clin North Am. 2006;37(2):223–32.

Femur Fracture

Fractures of the femoral shaft often can be treated non-operatively in children depending on age and displacement.

Overview

- In children <1 year, consider child abuse (up to 80%)
- Common mechanism in toddlers: falls from climbing
- Usually higher energy mechanisms in older children: MVA, ATV, or bicycle accidents
- In the absence of trauma, may consider neurologic/pathologic bone conditions
    - Cerebral palsy
    - Osteogenesis Imperfecta (Fig. 1)
    - Tumor: Aneurysmal bone cyst, fibrous dysplasia, nonossifying fibroma (Fig. 2)

History

- History of trauma?
- Mechanism of injury?
- Prior history of long bone fractures?

M.C. Makhni et al. (eds.), *Orthopedic Emergencies*,
DOI 10.1007/978-3-319-31524-9_107

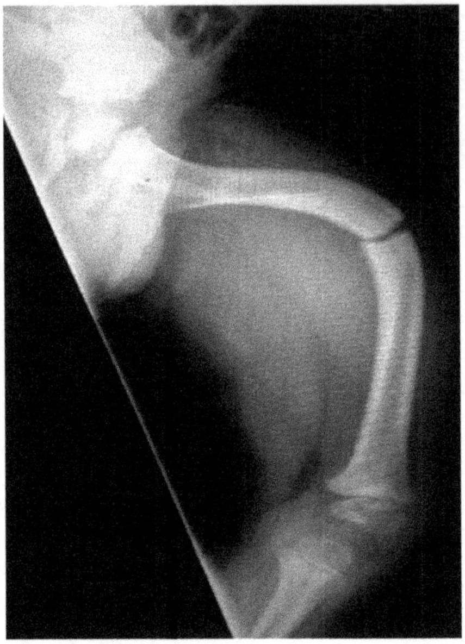

Fig. 1 Osteogenesis imperfecta femur fracture

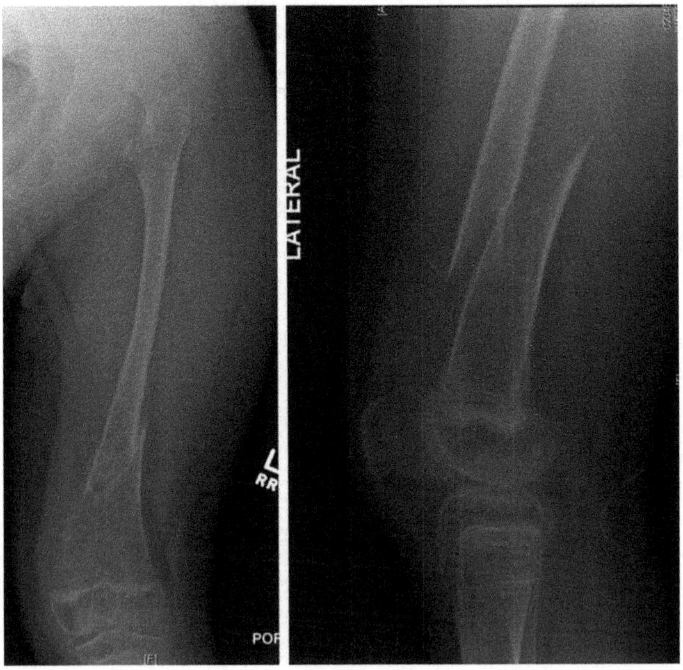

Fig. 2 Femoral shaft fracture

Physical Exam

- Full trauma survey (often done in conjunction with general surgery)
- Skin intact
- Shortening, malrotation, deformity
  - "Telescope" test—does fracture shorten >2 cm with gentle longitudinal pressure (perform with fluoroscopy under sedation)
- Distal neurovascular exam (Appendix A: LE neuro exam)

Diagnosis

Imaging

- XRs: AP pelvis, AP, and cross-table lateral of hip, femur, knee
- Consider contralateral side imaging for comparison/pre-op planning
- Skeletal survey (especially in young children with suspicion for child abuse)

Classification

Descriptive, similar to adult fractures: location, extent, comminution, displacement
OTA/AO 32

32A: simple
32B: butterfly/wedge
32C: complex/segmental

Treatment

Non-operative

- Gold standard for most fractures in children <6 years old
- Spica casting—most frequently done in the OR, may be immediate or delayed
  - Negative telescope test → immediate
  - Positive telescope test → skeletal traction and delayed casting

Surgery

- Usually done in first 24–48 h after injury
- **Treatment:**
  - External fixation
  - IM nailing (flexible vs. rigid)
  - Plating (submuscular vs. compression)
- **Indications:** older children, high-energy (comminuted/displaced) fractures, open fractures, neurovascular compromise, associated injuries, proximal or distal fractures

References

Anglen JO, Choi L. Treatment options in pediatric femoral shaft fractures. J Orthop Trauma. 2005;19(10):724–33.

Anglen JO, Flynn JM. Pediatric femoral shaft fractures. Orthop Knowl Online J. 2005.

Yandow SM, Archibeck MJ, Stevens PM, Shultz R. Femoral-shaft fractures in children: a comparison of immediate casting and traction. J Pediatr Orthop. 1999;19(1):55–9.

Distal Femur Physeal Fracture

A fracture of distal femur often involves the physis and may lead to growth disturbance and/or deformity.

History

- Are you able to bear weight?
- Mechanism of injury?
- Do you have numbness and tingling below your knee?

Physical Exam

- Skin integrity
- Deformity/Shortening
- Knee effusion/ thigh swelling
- Assess for tenderness at distal femur and throughout hip and LE
- Other injuries and signs of child abuse *IMPORTANT*
- ROM (hip, knee, ankle, LE ROM)
- Varus and valgus stress test (often helpful to examine knee stability when sedated, due to guarding of extremity in acute setting due to pain)
- LE neuro exam (Appendix A)
  - Check pulses distally for evaluation of popliteal artery injury

M.C. Makhni et al. (eds.), *Orthopedic Emergencies*,
DOI 10.1007/978-3-319-31524-9_108

Diagnosis

Imaging

- Knee, Femur, and Hip Xrays: r/o other knee and hip injuries *IMPORTANT* (Fig. 1)
- MRI: confirm physeal fracture when questionable on radiograph

Treatment

Nonoperative

- Physeal Injury: nondisplaced fractures only
  - Long leg cast
  - Non-weightbearing

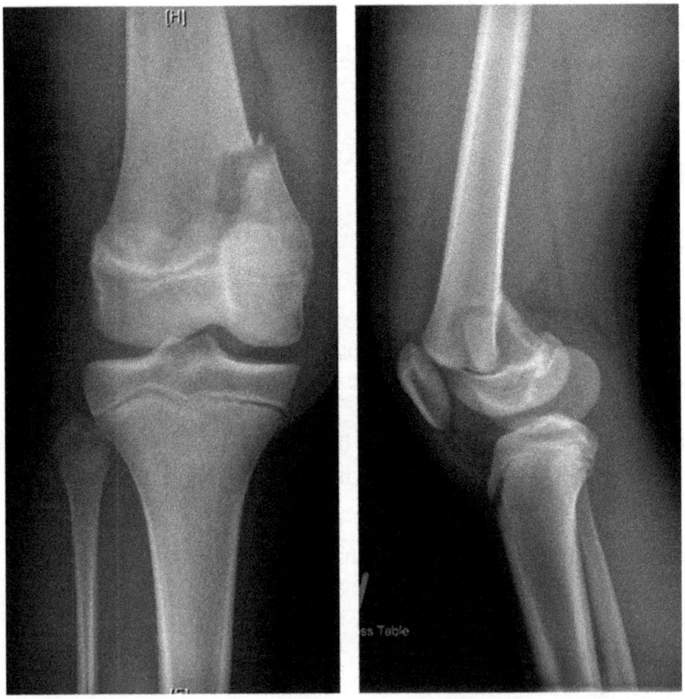

Fig. 1 Salter Harris 2 fracture of distal femur

Surgical

- **Treatment:**
  - Admit for surgical fixation
  - Displaced Salter Harris I or II → closed reduction percutaneous pinning or lag screw fixation
  - Displaced Salter Harris III or IV → ORIF to reduce articular surface
- **Indications:** Displaced physeal fracture (Salter Harris I, II, III, and IV)

References

Edwards PH Jr, Grana WA. Physeal fractures about the knee. J Am Acad Orthop Surg. 1995;3(2):63–9.

Flynn JM, Schwend RM. Management of pediatric femoral shaft fractures. J Am Acad Orthop Surg. 2004;12:347–59.

Kocher MS et al. Treatment of pediatric diaphyseal femur fracture. J Am Acad Orthop Surg. 2009;17(11):718–25.

Tibial Eminence Fracture

Tibial eminence occurs in children from age 8–14 due to incomplete ossification of tibial eminence. It is analogous to an anterior cruciate ligament (ACL) tear in an adult.

History

- Do you have pain in your knee?
- Did you have knee swelling?
- Are you able to bear weight?

Physical Exam

- Knee effusion
- Limited knee ROM
- Positive anterior drawer test
- Ligamentous evaluation (associated injuries include meniscus and collateral ligament injuries) → likely challenging due to guarding
- LE neuro exam (Appendix A)

M.C. Makhni et al. (eds.), *Orthopedic Emergencies*,
DOI 10.1007/978-3-319-31524-9_109

Diagnosis

Imaging

- XR knee (Fig. 1):
  - AP, lateral, and oblique view of the knee
  - May obtain contralateral images for comparison
- CT: used to evaluate osteochondral fractures as well as periarticular fractures with comminution
- MRI: helpful to evaluate associated ligamentous and meniscus damages .

Mayers and McKeever Classification, Zaricznyj Modification

1. Type I—Non-displaced
2. Type II—Displaced anterior margin with intact posterior cortex

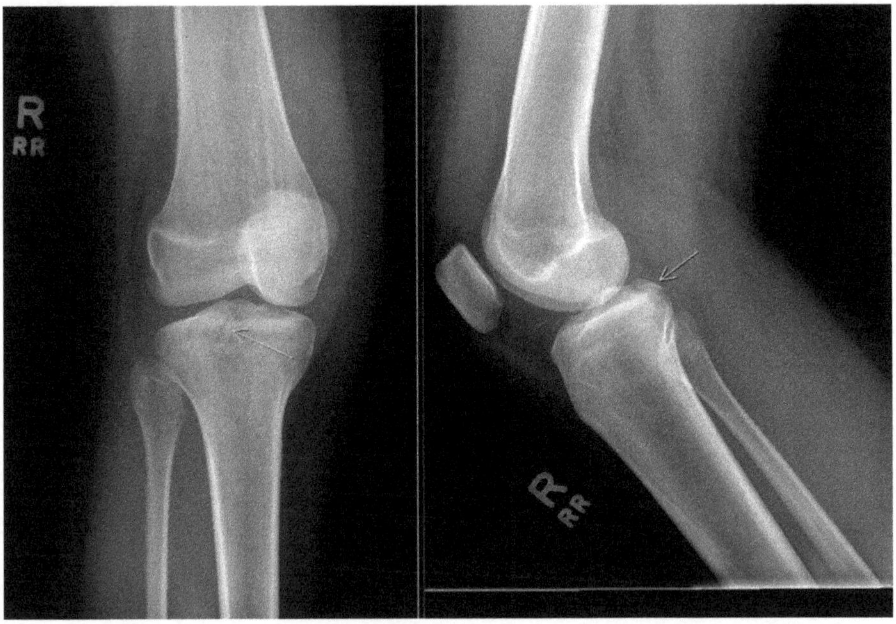

Fig. 1 Tibial spine

3. Type III—Completely displaced with no bony contact
   - IIIA: involve only ACL insertion
   - IIIB: involve entire intercondylar eminence
4. Type IV—Comminuted fracture

Treatment

Nonoperative

- Type I fractures → Immobilization
- Type II fractures → Close reduction and immobilization (controversial—could consider operative treatment to allow for early ROM)
- Immobilization consists of long leg splint, cylindrical cast, knee immobilizer, or Bledsoe brace locked in extension
- Follow up with orthopedic surgeon in 1 week with repeat radiograph to monitor possible displacement.

Surgical

- Treatment:
  - Open versus arthroscopic reduction and fixation (suture or screw fixation possible in most scenarios)
  - Fracture reduction with suture/screw fixation
  - Postoperative care include immobilization (typically 1–6 weeks), followed by protected early ROM and weight bearing
- Indications:
  - Type II and III that cannot be reduced
  - Type IV

References

Herman MJ, Martinek MA, Abzug JM. Complication of tibial eminence and diaphyseal fractures in children: prevention and treatment. J Am Acad Orthop Surg. 2014;22:730–41.

Lafrance RM, Giordano B, Goldblatt J, Voloshin I, Maloney M. Pediatric tibial eminence fractures: evaluation and management. J Am Acad Orthop Surg. 2010;19(7):395–405.

Zoints LE. Fractures around the knee in children. J Am Acad Orthop Surg. 2002;10:345–55.

Tibial Tubercle Fracture

A traction apophyseal avulsion fracture caused by the pull of the patellar tendon through the extensor mechanism (quadriceps). The failure is through the zone of hypertrophy of the physis.

Overview

- Mostly adolescents (13–16 years old), M>F
- Usually caused by violent contraction of quads
- Often sports related—basketball (jumping), football (being tackled), sprinting

History

- History of trauma?
- Length of symptoms?
- History of chronic symptoms/diagnosis of Osgood–Schlatter?

Physical Exam

- Skin intact
- Compartments soft
- Effusion (+)—inflammatory? hemarthrosis (recurrent anterior tibial artery)?
- Tender over anterior knee or throughout

M.C. Makhni et al. (eds.), *Orthopedic Emergencies*,
DOI 10.1007/978-3-319-31524-9_110

- LE ROM
  - Flexion/extension
  - Able to extend the knee against gravity *IMPORTANT*
- Associated injuries (stability to varus/valgus, Lachman)
- Distal neurovascular exam (Appendix, LE neuro exam)

Diagnosis

Imaging

- XR knee—AP, lateral, and oblique (best profile is with leg in slight internal rotation)
  - Assess for patella alta
- Consider contralateral views for comparison
- CT scan for evaluation of articular injury

Classification

Primary center: proximal tibial physis
Secondary center: apophysis (tibial tubercle)

Watson–Jones (with Ogden modification) (Fig. 1)

Type I: fracture of secondary center near patellar tendon insertion

- A: minimally displaced
- B: hinged forward

Type II: fracture propagates to coalescence of primary and secondary centers

- A: avulsed fragment centers on the proximal end of the tuberosity
- B: comminuted fragment, proximally displaced

Type III: fracture extends across primary center into the joint

- A: non-comminuted (Fig. 2)
- B: comminuted

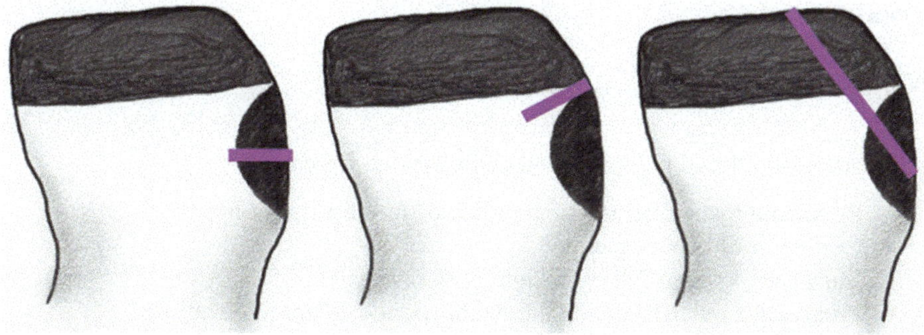

Fig. 1 Ogden classification

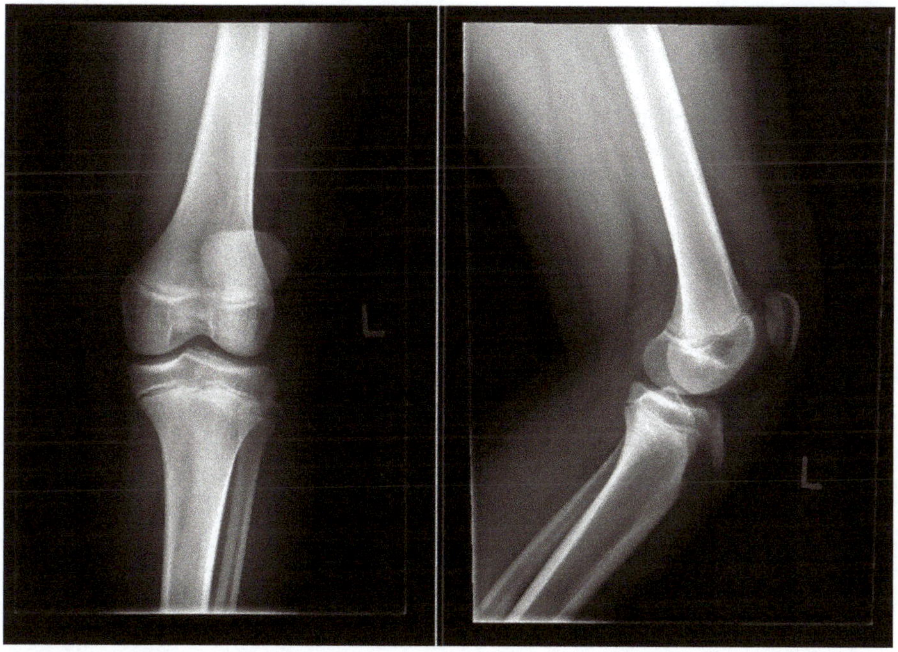

Fig. 2 Type III tibial tuberosity fracture

Treatment

Nonoperative

- **Treatment:** Closed reduction and cylinder/long leg cast
  - Reduction maneuver: traction with knee in full extension
  - Casting: mold above patella
  - Must keep knee in full extension for 4–6 weeks
  - Progressive rehab of quads follow this period of immobilization
- **Indications:** non-displaced fractures (<2 mm) that do not involve the joint

Surgery

- **Treatment:** Closed reduction and percutaneous pinning vs. Open reduction internal fixation
- **Indications:** any displaced fractures, all type II/III

References

McKinney BI, Nelson C, Carrion W. Apophyseal avulsion fractures of the hip and pelvis. Orthopedics. 2009;32(1):42.

Mosier SM, Stanitski CL. Acute tibial tubercle avulsion fractures. J Pediatr Orthop. 2004;24(2):181–4.

Zionts LE. Fractures around the knee in children. J Am Acad Orthop Surg. 2002;10(5):345–55.

Toddler's Fracture

These low-energy tibial shaft fractures are often spiral and non-displaced, and arise from low energy falls in newly walking toddler; they are almost always treated non-operatively. If they are seen in younger children who are not yet walking, they can be suspicious of possible child abuse.

History

Is the child walking independently? For how long?
Has the child had preceding leg pain or been walking with a limp before this injury?
Does the child (or anyone in the family) have metabolic bone disease?
Has the child had a fever?
Has the child had any recent trauma to the hip or legs, or any recent falls?

Physical Exam

Assess for bruising, tenderness, swelling along leg
Ambulation with limp, or refusal to bear weight
Rule out compartment syndrome—low likelihood as compared to traumatic fractures of the tibia and/or fibula
Rule out infection in hip and lower extremity joints and bones, and check for painless passive range of motion of joints

M.C. Makhni et al. (eds.), *Orthopedic Emergencies*,
DOI 10.1007/978-3-319-31524-9_111

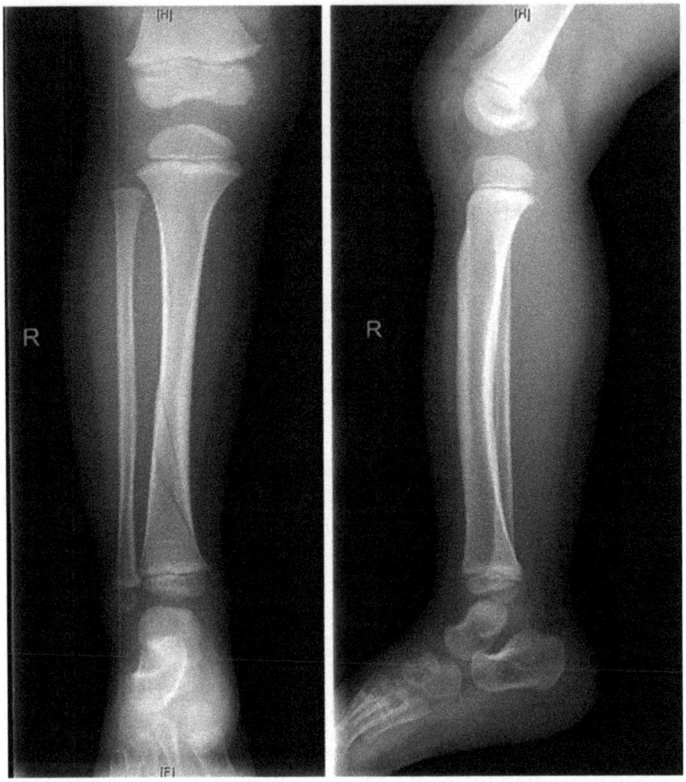

Fig. 1 Toddler's fracture

Diagnosis

Rule out underlying metabolic bone disease (i.e., osteogenesis Imperfecta, metaphyseal dysplasia, phosphate metabolism disorders)

Imaging

XR tibia–fibula (Fig. 1)

- Spiral, non-displaced
- May appear very faint and almost unnoticeable on plain XR
- Often distal ½ of tibia—proximal tibia fracture suspicious of abuse!

XR ankle, knee

Treatment Plan

Nonoperative

Long leg cast for alignment and rotational control
Non-weight bearing
3–4 weeks

Surgery

Rare for Toddler's fractures
Indicated for traumatic tibia fractures that are:

- Open
- Associated with compartment syndrome
- Have unacceptable shortening or angulation after closed reduction

Reference

Mashru RP, Herman MJ, Pizzutillo PD. Tibial shaft fractures in children and adolescents. J Am Acad Orthop Surg. 2005;13(5):345–52.

Ankle Fractures

May occur in similar patterns to adult fractures as children age and get physeal closure. Several unique types merit special consideration in the pediatric patient.

Salter-Harris I/II Fracture of Distal Fibula/Tibia

- Almost universally treated non-operatively
- Short leg cast immobilization
- Caution when reducing SHII fractures of the ankle so as not to damage the physis (Fig. 1)

Tillaux Fracture

SHIII fracture of anterolateral distal tibia epiphysis. A "transitional" fracture that occurs because of the central->medial->lateral order of ossification in the distal tibial physis.

Overview

- Often patient age 12–14
- Usually due to an external rotation force
- Caused by avulsion of the AITFL (anterior inferior tibiofibular ligament)

M.C. Makhni et al. (eds.), *Orthopedic Emergencies*,
DOI 10.1007/978-3-319-31524-9_112

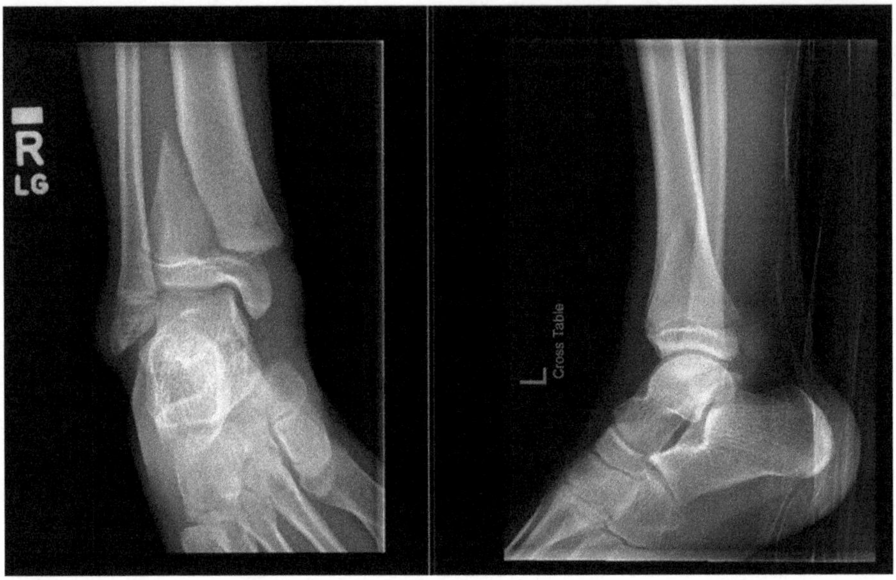

Fig. 1 Ankle fracture—SH2 distal tibia

History

- Tender over medial/lateral/posterior malleoli?
- Tender proximally near knee?
- Mechanism of injury?

Physical Exam

- Effusion
- LE ROM
- LE neuro exam (Appendix A)

Diagnosis

Imaging

- Look for SHIII fracture of anterolateral distal tibia epiphysis
- XR ankle: AP, lateral, and mortise (Fig. 2)
- XR tib-fib: AP and lateral
- CT scan may be required to fully characterize fracture (usually post-reduction and casting) to determine the residual degree of displacement. CT also helps with preoperative planning when fixation is required (Fig. 3)

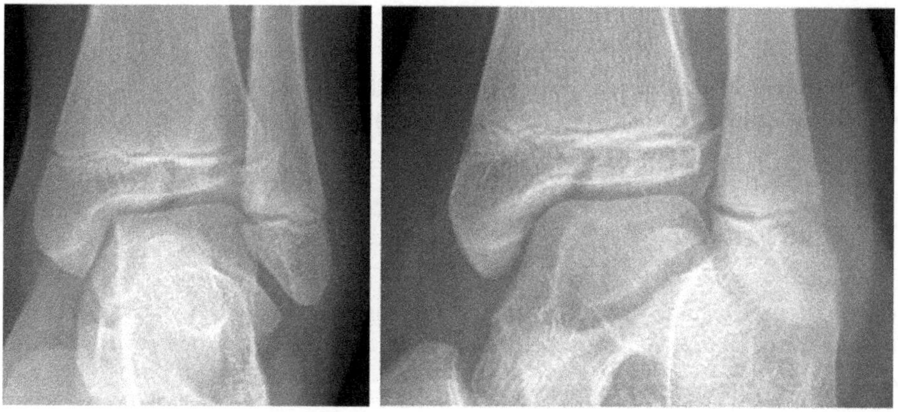

Fig. 2 Tillaux fracture XR

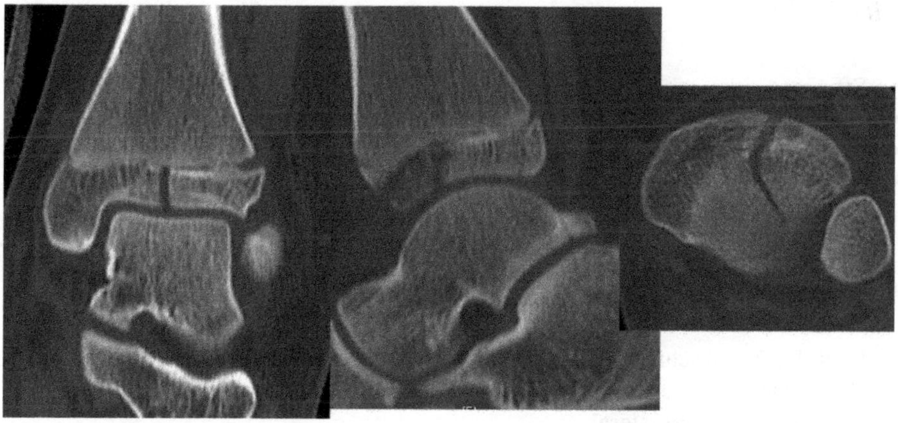

Fig. 3 Tillaux fracture CT

Treatment

Non-operative

- **Treatment:** Closed reduction
  - Often done under sedation
  - Internal rotation of foot (to counteract mechanism of injury)
  - Long leg cast × 4 weeks, transition to short leg cast × 2–3 weeks
- **Indications:** non-displaced <2 mm of articular displacement, or extra-articular fractures

Surgery

- **Treatment:** Closed versus open reduction and internal fixation
- **Indications:** More than 2 mm of displacement post-reduction

Triplane Fracture

Defined by a complex pattern involving the sagittal, axial, and coronal planes. Distinguished from a tillaux by the presence of fracture in the posterior distal tibial metaphysis.

Overview

Physical Exam

- Effusion
- Tender over medial/lateral/posterior malleoli? Tender proximally near knee?
- LE ROM
- LE neuro exam (Appendix A)

Diagnosis

- Look for 2–4 fracture fragments: (1) posterior, (2) medial, (3) tibial metaphysis
- XR Ankle: AP, lateral, and mortise
- XR tib-fib: AP and lateral
- SHIII fracture on AP (Figs. 4 and 5)

Treatment

Non-operative

- Treatment: Closed reduction
    - Often done under sedation
    - Axial traction on ankle and rotation of the foot
        - For medial fractures—position foot in external rotation
        - For lateral fractures—position foot in internal rotation
- Indications: Non-displaced (<2 mm of articular displacement)

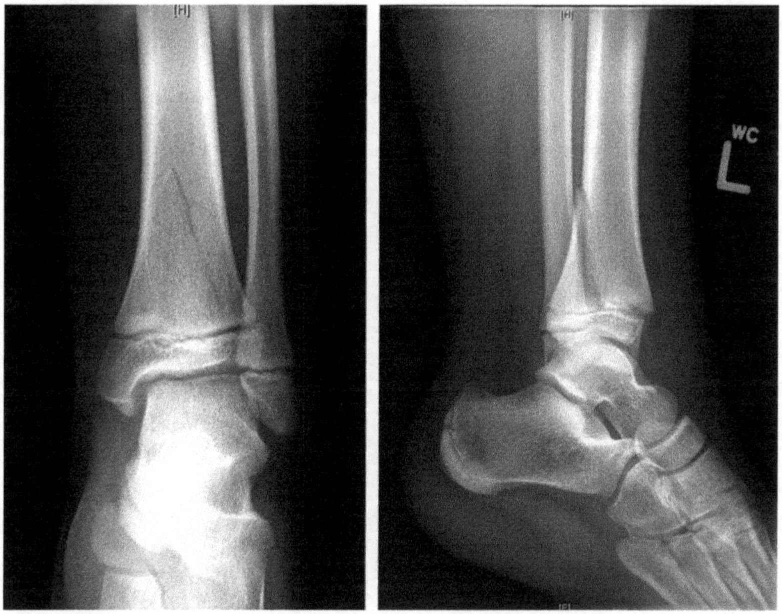

Fig. 4 Triplane fracture XR

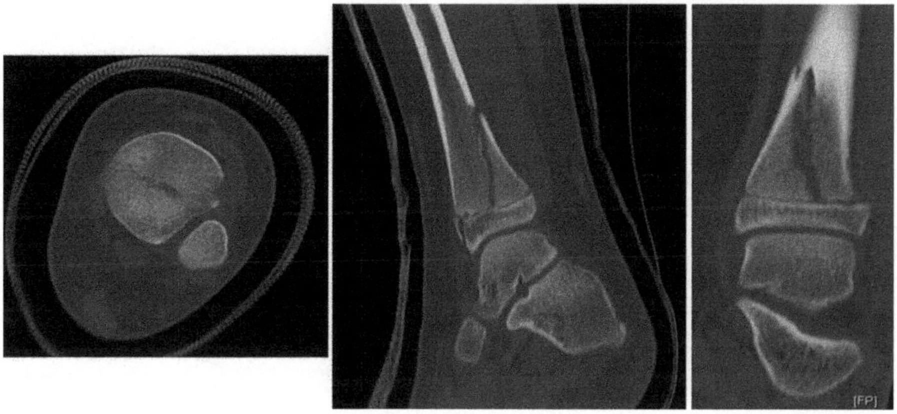

Fig. 5 Triplane fracture CT

Surgery

- **Treatment:** Closed versus open reduction and internal fixation
  - Ephiphyseal screw placed parallel to the physis
- **Indications:** more than 2 mm of displacement

References

1. Kay RM, Matthys GA. Pediatric ankle fractures: evaluation and treatment. J Am Acad Orthop Surg. 2001;9(4):268–78.
2. Blackburn EW et al. Ankle fractures in children. J Bone Joint Surg Am. 2012;94(13):1234–44.

Part IX
Emergency Sideline Management of Athletic Conditions

Jeremy Alland and Sonya Makhni

Concussion 505

Heat Illness 507

Exercise-Associated Hyponatremia (EAH) 509

Sudden Cardiac Arrest (SCA) 511

Asthma 513

Frostbite 515

Concussion

- Suspect with any type of head injury
- Remove from game for full evaluation
- Symptoms may not appear immediately—important to reexamine frequently
- Clinical Manifestations:
  - Symptoms—somatic (i.e., headache), cognitive (i.e., altered mental status), emotional
  - Physical signs—(LOC, amnesia)
  - Behavioral changes
  - Cognitive impairment
  - Sleep disturbances
- Clinical diagnosis and Evaluation
  - All tools are used as objective data to assist diagnosis (i.e., SCAT-3)
  - Diagnosis based on symptoms checklist, cognitive evaluation including orientation, past and immediate concentration, new learning and concentration, balance tests, and neurologic examination
    - Balance testing is sensitive, not specific—must account for sideline factors that would affect balance (surface, cleats, etc.)
- Increased risk with: female, contact sports, or prior history of concussion
- Return to Play (RTP) Guidelines
  - No same-day RTP with concussion diagnosis
  - (1) Patient must be completely asymptomatic at rest prior to returning to any activity
    - Symptom evaluation ± computerized neurocognitive testing immediately following injury and serially
    - Emphasize accurate symptom reporting

M.C. Makhni et al. (eds.), *Orthopedic Emergencies*,
DOI 10.1007/978-3-319-31524-9_113

- (2) Asymptomatic with both physical and cognitive exertion
  - Gradually progress return to activity in a stepwise fashion once patient is asymptomatic at rest
  - Should symptoms return at any point during return to exertion, patient should return to last level of exertion where he/she was asymptomatic
- (3) Athlete must return to baseline or normative values on neurocognitive testing

References

Concussion in Sport Group. SCAT3 sport concussion assessment tool. 3rd ed. Br J Sports Med. 2013.

Harmon KG et al. American Medical Society for Sports Medicine position statement: concussion in sport. Br J Sports Med. 2013;47:15–26.

McCrory P et al. Consensus statement on concussion in sport: the 4th international conference on concussion in sport held in Zurich, November 2012. Br J Sports Med. 2013;47:250–8.

Reddy CC, Collins MW. Sports concussion: management and predictors of outcome. Curr Sports Med Rep. 2009;8(1):10–5.

Heat Illness

- Clinical Manifestations
  - Spectrum from heat cramps to heat exhaustion to heat stroke
  - Highest risk with wet bulb temperature >82 °F, high-intensity exercise, and/or strenuous exercise for greater than 1 h
- Cramps
  - Treat with hydration (salts) and full-length stretching
  - Severe or unrelenting—can use diazepam or midazolam
- Heat Exhaustion
  - Tachycardia, fatigue, mild confusion, dizziness
  - Temperature <104 °F rectally
  - Remove clothing, asked to lie supine with legs elevated, apply ice bags to major arteries (axilla, inguinal), remove from heat, use a fan, hydrate (oral preferred), spray with water
- Heat Stroke
  - Temperature >104 °F rectally with signs of end organ damage, usually altered mental status
  - Medical emergency, life-threatening
  - MUST get rectal temperature
  - Immediate cold water immersion
  - Hydration
  - Remove from immersion around 102 °F

M.C. Makhni et al. (eds.), *Orthopedic Emergencies*,
DOI 10.1007/978-3-319-31524-9_114

- Return to competition
  - At least 7 days off
  - Repeat exam and labs in 1 week
  - When cleared, use 2 week heat acclimatization protocol starting in cool environment

Reference

Armstrong LE, Casa DJ, Millard-Stafford M, Moran DS, Pyne SW, Roberts WO. Exertional heat illness during training and competition. Med Sci Sports Exerc. 2007;39(3):556–72.

Exercise-Associated Hyponatremia (EAH)

- Clinical Manifestations
  - Symptoms include lightheadedness, nausea, vomiting, headache, altered mental status.
  - Suspicion increases if weight gain during exercise and symptoms above (versus heat illness)
  - Severe cases can cause cerebral edema and can lead to seizures (EAH encephalopathy)
- Higher risk in endurance athletes, military, extreme conditions, excessive training
- Risk factors include:
  - Overdrinking (especially hypotonic solutions)
  - Exercise >4 h
  - Inadequate training
  - High or low BMI
- General diagnosis is Na level <135
- Treatment
  - Mild/Moderate
    - Observation, restrict hypotonic fluids until urinating freely
    - Give oral hypertonic fluids (i.e., broth, HTS with crystal light or Kool-Aid packets, concentrated bouillon)
  - Severe (AMS, encephalopathy)
    - Emergency, transfer to ED ASAP
    - Needs IVF, likely 3 % NS

M.C. Makhni et al. (eds.), *Orthopedic Emergencies*,
DOI 10.1007/978-3-319-31524-9_115

Reference

Hew-Butler T, Rosner MH, Fowkes-Godek S, Dugas JP, Hoffman MD, Lewis DP, Maughan RJ, Miller, KC, Montain SJ, Rehrer NJ, Roberts WO, Rogers IR, Siegel AJ, Stuempfle KJ, Winger JM, Verbalis JG. Statement of the third international exercise-associated hyponatremia consensus development conference, Carlsbad, California, 2015. Clin J Sport Med. 2015;25(4): 303–20.

Sudden Cardiac Arrest (SCA)

- Clinical Manifestations
  - Suspect in ANY athlete who collapses or loses consciousness
  - Myoclonic jerks or seizure-like activity is common after collapse of SCA and should not be mistaken for seizure
- New CPR guidelines recommend CAB (circulation, airway, breathing)
  - Chest compressions more important than breaths
- CPR should be started immediately if no pulse is felt
  - 30 compressions, followed by two rescue breaths
  - Minimize any time without compressions
- In young healthy athletes, SCA is often related to arrhythmia
  - Apply AED as soon as possible—the goal is 3–5 min from time of collapse to time of first shock
- Have someone call EMS

Reference

Casa DJ, Guskiewicz KM, Anderson SA, Courson RW, Heck JF, Jimenez CC, McDermott BP, Miller MG, Stearns RL, Swartz EE, Walsh KM. National Athletic Trainers' Association position statement: preventing sudden death in sports. J Athl Train. 2012;47(1):96–118.

M.C. Makhni et al. (eds.), *Orthopedic Emergencies*,
DOI 10.1007/978-3-319-31524-9_116

Asthma

- Clinical Manifestations:
  - Wheezing, shortness of breath, chest pain, chest heaviness, coughing, cyanosis, difficulty speaking, difficulty recovering from exertion
  - If retaining CO_2: confusion, drowsiness
- Diagnosis on sideline can be clinical with symptoms
  - Check peak flow meter
- Recognize exacerbating factors
  - Smoking (firsthand and secondhand)
  - Allergies
- Treatment
  - Short-acting bronchodilator (i.e., albuterol)
    - Best with inhaler and spacer
      - Rapid sequential administration of two puffs until feeling better
      - If no improvement with three administrations, transfer to facility
    - Supplemental O_2 as needed
    - Failure to resolve symptoms should warrant consideration for 911/EMS activation

Reference

Casa DJ, Guskiewicz KM, Anderson SA, Courson RW, Heck JF, Jimenez CC, McDermott BP, Miller MG, Stearns RL, Swartz EE, Walsh KM. National Athletic Trainers' Association position statement: preventing sudden death in sports. J Athl Train. 2012;47(1):96–118.

M.C. Makhni et al. (eds.), *Orthopedic Emergencies*,
DOI 10.1007/978-3-319-31524-9_117

Frostbite

- Causes
  - Occurs at temperatures <32 °F
  - Natural physiology of body shunts blood from distal extremities to keep central organs warm, and therefore, will present distal and progress proximally.
  - Wet skin cools faster, and therefore sweating increases risk. Try to keep covered and dry with special apparel. Remove wet clothing promptly.
- Clinical Manifestations
  - Frostnip—superficial skin freezes, no cell damage
  - Mild frostbite—skin and subcutaneous tissues freeze
  - Severe frostbite—below subcutaneous tissue (muscles, tendons, bones)
  - Symptoms
    - Edema, redness or mottled gray skin appearance, stiffness, and transient tingling or burning
    - Deep (severe): hard tissue, vesicles, numbness
- Treatment
  - To rewarm, the affected tissue should be immersed in a warm (98 °F–104 °F [37 °C–40 °C]) water bath
  - Remove any constrictive clothing and submerge the entire affected area.
  - The water will need to be gently circulated, and the area should be immersed for 15–30 min.
  - Thawing is complete when the tissue is pliable and color and sensation have returned.
  - Rewarming can result in significant pain, so a physician may prescribe appropriate analgesic medication.
  - AVOID: friction massage, dry heat, steam heat; do NOT open vesicles
  - Once rewarming is started, tissue can NOT refreeze again (as this causes tissue necrosis)

M.C. Makhni et al. (eds.), *Orthopedic Emergencies*,
DOI 10.1007/978-3-319-31524-9_118

References

Cappaert TA, Stone JA, Castellani JW, Krause BA, Smith D, Stephens BA. National Athletic Trainers' Association position statement: environmental cold injuries. J Athl Train. 2008;43(6):640–58.

Castellani JW, Young AJ, Ducharme MB, Giesbrecht GG, Glickman E, Sallis RE. Prevention of cold injuries during exercise. Med Sci Sports Exerc. 2006;38(11):2012–29.

Appendix A
Physical Exam Overview

Danica Vance and Maggie Wright

Distal Extremity Exam 518
Spine Exam 519
Shoulder Exam 526
Elbow Exam 528
Wrist Exam 531
Hand Exam 536
Hip Exam 542
Knee Exam 544
Foot and Ankle Exam 549
References 554

M.C. Makhni et al. (eds.), *Orthopedic Emergencies*,
DOI 10.1007/978-3-319-31524-9

Initial evaluation guided by Advanced Traumatic Life Support protocol (ATLS)

- A: Airway
- B: Breathing
- C: Circulation
- D: Deficits
- E: Exposure/Environment

  Physical exam of all affected systems
  See Chap. "***Initial Trauma Evaluation***" for more details

Distal Extremity Exam

Upper Extremity

Motor

Radial nerve: MCP extension, thumb abduction/extension.
Median nerve: finger flexion, thumb flexion/opposition.
Ulnar: interosseous muscles.

Sensory

Radial nerve: dorsal web space between thumb and index finger.
Median nerve: radial border of tip of index finger.
Ulnar nerve: palmar side of tip of little finger.

Lower Extremity

Motor

Deep peroneal nerve.

  Tibialis anterior—foot inversion/dorsiflexion.
  EHL—great toe dorsiflexion.

Superficial peroneal: peroneal muscles → foot eversion.
Tibial: Gastrocnemius—plantarflexion.

Sensory

Deep peroneal nerve: 1st dorsal webspace.
Superficial peroneal nerve: dorsal foot.
Tibial nerve: plantar foot.
Saphenous nerve: medial foot.
Sural nerve: lateral foot.

Spine Exam

Inspection

- Scars: location, surgical or traumatic, healing.
- Skin abnormalities (cafe-au-lait spots, dimple/hair over spine).
- Muscle atrophy.
- Spinal deformity.

Gait

- Wide-based, unsteady gait (myelopathy).
- Foot drop (weakness of TA or EHL, nerve root compression L4–L5).
- Flatfoot/loss of push off (weakness in gastrocnemius–soleus, nerve root compression S1–S2).
- Abductor lurch (possible weakness of gluteus medius, nerve root compression of L5).

Palpation

- Useful landmarks:
  - T4: Level of the nipples.
  - T7: Xiphoid process/inferior sternum.
  - T10: Level of umbilicus.
- Bony palpation.
  - Starting at occiput, palpate spinous processes from C2 down to sacrum, checking for any tenderness or step off deformity consistent with a spondylolisthesis/fracture.
- Soft tissue/paraspinal muscles.

Range of Motion

Cervical Spine

- Flexion: 75°—"chin to chest."
- Extension: 60°—"look up at ceiling."
- Lateral flexion: 20°–45°—"ear to shoulder."
- Rotation: 70–90°—"chin to shoulder, with shoulder stabilization."

Thoracic Spine

Limited range of motion due to rib stabilization.

Lumbar Spine:

- Flexion: 45–60°—"toe touch with straight legs."
- Extension: 20–30°.
- Lateral flexion: 10–20—"bend to each side."
- Rotation: 5–15°—stabilize the hip.

Neurovascular

- Motor testing: Assessed using a 0–5 grading scale
- Sensory: Dermatomal.
- Reflexes: Assessed using a 0–4+ grading scale.
- ***Motor/Sensory/Reflexes***
  - Cervical
    - C5: Deltoid and biceps/upper lateral arm and elbow/biceps
    - C6: Biceps, wrist extension/lateral forearm, thumb and index finger/ brachioradialis
    - C7: Triceps, wrist flexors, long finger extension/middle fingers/triceps
    - C8: Digital flexors/little and ring finger/none
    - T1: Interossei muscles/medial arm/none
  - Lumbar
    - L3: Iliopsoas/anterior and medial thigh/none
    - L4: Quadriceps/medial leg and ankle/patellar tendon.
    - L5: Gluteus medius, Tibialis anterior and Extensor hallucis longus/dorsal foot and 1st web space/none.
    - S1: Gastrocnemius-soleus/lateral and plantar foot/Achilles tendon.
    - S2–4: Anal sphincter/perianal sensation/bulbocavernosus.

Additional Tests:

- Rectal exam
  - Rectal tone.
  - Presence of normal "anal wink."
- Bulbocavernosus reflex.
  - Anal sphincter contraction in response to squeezing glans penis or tugging Foley.
  - If reflex absent (acute injury), cannot determine if neurologic injury permanent.
  - Return of reflex marks end of spinal shock.

- **Cervical**
  - **Babinski sign:** Run stick/pointed object along plantar foot; upgoing big toe (patient above 1 year of age) indicative of upper motor neuron injury/myelopathy (Fig. A.1).
  - **Brudzinski:** With patient supine and neck flexed, flex the hip; reduction of symptoms with hip flexed indicative of meningitis (Fig. A.2).
  - **Distraction test:** With patient supine and neck stabilized, apply a distraction force; relief of symptoms indicative of foraminal compression of nerve root.
  - **Hoffman's sign:** Flicking the distal phalanx of the middle finger into flexion of the DIPJ; pathologic if thumb IPJ flexes indicating myelopathy (Fig. A.3).
  - **Kernig's sign:** With patient supine, flex neck; radiating pain with neck flexion indicative of meningitis (Fig. A.4).

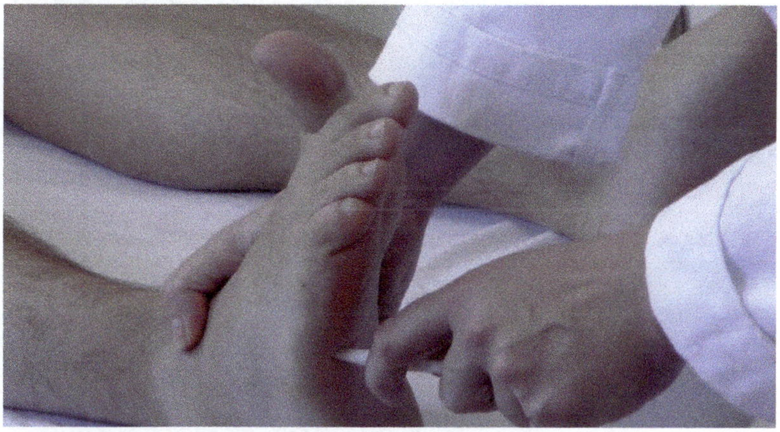

Fig. A.1 Babinski sign

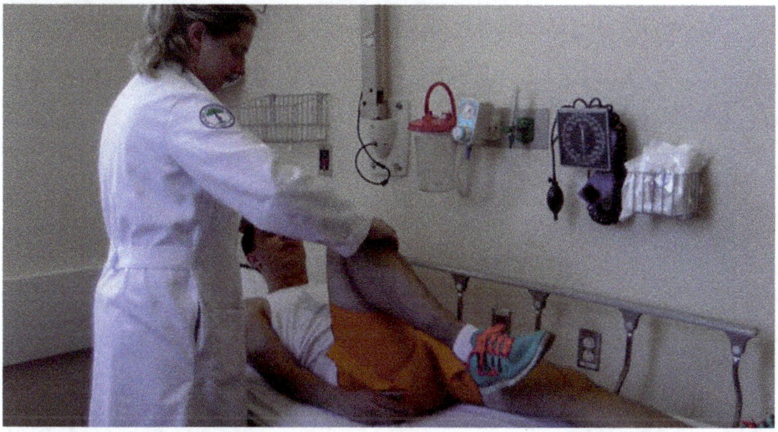

Fig. A.2 Brudzinski sign

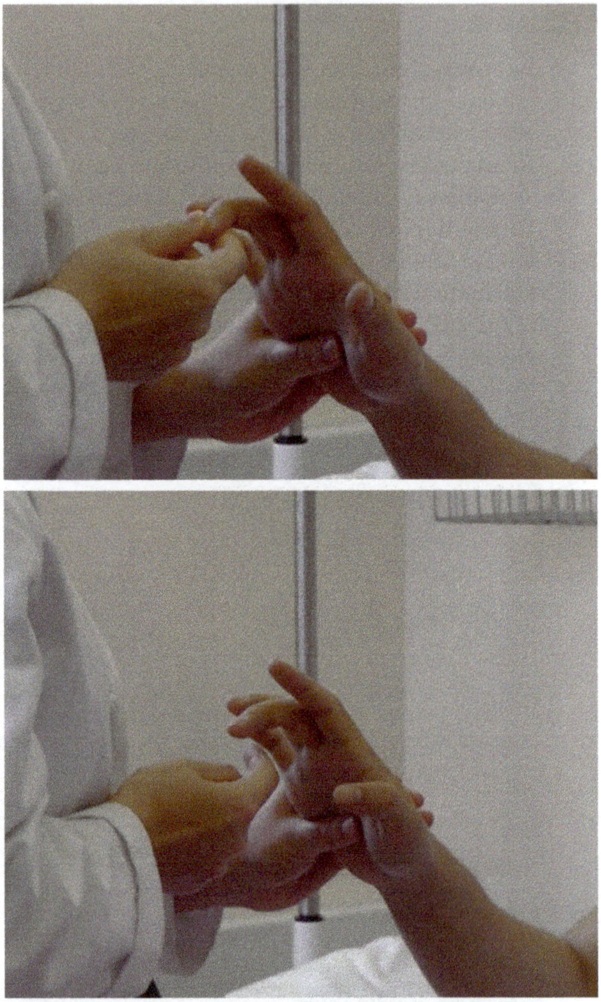

Fig. A.3 Hoffman's sign

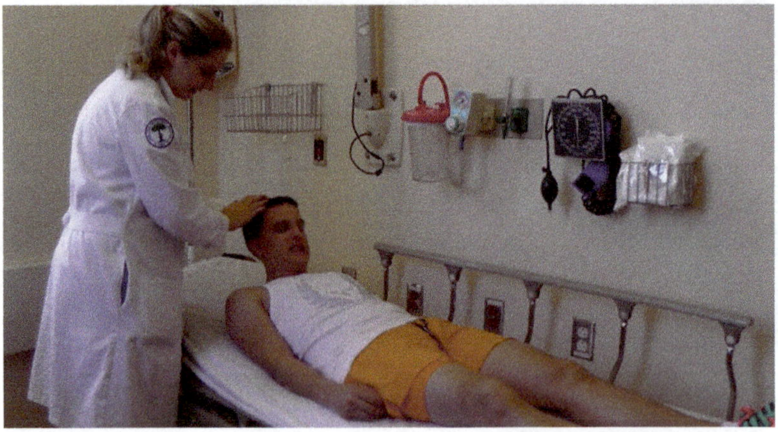

Fig. A.4 Kernig's sign

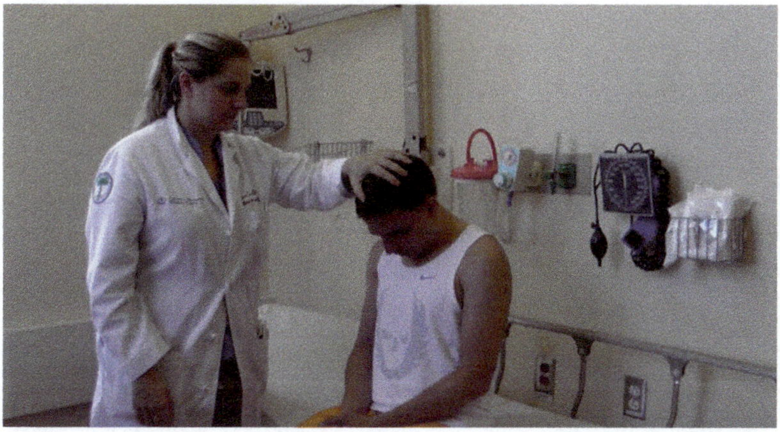

Fig. A.5 Lhermitte's sign

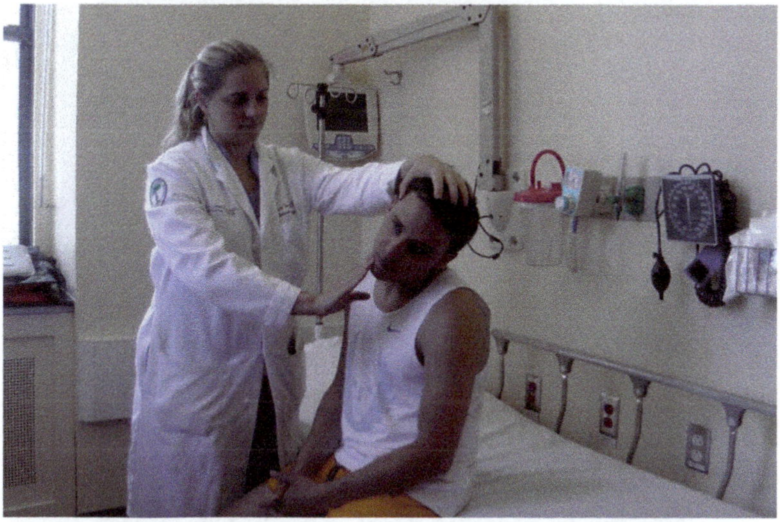

Fig. A.6 Spurling's maneuver

- **Lhermitte's sign:** With neck flexed apply axial load to cervical spine; electric/shock like sensation down trunk/extremities indicative of possible cervical disc disease/herniated disc/cervical spondylosis/MS (Fig. A.5).
- **Spurlings maneuver:** With neck flexed and rotated toward affected side, apply axial load; radiating pain down affected side indicative of nerve root compression; can help differentiate between neck and shoulder related pain (Fig. A.6).
- **Arm abduction relief sign**: In seated position, have patient place arms on top of their head; reduction of symptoms (Fig. A.7).

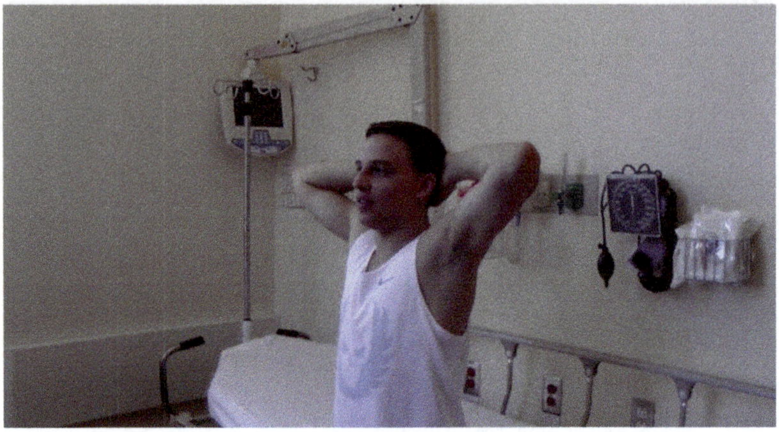

Fig. A.7 Arm abduction relief sign

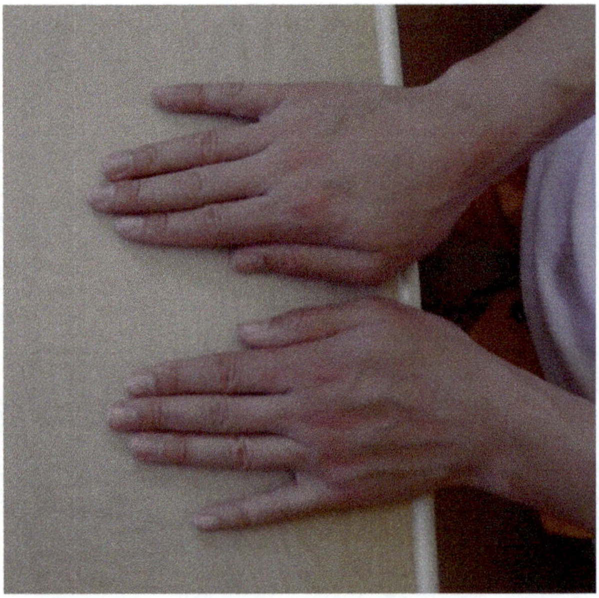

Fig. A.8 Finger escape sign

- ◦ **Finger escape sign:** The patient holds their fingers extended and adducted; the two ulnar digits will be flexed and abducted usually in less than 1 min in patients with cervical myelopathy (Fig. A.8).

- <u>**Lumbar**</u>
  - ◦ **Bowstring:** With patient supine, perform an SLR until pain is felt; once pain is felt have patient flex the knee slightly to relieve the pain and then apply pressure to popliteal fossa; radiating pain with popliteal pressure indicative of sciatic nerve pathology.

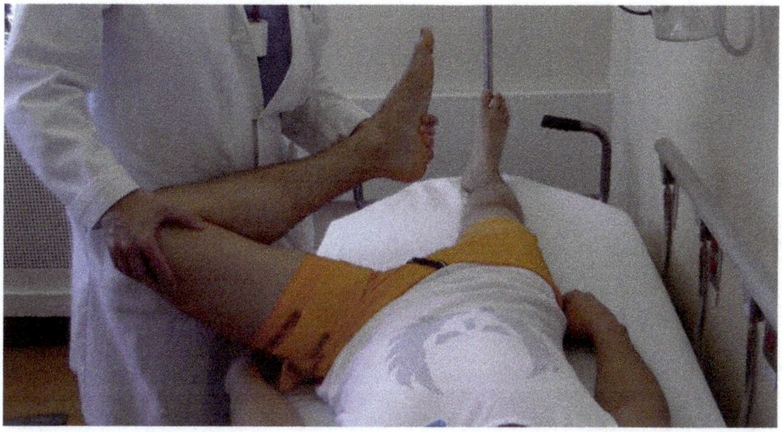

Fig. A.9 FABER sign

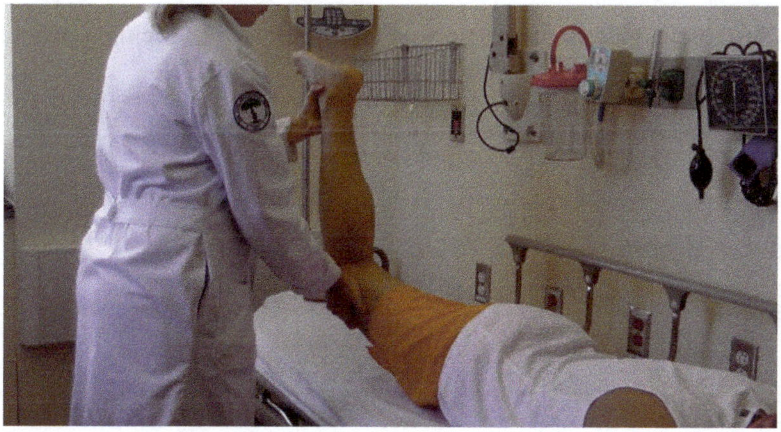

Fig. A.10 Femoral nerve stretch test

- **FABER:** (**Fl**exion, **AB**duction, **E**xternal **R**otation) With patient supine, place leg in figure four position; anterior hip pain/groin pain indicative of hip conditions; lower back pain/posterior pelvic pain indicative of sacroiliac joint conditions (Fig. A.9).
- **Femoral nerve stretch test:** With patient prone and knee flex, passively hyperextend the hip; anterior thigh pain indicative of L2–L4 nerve root compressions (Fig. A.10).
- **Straight-leg raise test (SLR):** With patient supine, flex hip; radiating lower extremity pain between 30° and 70° indicative of radiculopathy (Fig. A.11).
  - **Lasegue's Sign:** While performing straight-leg raise, dorsiflex foot; worsening/aggravated pain with ankle dorsiflexion indicative of radiculopathy.

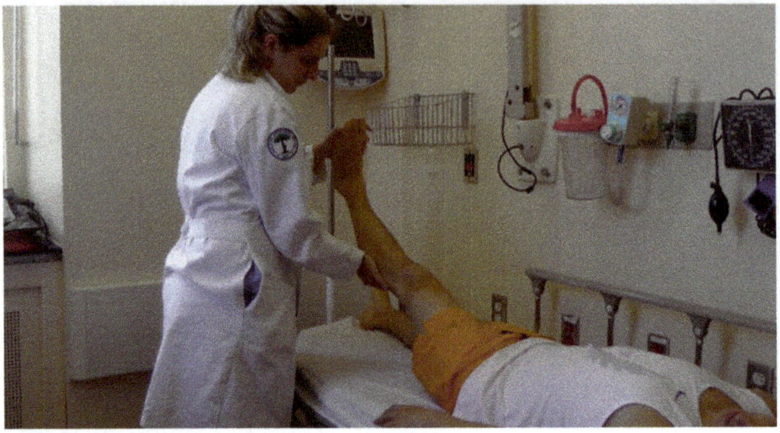

Fig. A.11 Straight leg raise

- **Sustained ankle clonus:** rapidly flex and extend ankle. Multiple beats of clonus indicative of upper motor neuron injury.
- **Waddell's signs:** Presence of >3 signs indicate possible non-organic causes of pain that may cause patient to respond poorly to treatment.

Shoulder Exam

Inspection

- Deformity, swelling/ecchymosis, skin integrity, resting position of arm, muscle tone.
  - Skin tenting → clavicle fracture, AC separation.
  - Flattened shoulder in flexion/IR → dislocation.

Palpation

- Bony palpation
  - Clavicle, AC joint → tenderness or crepitus indicating fracture or separation.
  - Humeral head (greater/lesser tuberosity) → fracture vs rotator cuff.
- Soft tissue palpation
  - Biceps tendon → tendonitis vs. tear (hook test for tear distally).

Range of Motion

- Decreased due to fracture/pain, osteoarthritis, rotator cuff tear.
- Normal values:
  - Forward flexion 0–180.
  - Abduction 0–180.
  - Internal rotation—note level reached on back, mid thoracic normal.
  - External rotation—0–60.

Neurovascular

- Axillary nerve—Important to test in proximal humerus fractures and shoulder dislocations.
  - Motor—deltoid, can have patient fire posterior fibers and push elbow back if too painful/unable to abduct.
  - Sensory—over lateral shoulder.
- Radial nerve—Important to test in humeral shaft fractures, especially middle third fractures.
  - Motor—triceps extension may be painful, can do wrist/finger extension distally.
  - Sensory—dorsal aspect of hand and forearm.
- Median/ulnar nerves—test distally if suspicion for brachial plexus injuries (i.e., clavicle fracture or shoulder dislocation).

Special Tests

- Impingement
  - Neer—pain in passive forward flexion.
  - Hawkins—arm held in abduction with pain in passive internal rotation.
- Rotator cuff—includes a resistance and lag sign for each muscle.
  - Jobe empty can/drop arm—supraspinatus, resisted forward flexion and forward flexion lag.
  - Resisted external rotation and arm held in external rotation—infraspinatus.
  - Hornblower—ER lag sign in abduction, isolates teres minor.
  - Lift off/lift off lag-arm behind back to isolate subscapularis.
- Biceps/labral pathology.
  - O'Briens—forward flex to 90 and adduct 10°, pain in pronation > supination with SLAP tears.

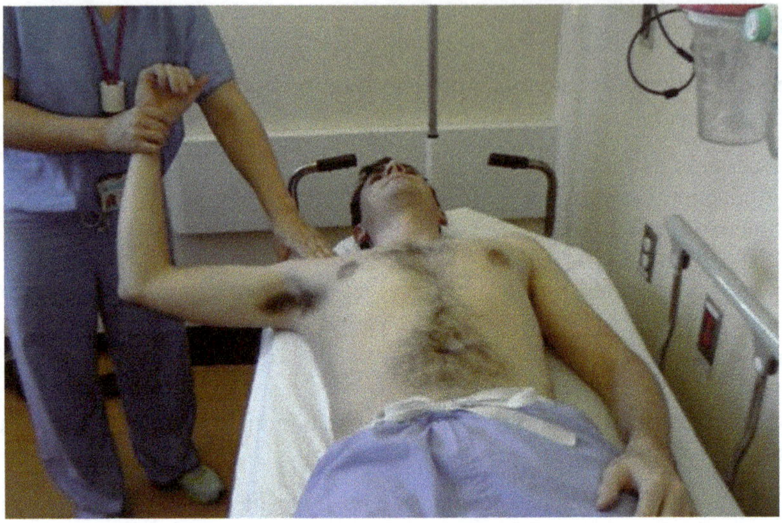

Fig. A.12 Apprehension test

- Speed-pain with resisted flexion of shoulder → biceps tendinitis
- Yergasons—pain with resisted supination → biceps tendinitis.

- Instability
  - Apprehension—pain and apprehension in abduction/external rotation (Fig. A.12). Patient should feel relief of symptoms when posteriorly directed force placed on shoulder.
  - Load and shift—axial load and anterior/posterior translation-movement increased with instability.
- AC pathology
  - Cross body adduction-pain at AC with passive adduction.

Elbow Exam

Inspection

- Check alignment/deformity, positioning
  - Nursemaid's elbow (peds)—arm held slightly flexed and pronated.
  - Posterolateral dislocation—arm held in fixed flexion.
  - Popeye sign—biceps tendon rupture.

- Check skin—erythema, ecchymosis, lacerations.
  - Olecranon bursitis will have focal swelling/erythema over only the olecranon.
  - Erythema, warmth in septic olecranon bursitis.

Palpation

- Bony Palpation
  - Medial epicondyle
  - Lateral epicondyle, radial head.
  - Olecranon.
- Soft tissue palpation
  - Anterior structures—biceps tendon
  - Medial structures—UCL, ulnar nerve in cubital tunnel.
  - Lateral structures—LUCL/LCL
  - Posterior structures—triceps tendon.

Range of Motion

- Pronation/supination—isolate elbow to make sure not cheating and moving through shoulder.
  - Normal range 70–70.
  - Important to test in radial head fracture to make sure no block to motion.
- Flexion/extension—may be limited by pain or mechanical block.
  - Normal is 0–150°.

Neurovascular

- Musculocutaneous nerve
  - Resisted elbow flexion and resisted supination (biceps).
- Radial nerve
  - Motor with resisted elbow extension (triceps) or if painful due to elbow injury can be tested distally with resisted wrist extension.
  - Sensory with posterior arm and radial aspect of forearm.

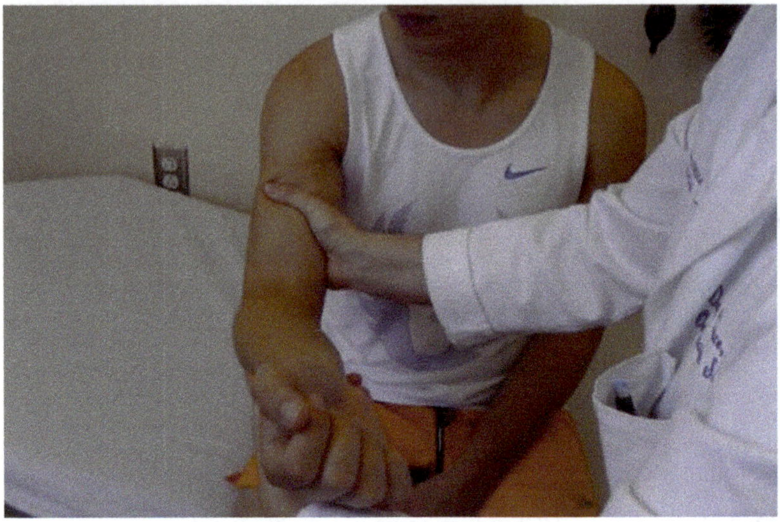

Fig. A.13 Varus stress

- Median nerve—can be affected by injuries to the medial aspect of the antecubital fossa (i.e., peds supracondylar fractures or anterior elbow dislocation).
  - Motor tested with resisted pronation (pronator teres) or more distally if pronation painful with resisted wrist or finger flexion (flexor digitorum superficialis and profundus [AIN]).
  - Sensory tested distally over palmar first to third fingers.
- Ulnar nerve—runs in cubital tunnel in medial aspect of elbow, important to test with fractures or soft tissue injuries to the medial aspect of the elbow.
  - Motor can be tested distally with finger abduction (interossei).
  - Sensory can be tested distally over palmar aspect of fourth and fifth fingers.
- Brachial, radial pulses and capillary refill important to test to confirm no compromise distal to elbow injuries.

Special Tests

- Varus and valgus stress tests: apply valgus or varus force to elbow to confirm integrity of UCL and LUCL, respectively. Important to test after trauma/elbow dislocation to test elbow stability (Figs. A.13 and A.14).
- Tinel's sign—Tapping over cubital tunnel medially with pain down medial arm → ulnar nerve entrapment.
- Hook test—hook index finger around distal biceps tendon to confirm that it is not ruptured if worried about biceps tendon rupture (Fig. A.15).

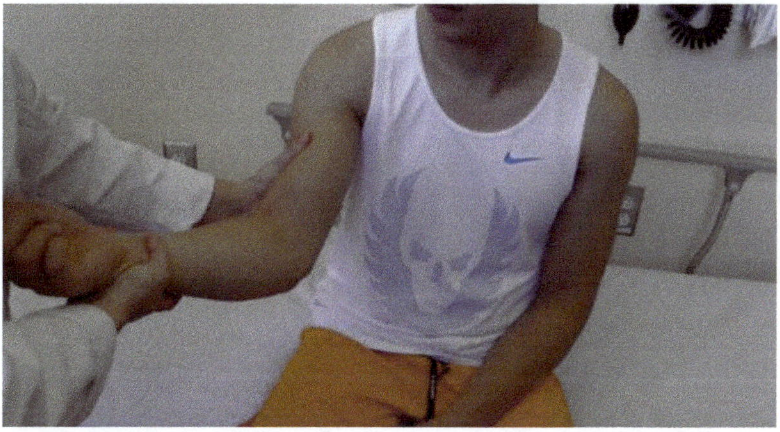

Fig. A.14 Valgus stress

Wrist Exam

Inspection

- Deformity.
- Swelling.

Palpation

- Bony Palpation
  - Two rows of carpal bones;
    - Proximal row: (from radial to ulnar side) scaphoid, lunate, triquetrum, and pisiform
      - Scaphoid: anatomical snuff box
      - Lunate: between radius and capitate; has ECR lying over it
      - Triquetrum: palpate with radial deviation of the hand.
      - Pisiform: hard to palpate, usually incorporated within FCU.
    - Distal row: trapezium, trapezoid, capitate, and hamate.
      - Trapezium: just distal to scaphoid, best palpated with thumb extension and flexion.
      - Capitate: medial to Lister's tubercle.
      - Hook of hamate: sometimes involved in fractures, lateral border of Guyon's tunnel which holds ulnar nerve and artery.

  - Radial styloid process
  - Ulnar styloid process
  - Anatomical snuff box: seen best with thumb extension, located just distal to radial styloid; tenderness in this area concerning scaphoid fracture
  - Lister's tubercle

- Soft tissue palpation:
  - First dorsal extensor compartment: located radially to anatomical snuff box
    - Contains EPL and EPB
    - Finkelstein's test (De Quervain's disease)
  - TFCC: Triangular fibrocartilage complex.
    - Made of dorsal and volar radioulnar ligaments.
    - Fovea sign: tenderness at soft spot between the ulnar styloid and FCU tendon.
    - Pain with ulnar or radial deviation of wrist.

Range of Motion

- Flexion/extension: 80/70.
- Radial deviation: 20°.
- Ulnar deviation: 30°.
- Supination/pronation.

Motor

- Wrist extension: C6; radial nerve.
  - Patient extends wrist against resistance
  - Primary wrist extensor muscles: ECRL, ECRB, ECU
- Wrist flexion: C7
  - Make fist and flex wrist against resistance
  - Primary wrist flexors: primarily FCR: median nerve (C7), FCU: ulnar nerve (C8)

Special Tests

- Durkan carpal compression: pressure on median nerve at carpal tunnel: Positive test=reproduction of symptoms indicating CTS (Fig. A.16).
- Phalen test: Flex both wrists and hold together. Positive test=reproduction of symptoms indicating CTS (Fig. A.17).

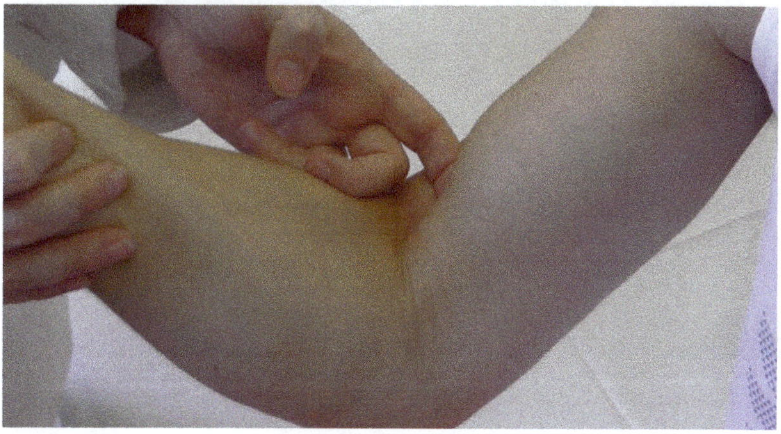

Fig. A.15 Hook test

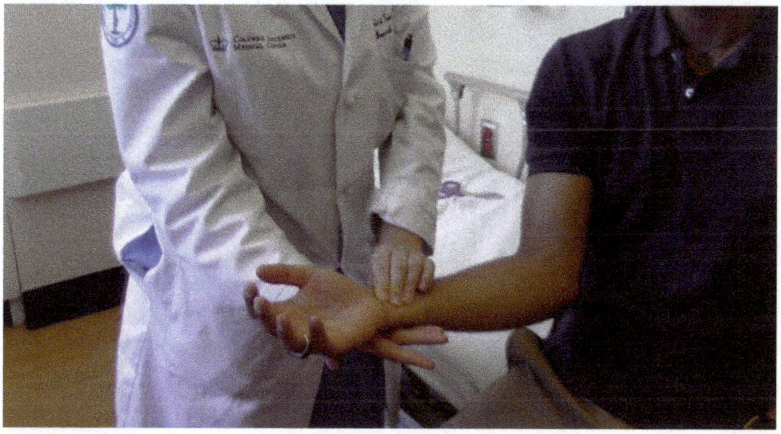

Fig. A.16 Durkan test

- Tinel sign: Tap the volar wrist over the carpal tunnel. Positive test = reproduction of symptoms indicating CTS (Fig. A.18).
- Finkelstein test: make a fist with thumb inside the fist and have the wrist ulnar deviated; positive if elicits sharp pain (Fig. A.19).
- Piano key: stabilize the ulna and translate radius dorsal and volar; compare to contralateral side. Positive test = increase laxity on injured side indicating possible DRUJ injury (Fig. A.20).
- Watson test: from the palmar side apply dorsal pressure on the scaphoid while moving the wrist from ulnar to radial deviation: Positive test = clunk or clicking of scaphoid over the distal radius indicating scapholunate dissociation (Fig. A.21).
- Allen test: occlude radial and ulnar arteries, have patient pump fist and release one artery only: Positive test = delay in blood return to the palm indicates artery compromise (Fig. A.22).

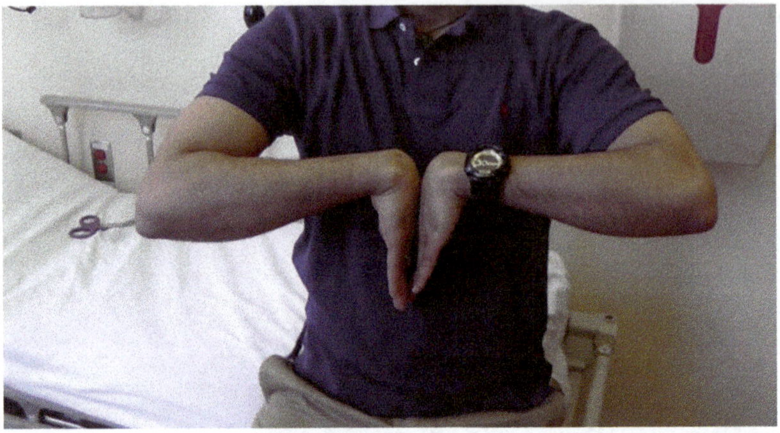

Fig. A.17 Phalen test

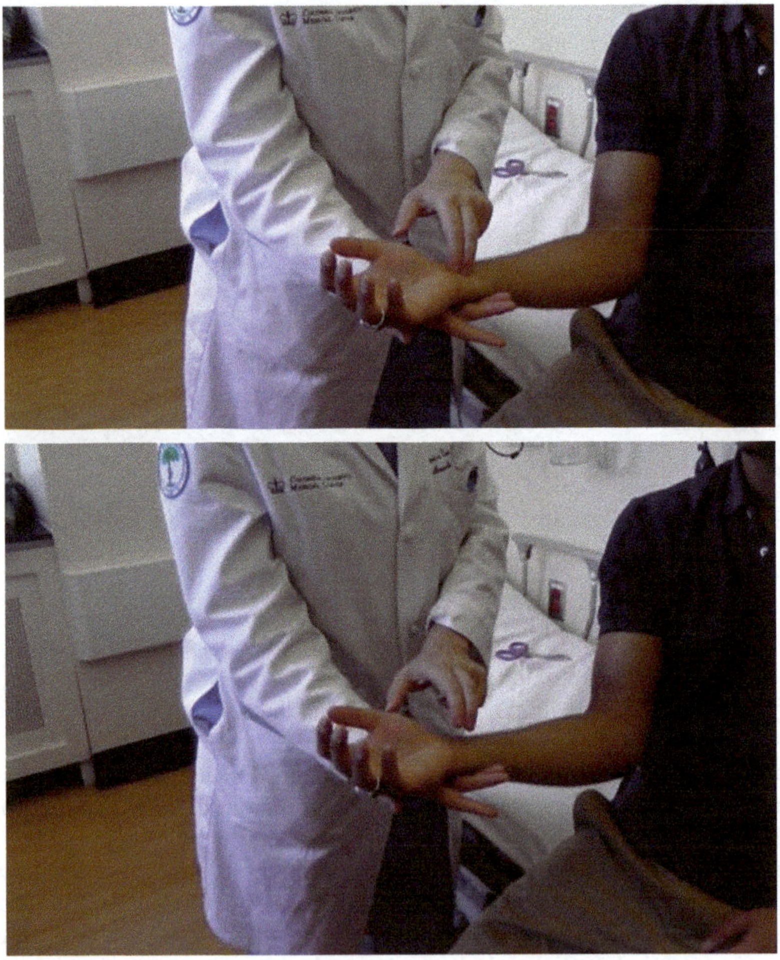

Fig. A.18 Tinel

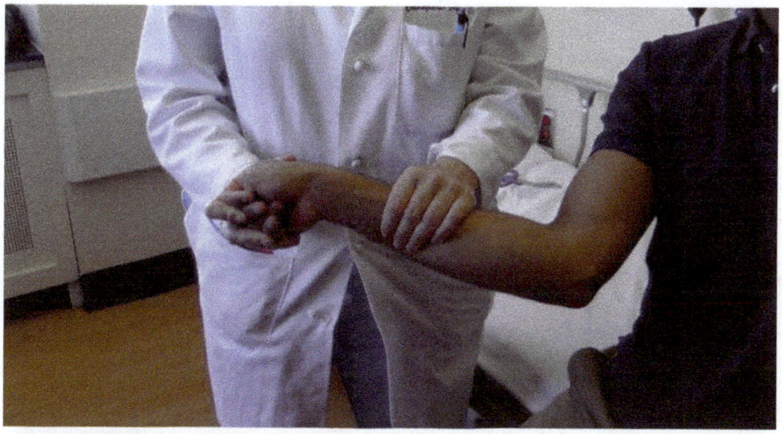

Fig. A.19 Finkelstein

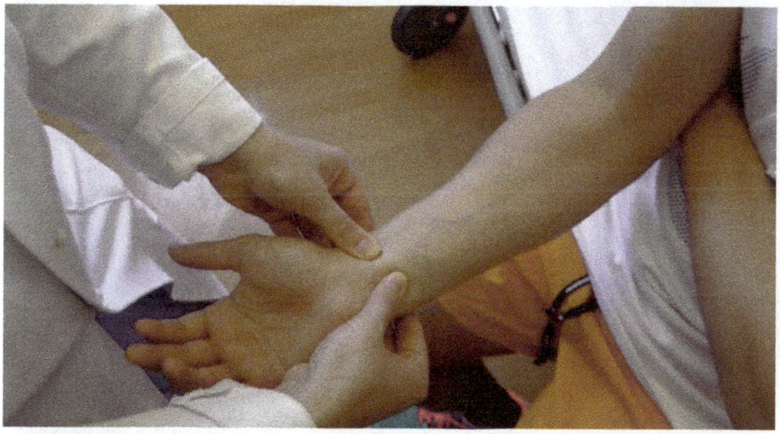

Fig. A.20 Piano key

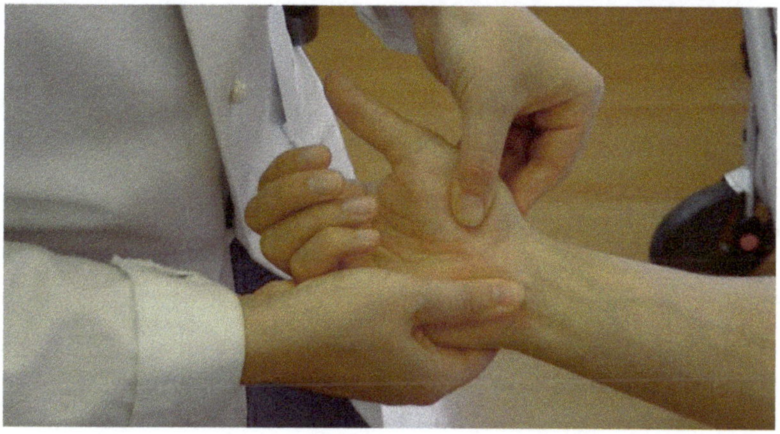

Fig. A.21 Watson test

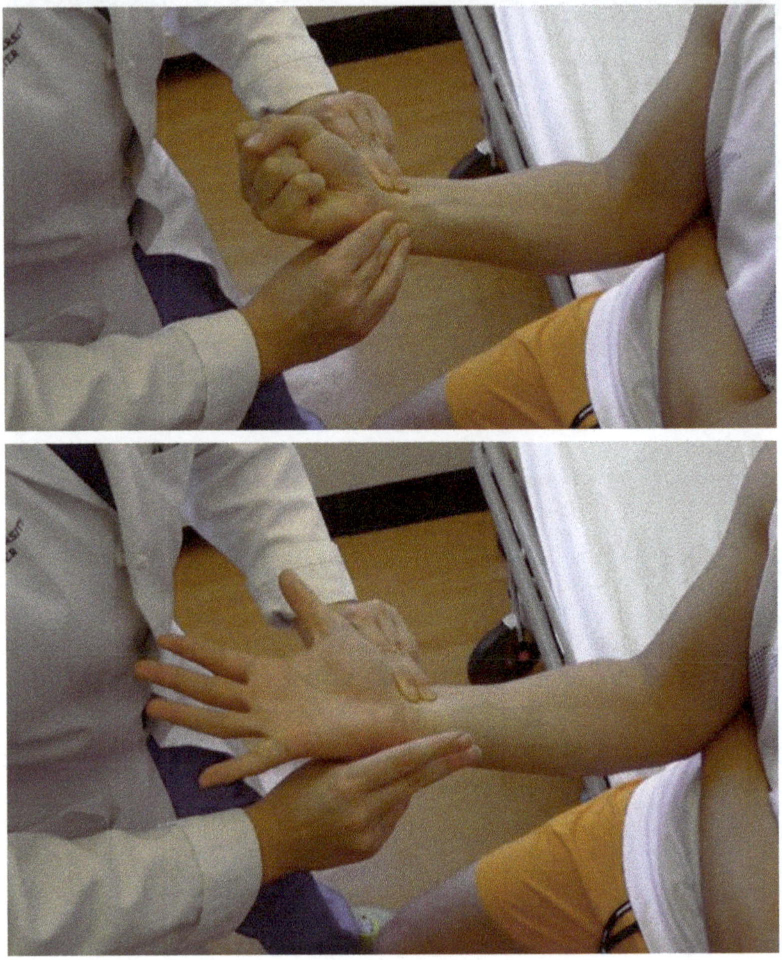

Fig. A.22 Allen test

Hand Exam

Inspection

- Deformity
  - Fracture
  - RA (ulnar deviation, swan neck, boutonniere deformity)

- Swelling
- Color
  - Vascular injury
  - Infection
- Finger position
    - Normal cascade: with wrist in slight extension and fingers at rest, fingers should be held in less flexion from first to fifth digit
    - Flexed finger: Dupuytren's contracture, trigger finger
    - Rotation of digit: fracture, malunion
  - Muscle wasting
    - Thenar eminence: median nerve injury
    - Hypothenar eminence: ulnar nerve injury

Range of Motion

- First to fourth finger
  - MCP: flexion, 90; extension, 0; adduction/abduction, 0–20
  - PIP: flexion, 110; extension: 0.
  - DIP: flexion, 65; extension: 0.
- Thumb:
  - CMC: flexion, 50; extension, 50; adduction/abduction, 0/70.
  - MCP: flexion, up to 90; extension, up to 0.
  - IP: flexion, up to 90; extension, up to 0.
  - Opposition: touch thumb to small finger base.

Neurovascular

- Motor
  - Radial nerve (PIN) (C7)
    - Finger MCP extension: extensor digitorum
    - Thumb abduction/extension: APL/EPL
    - To test radial nerve function, ask patient to make a thumbs up and hold the thumb in position against resistance
  - Median nerve/AIN (C8)
    - Finger PIP: FDS
    - Index finger DIP: FDP
    - Thumb IP flexion: FPL

    - Thumb opposition (motor recurrent nerve): APB, OP
    - To test median nerve function ask patient to make an "O"-shaped "ok sign" and hold against resistance
  - Ulnar nerve (T1)
    - Finger abduction: Interosseous muscles
    - Thumb adduction: Adductor pollicis
    - To test ulnar nerve function ask patient to spread fingers far apart (abduct) and hold against resistance
  - Simple way to test motor function in children: "paper, rock, scissors"
    - Paper: Radial nerve (MCP extension, Thumb abduction/extension)
    - Rock: Median nerve (finger flexion, thumb flexion/opposition)
    - Scissors: Ulnar (interosseous muscles)
- Sensory
  - Radial nerve: dorsal web space between thumb and index finger
  - Median nerve: radial border of tip of index finger
  - Ulnar nerve: palmar side of tip of little finger
- Vascular
  - Capillary refill: pinch finger, blood/color should return in less than 2 s

Special Tests

- Flexor digitorum superficialis test: hold all fingers in extension except finger being tested. Ask patient to flex the PIP of free finger; inability to perform indicates FDS injury (Fig. A.23)
- Flexor digitorum profundus test: hold MCP and IP joints in extension and ask patient to flex DIP of finger being tested; inability to perform indicated FDP injury (Fig. A.24)
- Froment's sign: patient is asked to hold a piece of paper between thumb and index finger (pinch grip) while examiner tries to pull the paper out; difficulty holding on to paper indicates possible ulnar nerve palsy (Figs. A.25 and A.26).
- CMC grind test: examiner grips patient's thumb metacarpal bone and places rotational and gentle axial forces by moving it in a circle; sharp pain indicates arthritis at the CMC joint
- Thumb instability test: Examiner holds thumb at metacarpal and then places valgus (UCL) and varus stress (RCL) to the MCP joint. Examiner should determine whether there is endpoint with each stress; pain with valgus stress indicates UCL injury (Skier's thumb), while pain with varus indicates RCL injury (Figs. A.27 and A.28)

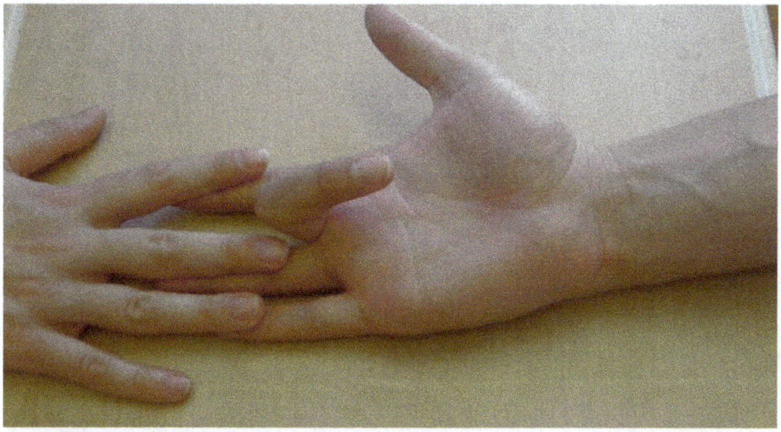

Fig. A.23 Flexor digitorium superficialis test

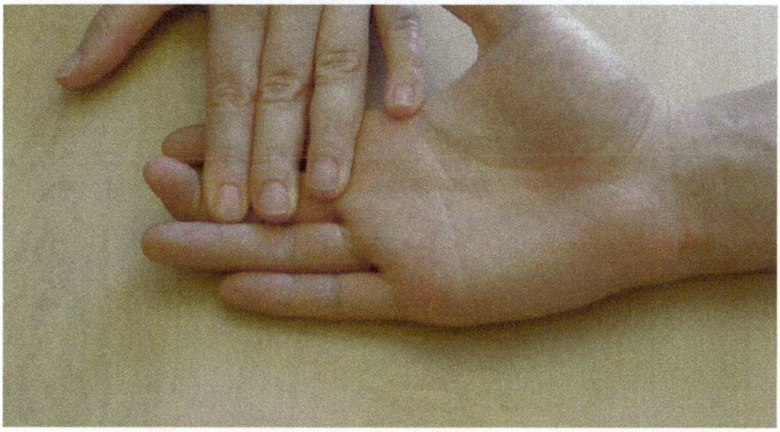

Fig. A.24 Flexor digitorum profundus test

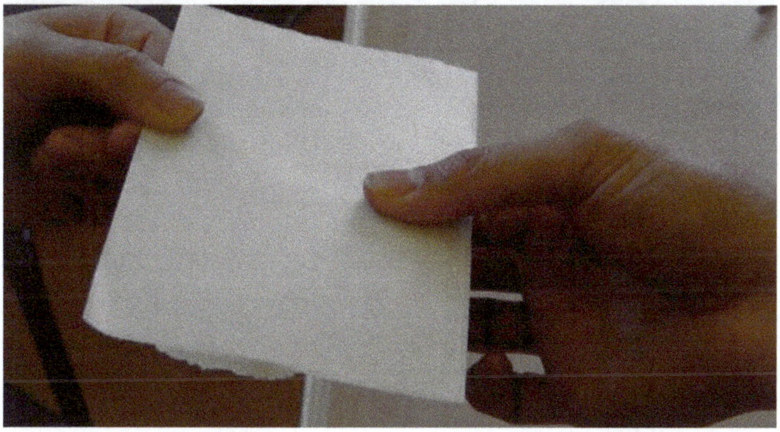

Fig. A.25 Negative Froment's sign

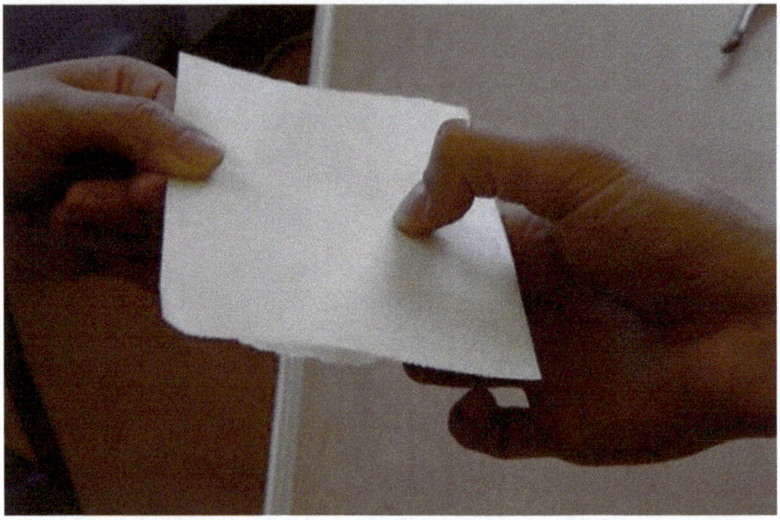

Fig. A.26 Positive Froment's sign

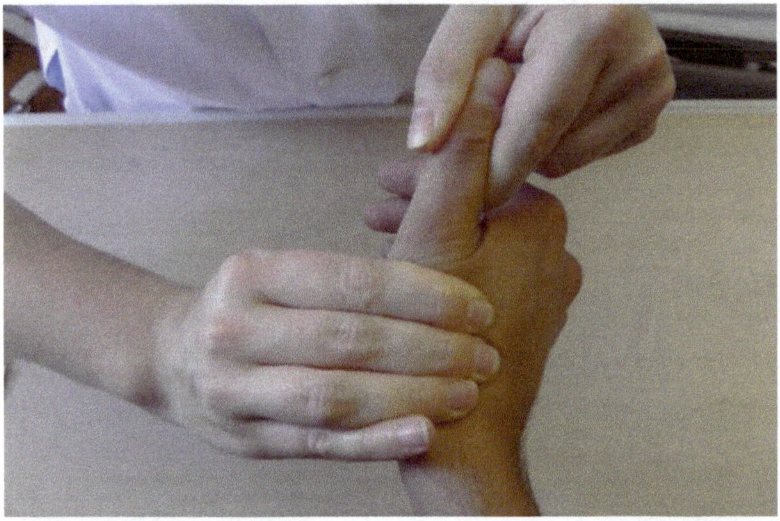

Fig. A.27 Thumb RCL instability test

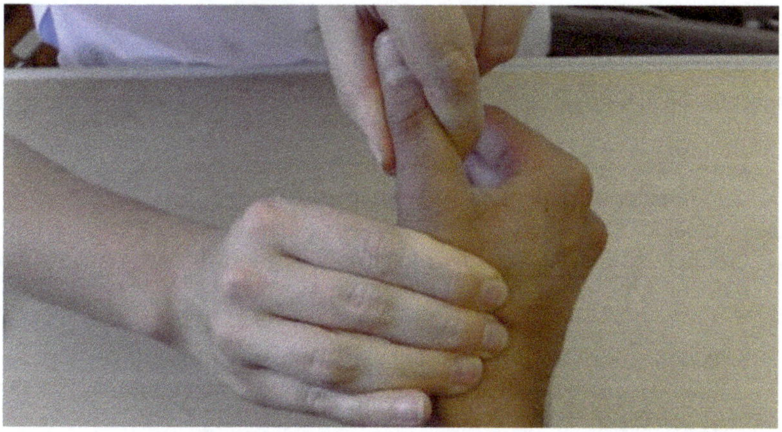

Fig. A.28 Thumb UCL instability test

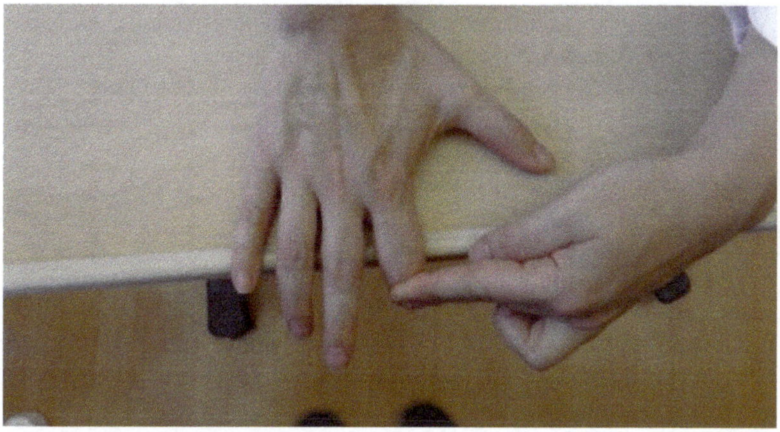

Fig. A.29 Elson test

- Elson test: Patient places finger over edge of table with PIP flexed at 90°. Examiner places finger on middle phalanx to provide resistance and asks patient to extend finger against resistance; inability to perform extension of PIP against resistance or hyperextension of DIP indicates central slip rupture (Fig. A.29)

Hip Exam

- Inspection—Gait, positioning, deformity, skin integrity, swelling, ecchymosis
  - Positioning
    - Shortened, externally rotated → hip fracture
    - Adducted, flexed, internally rotated → posterior dislocation
    - Abducted, flexed, externally rotated → anterior dislocation (uncommon)
  - Gait
    - Coxalgic—lean towards affected side while weight bearing → OA
    - Antalgic—decreased stance phase on affected side, common in knee and foot disorders
    - Trendelenburg—hip opposite the affected side drops when weight bearing on affected side → abductor weakness
- Palpation
  - ASIS → pain just medial can be due to meralgia paresthetica (LFCN pain)
  - Iliac crest → pain after direct trauma due to hip pointer
  - Ischial tuberosity → painful with hamstring tendonitis or rupture
  - SI joint → pain with sacroiliitis
  - Greater trochanter → pain with bursitis
  - TFL/IT band → pain distally with ITB syndrome
- Range of motion
  - Important to range hip with knee pain complaints, as hip pain is often referred to the knee
  - Limited ROM can occur with OA (often IR decreased first), FAI, fracture. Consider septic or inflammatory arthritis in patients (esp children) with acute/atraumatic decrease in ROM
    - Flex/extension: 0–130 flexion and 0–20 extension (can test ext with patient in lateral or prone position)
    - Abduction/adduction—0°–45° abduction, 0–25° adduction
    - Internal/external rotation—0–30 internal rotation, 0–50 external rotation (can test with patient supine and knee flexed)
- Neurovascular—Stabilize pelvis to prevent pelvic motion when testing hip strength and ROM.
  - Obturator nerve
    - Motor: Hip adduction (adductor longus and magnus, gracilis)
    - Sensory: inferomedial thigh

- Superior gluteal nerve
  - Motor: Hip abduction or Trendelenburg gait (gluteus medius and minimus)
  - Sensory: none
- Inferior gluteal nerve
  - Motor: Hip extension or rise from chair (gluteus maximus)
  - Sensory: none
- Femoral nerve
  - Motor—Resisted hip flexion or knee extension (iliopsoas and quads)
  - Sensory—Anteromedial thigh and leg
- Sciatic nerve
  - Motor: Resisted knee flexion (hamstrings), can also test distally (see knee section)
  - Sensory: Test distally (see knee section)
- **Important to test distal neurovascular function (see knee/foot and ankle sections) with any trauma to the hip and thigh, especially femur fractures

- Special tests
  - Pelvic compression—compress pelvis A-P and laterally to assess stability and pain, especially important after severe trauma if possible pelvis fracture.
  - Hip Fracture Exam
    - Log roll—pain in hip with IR/ER rolling of distal leg → hip fracture, OA
    - Heel strike—pain in hip with axial strike of heel → hip fracture
  - FABER—flexion, abduction, and external rotation → can reproduce pain with intra-articular pathology (OA) or in the SI joint with sacroiliitis (Fig. A.9).
  - FADIR—pain with flexion, adduction, and internal rotation → FAI.
  - Thomas—flexion of knee and hip with patient supine, elevation of opposite leg → hip flexor tightness.
  - Ober—abduct and extend hip, if hip remains abducted in extension → ITB tightness.
  - Ortolani—anterior force on abducted hips → clunk indicates reducible hip that had been dislocated in infants.
  - Barlow—posterior force on adducted hips → clunk indicates subluxable/dislocatable hip in infants.
  - Galeazzi—look at height difference in knees with patient supine and hips and knees flexed → difference in infants indicates dislocated hip or shortened femur.

Knee Exam

Inspection

- Gait/Alignment
  - Excessive varus/valgus in standing or walking, note asymmetry
    - Genu valgum can increase risk for patellar instability or ACL injury
    - Genu varum can be result of arthritis, blount's disease in children
  - Can have posttraumatic deformity if history of prior fracture/injury, especially in children/adolescents with prior fractures through the physis
- Skin—swelling, ecchymosis, erythema, masses, lacerations
  - Erythema/swelling over entire joint → cellulitis vs. septic joint vs. inflammatory arthritis
  - Isolated swelling over patella → prepatellar bursitis
  - Prominence of tibial tubercle → Osgood–Schlatter's
- Patellar position
  - Patella alta—physiologic vs patellar tendon rupture
  - Patella baja—physiologic vs quad tendon rupture
  - Lateral position—subluxed vs dislocated acutely, could also be chronic cause of patellofemoral pain if tracking in lateral trochlea

Palpation

- Effusion/hemarthrosis of knee—common with arthritis and acute injuries (ACL tear, meniscal injury, intra-articular fracture)
- Anterior structures:
  - Joint line—pain with meniscal injury, arthritis
  - Patella—pain with fracture, pain along borders with attaching tendon/ligament rupture (i.e., patellar tendon, MPFL)
  - Patellar tendon/quad tendon—insufficiency/defect → rupture, pain in patellar tendon → tendonitis
  - Proximal tibia and tibial tubercle—pain with fracture or Osgood–Schlatter's (over tubercle)
- Posterior structures:
  - Joint line:
    - Mobile/tender mass along joint line → Baker's cyst
    - Pain—arthritis or meniscal injury

- Medial structures:
  - Medial joint line
  - MCL
  - Pes anserine insertion → pain or swelling with pes bursitis
- Lateral structures:
  - Lateral joint line
  - LCL
  - IT band
  - Proximal fibula—important to palpate with tibial and ankle fractures, as there may be a Maisonneuve injury
- Palpate all compartments of leg with any tibial plateau or other high-energy knee/tibial injury → Severe pain/tightness may indicate compartment syndrome!

Range of Motion

- Flexion/extension: Normal 0–130, AROM often limited by pain with acute trauma
  - Flexion may be limited by OA, effusion, or obesity (soft tissue)
  - Ext may be limited by OA or effusion
  - If extreme pain with minimal motion, consider septic arthritis
  - Note crepitus if likely OA
- External rotation: 10–15° tibial ER at terminal extension to stabilize joint

Neurovascular

- Femoral nerve (L2–4)
  - Motor: Resisted knee extension (quads), may not be able to perform if extensor mechanism is affected by injury
  - Sensory: Medial leg distal to knee (saphenous nerve is terminal branch)
- Tibial nerve (S1, branch of sciatic)
  - Motor: Resisted plantarflexion of foot and toes (posterior compartments of leg—gastrocnemius, soleus, posterior tibialis, FHL, FDL)
  - Sensory: Posterolateral leg and plantar aspect of foot
- Superficial peroneal nerve (L5, branch of sciatic and common peroneal)-important to test both peroneal nerves with proximal fibula injuries because the nerve courses around the fibular head

- Motor: Resisted foot eversion (peroneus longus and brevis)
- Sensory: Lateral leg and foot

- Deep peroneal nerve (L4, branch of sciatic and common peroneal)
  - Motor: Resisted foot dorsiflexion (anterior tib, EHL, EDL)
  - Sensory: First toe webspace

- Popliteal, dorsalis pedis, and posterior tibial artery pulses → palpate with every injury to assess pulses proximal and distal to injury, especially important following knee dislocation because arterial injury is common.

Special Tests

- Ligamentous Knee Exam
  - Lachman—tibia pulled anteriorly with knee in 30° flexion, laxity with ACL injury (Fig. A.30)
  - Anterior/Posterior drawer—Tibia moved anteriorly or posteriorly to femur at 90° of knee flexion, laxity with ACL or PCL injury, respectively (Fig. A.31)
  - Varus/Valgus knee stability
    - Tests LCL and MCL integrity
    - Important to test with isolated injuries and with tibial plateau fractures (Fig. A.32)

- Meniscus Exam
  - Apley's compression test—With knee at 90° flexion, compress and rotate tibia against femur and assess for pain or clicking → positive with meniscal tear (Fig. A.33)
  - McMurray test—Flex and extend knee with varus and ER forces, then with valgus and IR forces → pain with either of the forces indicates medial and lateral meniscal injuries respectively

- Straight leg raise—evaluate extensor mechanism, inability to perform could be due to quad tendon rupture, patellar fracture, or patella tendon rupture
- Patellar apprehension—push patella laterally in extended knee, evaluate instability/pain with lateral movement
- Patellar compression—compress patella in extended knee and through ROM, pain can indicate chondral injury or patellofemoral syndrome

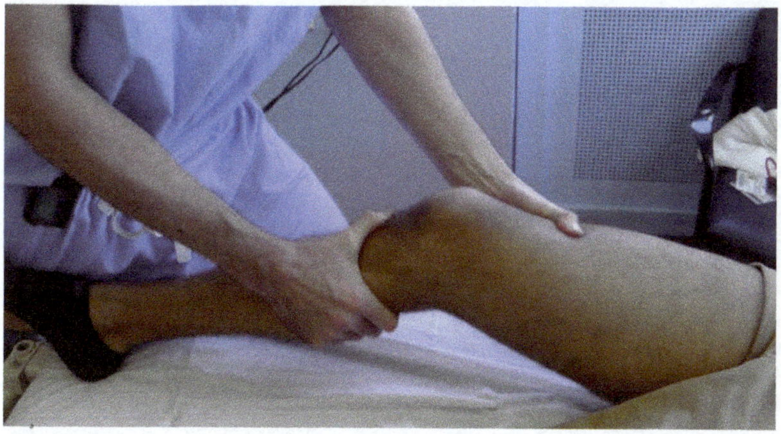

Fig. A.30 Lachman

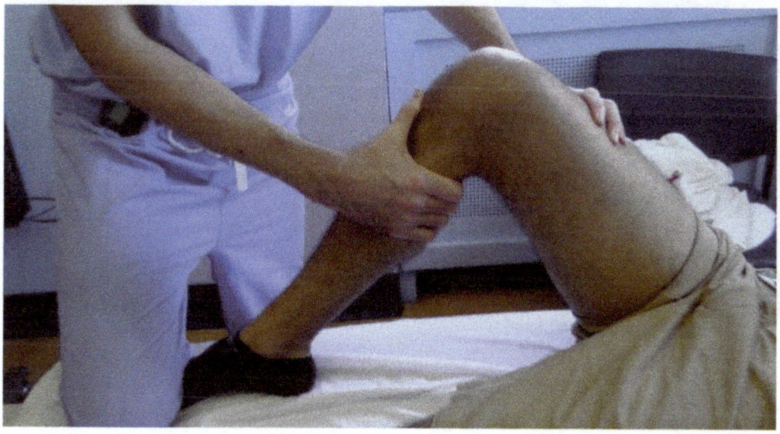

Fig. A.31 Anterior and posterior drawer test

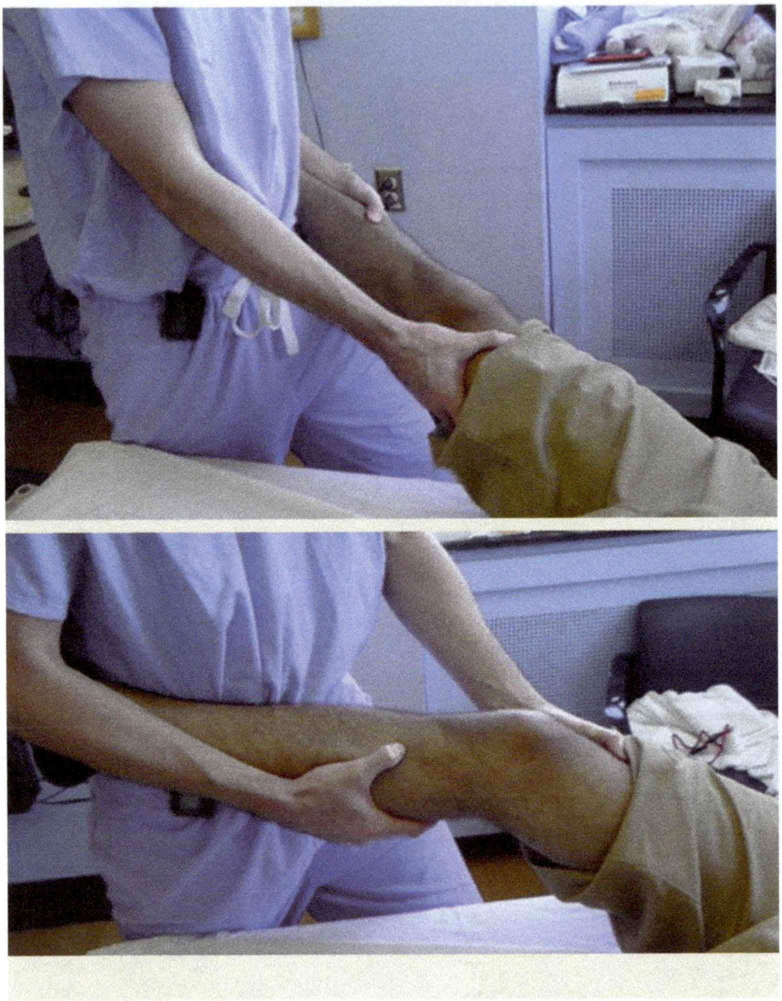

Fig. A.32 Varus/Valgus stress test

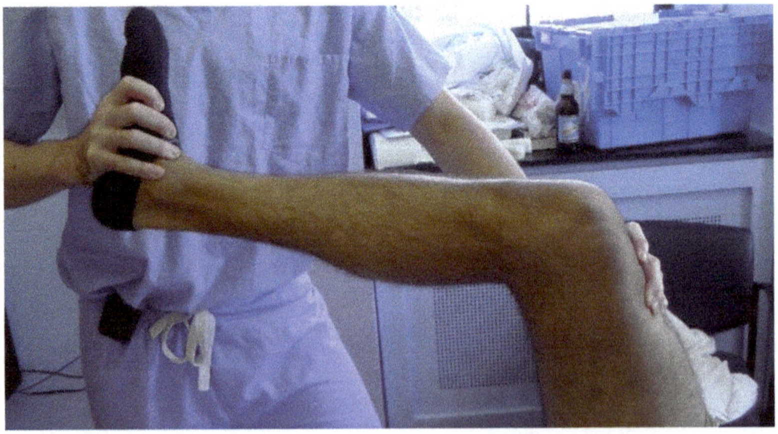

Fig. A.33 Apley's compression test

Foot and Ankle Exam

Inspection

- Begin by observing patient's stance and gait.
- Gait
  - Normal heel strike, toe-off gait, smooth and symmetrical
  - Limp
  - Antalgic gait
    - Shorter stance phase on injured side
    - Decreased walking velocity
  - "Steppage gait" → increase use of hip flexors → weak dorsiflexors
  - Foot slap → weak dorsiflexors
  - Gait tests
    - Heel walk → dorsiflexor strength
    - Toe walk → plantar flexor strength → Achilles tendon injury, nerve injury
    - Lateral foot walking → inversion strength → TP injury, nerve injury
- Stance (weight-bearing)
  - Posterior view
    - Normal ankle position is in slight valgus 5°–10°
    - Increase valgus deformity → tarsal coalition, planovalgus, PTT dysfunction, advanced RA, pilon fracture malunion
    - Varus deformity → neurologic disease
    - "Too many toes sign" → >1.5/2 toes visible from behind as a result of abduction of the forefoot and/or valgus angulation of hindfoot. Often result of PTT dysfunction.
    - Achilles tendonitis → "pump bump" → tender nodule at insertion site of Achilles tendon
  - Anterior view
    - Deformities
      - Hallux valgus
      - Hammertoes
      - Mallet toe
  - Medial view
    - Medial arch:
      - Normal apex height → 1 cm
      - Pes planus "flat foot" → PTT dysfunction, RA, Achilles tendon contraction, tarsal coalition, congenital
      - Pes cavus " high arch" → idiopathic, congenital, neurologic

    - Flexible: normal arch when non-weight bearing
  - Plantar view
    - Ulcers
    - Callus
- Skin
  - Color
    - Pallor → vascular disease
    - Congestion → venous insufficiency
- Swelling
  - Fracture, sprain, contusion
  - Medial side → deltoid ligament injury, medial malleolus injury
  - Lateral side → lateral malleolus injury, CFL injury, peroneal tendons
  - Posterior aspect → retrocalcaneal bursitis, Achilles tendinitis
- Shoe-wear

  Overpronation → more medial wear
  Oversupination → more lateral wear
  Narrow toe box → hallux valgus

Palpation

- Bony Palpation
  - Lateral malleolus → fracture
  - Medial malleolus → fracture
  - Calcaneus/heel → posterior → bursitis, spur, plantar surface → plantar fasciitis, anterior palpation → fracture,
  - Lateral aspect of talus → fracture
  - Sinus tarsi → soft spot on lateral hindfoot → subtalar joint pathology
  - Midfoot → fractures, Lisfranc joint, arthritis
  - MTP joints. First metatarsal-phalangeal joint and head of first metatarsal → bunion, metatarsalgia
  - Plantar surface → sesamoid bones of 1st MTP → sesamoiditis, fracture, AVN
- Soft Tissue Palpation
  - Medial ankle
    - Deltoid ligaments → sprain
    - PTT → directly posterior to medial malleolus → tendinitis, tear

    - lateral ankle
        - ATFL (anterior-lateral), CFL, PTFL → sprain
        - peroneal tendons → tendinitis, tear
    - Dorsum of the foot
        - Anterior tibialis tendon → medial aspect of ankle/foot → tendon pathology
        - EHL → lateral to Anterior tibialis tendon extending to 1st toe
    - Achilles tendon → tendinitis, Achilles rupture if defect present

Range of Motion

- Ankle: stabilize subtalar joint
    - dorsiflex/plantarflex → 20°/50°
- Subtalar: stabilize tibia
    - inversion/eversion → 5–10°/ 5°
- Forefoot: stabilize heel/hind foot and moved forefoot medially and laterally
    - abduction/adduction → 10°/20°
- Big toe
    - MTP joint: extension/flexion → 70°/45°
    - IP joint: extension/flexion → 0°/90°
- Lesser toes
    - MTP joint: extension/flexion → 40°/40°
    - PIP joint: extension/flexion → 0°/30°
    - DIP joint: extension/flexion → 30°/60°

Neurovascular

- Motor
    - Deep peroneal
        - (L4): tibialis anterior → foot inversion/dorsiflexion
        - (L5): EHL → great toe dorsiflexion
    - Tibial (S1): gastrocnemius → plantarflexion
    - Superficial peroneal: peroneus muscle → foot eversion

- Sensory
  - Saphenous (L4) → medial foot
  - Tibial (L5) → plantar foot
  - Superficial peroneal → dorsal foot
  - Deep peroneal (L5) → 1st dorsal webspace
  - Sural (S1) → lateral foot

Special Tests

- Anterior drawer test: stabilize the tibia proximal to the ankle and while holding the heel translate the ankle forward/anterior. compare to contralateral side. Positive test → increase laxity indicative of possible lateral ligament (ATFL) injury (Fig. A.34).

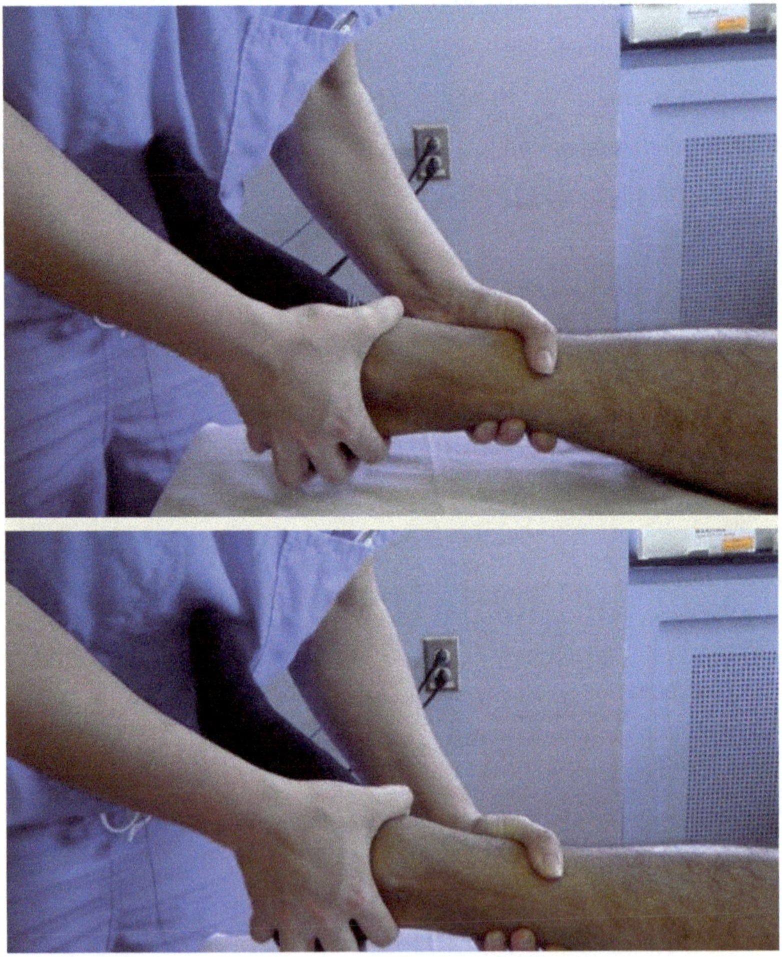

Fig. A.34 Ankle anterior drawer test

- Compression test/Mudler's sign: Squeeze the foot at the metatarsal heads. Positive test → pain/numbness/tingling indicative of interdigital neuroma.
- External rotation test: stabilize the tibia above ankle with knee flexed at 90° and externally rotate foot. Positive test → pain at ankle indicative of syndesmosis injury or deep deltoid injury.
- Eversion test: stabilize tibia and evert foot. Positive test → increase laxity indicative of deltoid ligament injury
- Heel rise: standing, rise up on toes. heel should go into varus. Positive test → no heel varus indicative of PTT dysfunction, fixed deformities
- Jack test: Can distinguish between flexible and rigid flat foot. While patient is standing, dorsiflex the big toe and observe whether there is a change in height of the medial arch. Flexible → dorsiflexion of big toe results in increase medial arch. Rigid → no change in medial arch height.
- Squeeze test: squeeze tibia and fibula together at mid-shaft. Positive test → pain at ankle indicative of syndesmotic injury
- Silfverskiold test: improved ankle dorsiflexion with knee flexed compared to extension → gastrocnemius tightness equivalent ankle dorsiflexion with knee flexed and extension → Achilles tendon
- Talar tilt: stabilize tibia above ankle, dorsiflex and invert foot. Positive test → laxity of ligaments indicative of superficial deltoid ligament injury
- Thompson's test: while patient prone, squeeze calf. Positive test → absent foot plantarflexion indicative of Achilles tendon rupture (Fig. A.35)
- Tinel's sign: tap nerve posterior to medial malleolus. Positive test → tingling/paresthesias indicative of tibial nerve entrapment.

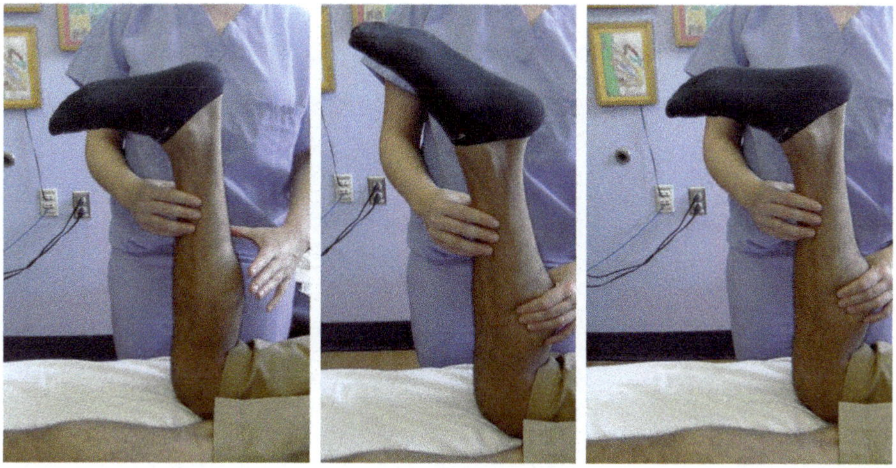

Fig. A.35 Thompson test, (far left): Neutral position, (middle): Negative Thompson test, (far right): Positive Thompson test

References

(1) Rapid Orthopedic Diagnosis.
(2) Netter's Concise Orthopaedic Anatomy.
(3) Clinical Examination in Orthopedics. Springer-Verlag London Limited 2012.
(a) Examination of wrist and hand. K Mohan Iyer.
(4) Morgan WJ, Slowman LS. Acute hand and wrist injuries in athletes: evaluation and management. J AM Acad Orthop Surg. 2001;9(6):389–400.
(5) Skinner H. Current diagnosis & treatment in orthopedics. New York: McGraw-Hill; 2013, Blacklick: McGraw-Hill Companies, The [Distributor].
(6) Bono CM, Garfin SR. Spine. Philadelphia: Lippincott Williams & Wilkins; 2004.
(7) Young CC, Niedfeldt MW, Morris GA, Eerkes, KJ. Clinical examination of the foot and ankle. Prim Care Clin Office Pract 2005;32:105–32.
(8) Dapore JP. On field and clinic assessment. In: Philbin TM editor. Sports injuries of the foot. Evolving diagnosis and treatment (chapter 1). New York: Springer; 2014. P. 1–8.
(9) Thordarson DB. Foot and ankle. Lippincott William & Wilkins; 2004. P. 24–40.
(10) Miller review of orthopedics. 6th ed. Elsevier Saunders; 2012.

Appendix B
Procedure Guides

William Giles Stuart Mackenzie

General Principles of Casting and Splinting	560
Upper Extremity Immobilization	561
Lower extremity immobilization	576
Reduction Techniques:	583
Local Anesthesia and Blocks	591
Intra-articular Injections and Aspirations	593
Saline Load Testing	598
Skeletal Traction	600
Nail Bed Laceration Repair	601
Compartment Check with "Stryker Needle"	603
Gardner Wells Tongs Traction	604
References	606

M.C. Makhni et al. (eds.), *Orthopedic Emergencies*,
DOI 10.1007/978-3-319-31524-9

General Principles of Casting and Splinting

- Padding a cast or splint is a balance between protecting the soft tissues and maintaining immobilization. Under-padding will result in skin breakdown or frank ulceration, whereas over-padding will compress over several days, leading to a loose cast or splint.
  - The proximal and distal extents of the cast/splint should have a cuff of soft roll of 3–4 layers, with a minimum of 2 layers of padding spanning the two extremes.
  - Bony prominences (i.e., olecranon process) require attention and adequate padding. It is easiest to lay 3–4 layers of soft roll directly over bony prominence.
  - Padding may also constrict soft tissues and neurovascular structures. Sites of concern include antecubital and popliteal fossas. By bulking padding from these areas and being careful not to flex the joint once material has been applied, complications can be avoided.
- Both plaster and fiberglass harden exothermically and care must be taken to decrease risk of thermal injury to the patient.
  - Never use water above room temperature when working with fiberglass. There is significant risk of thermal injury to the patient.
  - It is safe to use warm water with plaster to speed up drying time, though only for the experienced practitioner. Any delay will mean unusable, half-hardened plaster.
  - Plaster slabs for splinting should be eight layers thick for upper extremity and ten layers thick for lower extremity.
  - When applying circumferential cast, advance along limb with 50 % overlap, providing two layers of casting material at every level. With final overwrap, the cast should be at least three layers thick.
- Some practitioners prefer to overwrap plaster splints with soft roll prior to wrapping with compressive bandage. This helps secure plaster slab and allows for compressive bandage to be removed more easily in future. Others skip this step to save time and materials.
- If you have an assistant, ask them to hold the injured extremity underneath the stockinette and padding. Holding on top will pull out the material and damage the finished result.
- If a cast or mold is unfamiliar or complicated, consider not wetting the fiberglass. This will allow longer working time and fiberglass will slowly harden. Water can be applied after application to speed up process.

Upper Extremity Immobilization

1. **Coaptation splint—**Over-the-shoulder splint to immobilize the shoulder and humerus.

   Materials:

   - 6″ stockinette (approximate length=patient's arm span), three rolls of 6″ soft roll, three rolls of 6″ plaster, three 6″ compressive bandages, 2″ tape, large sling.

   Steps:

   - Measure the length of the plaster slab from the axilla of affected arm, distal around elbow flexed to 90°, then up the lateral arm, over top of the shoulder to the level of the middle 1/3 clavicle.
   - Using this length, create a plaster slab eight layers thick.
   - Place five layers of soft roll over the plaster on the skin side, three layers over the backside.
   - Cut one end of stockinette down the middle approximately 24″, long enough to pull the remaining stockinette up into the axilla, and tie the two cut ends around the neck comfortably.
   - Wet the plaster slab and place soft roll as described on either side.
   - Reach through the stockinette and pull the padded slab up the level of the split.
   - Tie the two cut ends using a hitch, cinched at the level of the split, and then pull the stockinette-wrapped slab up into the patient's axilla.
   - Tie the cut ends of stockinette around the patient's neck, so the slab is now secured along medial aspect of the arm.
   - Wrap the remaining slab down around the elbow flexed to 90°, then up the outside of the arm and over the shoulder. (Fig. B.1).
   - Starting at the elbow, wrap the splint using 6" compressive bandage, moving proximally. Be sure to wrap all the way up to the axilla and over shoulder, covering the entire splint.
   - Secure the compressive bandage using 2″ tape.
   - Apply mold to the splint.
   - Once dried, place the arm in a large sling to keep the elbow flexed to 90°.
   - The stockinette may be left tied about the neck, or cut off for patient comfort.

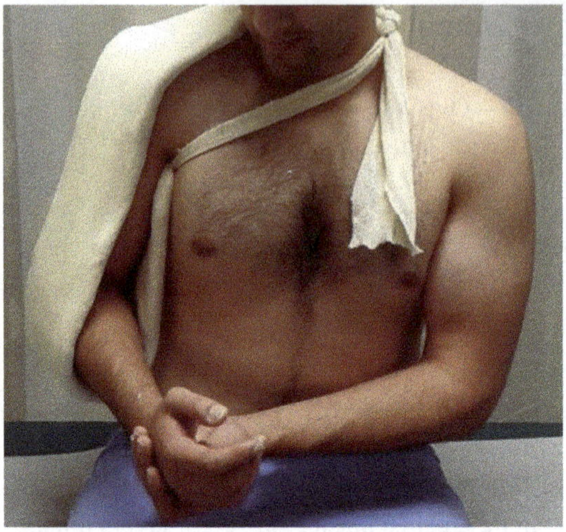

Fig. B.1 Coaptation splint with plaster slab located high in axilla, with elbow flexed to 90°, and extending all the way up and over the lateral shoulder

Alternatives:

- It is also possible to make this splint by first wrapping the affected arm in soft roll, and then applying plaster, though this technique can take longer and require an extra set of hand to hold your materials in place.
- The medial aspect of the slab should ideally extend proximal to the fracture site, though not so deep into the axilla as to risk skin breakdown.
- If the splint does not extend fully overtop of the shoulder, it will not effectively immobilize the joint.

Pearls:

- This splint is most commonly used for midshaft humerus fractures, which have a tendency to fall into varus angulation. By incorporating a valgus bump at the level of the medial elbow, angulation can be avoided. Try taping four 3″ compressive bandages together to create your bump. (Fig. B.2).

2. **Long arm splint—**Long splint used to immobilize distal humerus and elbow.

Materials:

- Three rolls of 4″ soft roll, three rolls of 4″ plaster, one roll of 4″ and 6″ compressive bandages, 2″ tape, sling.

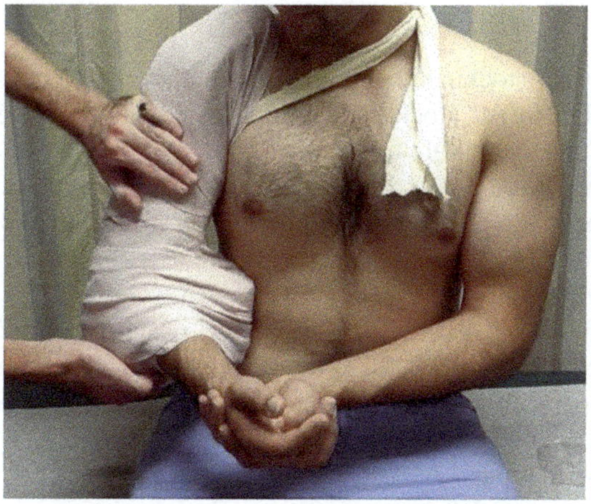

Fig. B.2 Coaptation splint with valgus bump in place at elbow, with a valgus mold being applied

Steps:

- Measure plaster slab from wrist to axilla with elbow at desired ` of flexion. Wrist can be immobilized according to injury. Measure side slab of plaster, can be placed medially or laterally, extending from midhumerus to midforearm with elbow flexed.
- Apply soft roll from wrist proximally to axilla. Place 3–4 layers of extra padding over posterior elbow.
- Wet plaster and place long plaster slab from wrist to axilla with elbow flexed and forearm in neutral rotation. Place side slab on medial or lateral aspect of elbow, whichever best suits the reduction, from midhumerus to midforearm.
- Wrap splint with compressive dressing.
- Secure with tape and apply mold.
- Place arm in sling.

Pearls:

- This splint should begin high on upper arm, but distal to axilla. Ensure proximal extent well padded to avoid soft tissue complications.

3. **Long arm cast**—Similar to principles of long arm splint above.

Materials:

- Two lengths of 3″ stockinette, three rolls of 4″ soft roll, one roll of 3″ fiberglass, two rolls of 4″ fiberglass.

Steps:

- Place length of stockinette about proximal upper arm with 4" of extra material at axilla. Roll 4″ stockinette onto affected hand from level of PIP joints to wrist. Cut a small hole for thumb.
- With elbow flexed at 90° and forearm in neutral rotation, roll on soft roll from midpalmar crease to three fingerbreadths distal to axilla. Tear a hole in the soft roll to allow for passage over thumb. Tear an extra piece of soft roll to cover first web space if necessary.
- Use a four-layer slab of 4″ soft roll to pad posterior elbow. Remove excess padding from antecubital fossa to prevent soft tissue impingement. Do not remove too much so that the antecubital fossa is uncovered and exposed directly to the fiberglass (Fig. B.3).
- Wet 3″ fiberglass and wrap once around the wrist and move distally, up to midpalmar crease. When passing through first webspace, use shears to cut transversely through 90% of material so only several strands of material remain, avoiding impingement in webspace. Stay clear of thenar eminence and MCP joints to allow full hand ROM. (Fig. B.4).
- Extend cast from wrist to three fingerbreadths distal to axilla using 4″ fiberglass. Advance 50% with each wrap. Ensure no further flexion of elbow during casting due to risk of compression of neurovascular structures by excess material.

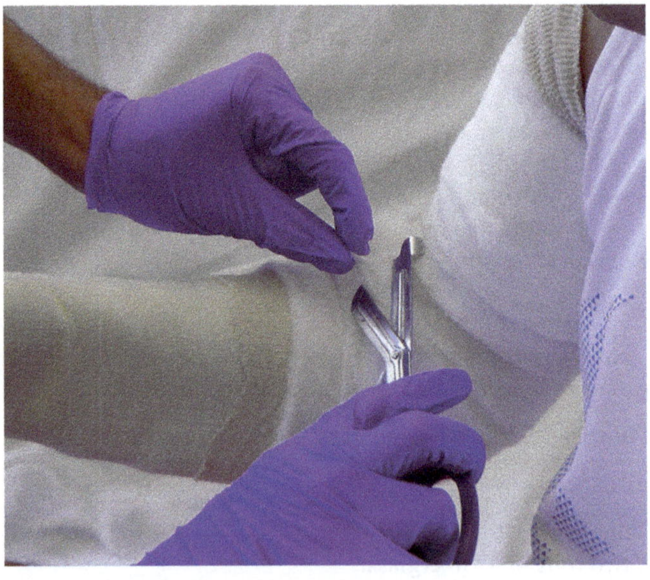

Fig. B.3 Removing soft roll from antecubital fossa

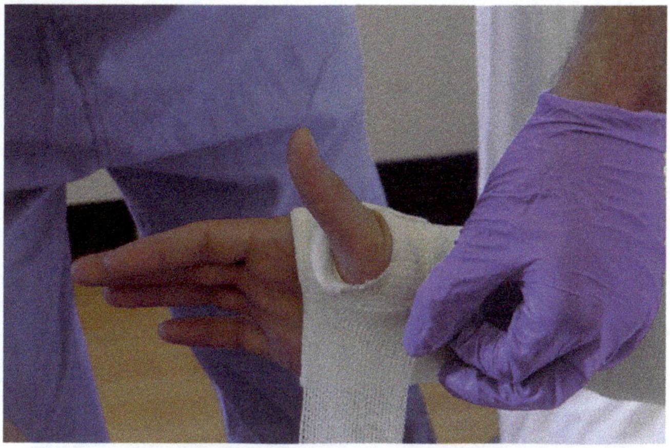

Fig. B.4 Leave only several strands of fiberglass in 1st webspace

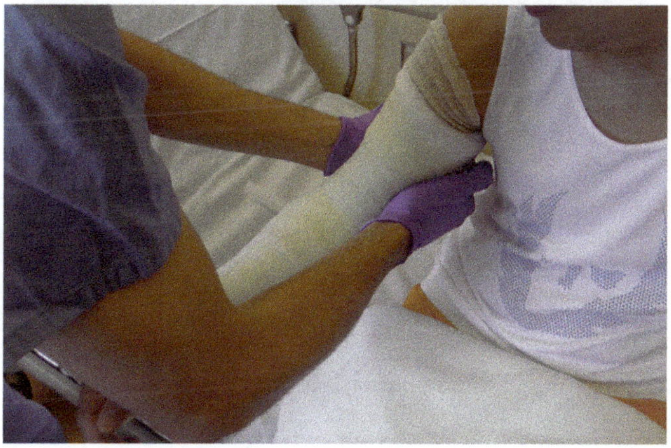

Fig. B.5 Applying supracondylar mold

- Cut thumbhole in distal stockinette and pull back over thumb and hand to create padded cuff at midpalmar crease. Fold proximal stockinette over to create padded cuff over proximal upper arm.
- Use fiberglass to apply final cast layer. Stay 1 cm from edge of cuff to protect soft tissues.
- In addition to reduction mold, apply interosseous mold to forearm, ensuring ovalization about forearm with cast index 0.8. Also consider supracondylar mold about elbow and palmar mold for well-fitting cast. (Fig. B.5).

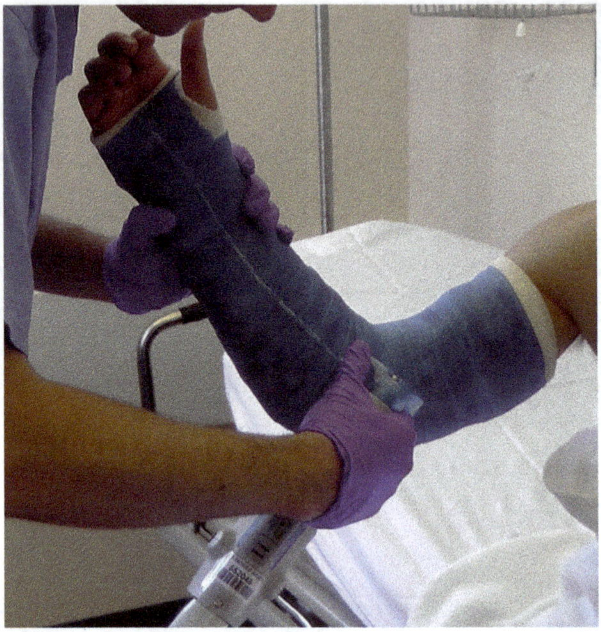

Fig. B.6 Bivalving cast

- Any for edema or compartment syndrome, the cast should be bivalved using a cast saw (Fig. B.6).
    - Cut down medial and lateral aspects of cast, using a cast spreader to ensure cast is fully released.
    - Loosely wrap in 4″ compressive bandage to protect cast.

Alternatives:

- Some providers prefer to first place a short arm cast, then rolling soft roll from forearm to axilla, and extending cast above elbow.

4. **Sugar tong splint**—Long forearm splint to immobilize elbow and wrist.

Materials:

- Two rolls of 4″ soft roll, two rolls of 4″ plaster, two rolls of 4″ compressive bandage, 2″ tape, sling.

Steps:

- Before reduction, measure out long plaster slab from midpalmar crease along volar forearm, proximally around posterior elbow flexed to 90°, and then back along dorsal forearm to metacarpal heads. Add 1–2″ of length to account for shrinking of plaster once wet.

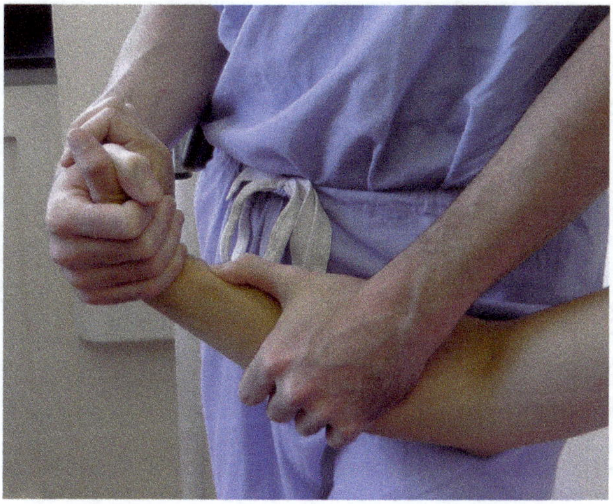

Fig. B.7 Hyperextension and axial traction are first applied to a Colles' fracture, followed by reduction with flexion through the fracture

- Reduction of a wrist fracture depends on the direction of deformity, as previously described. To achieve optimal reduction parameters, there are several steps:
  - The deformity must first be accentuated to unlock the fracture fragments.
  - Axial traction should be applied by gripping the patient's hand, while providing countertraction on the proximal forearm (Fig. B.7).
  - The deformity should then be reduced, while maintaining ulnar deviation of the wrist to bring the radius back out to length.
  - The reduction may then be assessed by palpation to feel for any bony step-off suggesting inadequate reduction.
  - If the reduction is unstable, an assistant may need to hold the wrist and forearm as the splint is placed.
- After reduction, roll on 4″ soft roll starting from the midpalmar crease of palm and progressing proximally to 4″ above elbow. Pad olecranon process well using an extra slab of padding 3–4 layers thick laid over posterior elbow (Fig. B.8).
- Wet plaster and apply at level of midpalmar crease along volar forearm, proximally around posterior elbow flexed to 90°, and then back along dorsal forearm to metacarpal heads (Fig. B.9).
- Fold wet plaster off of thenar eminence. Ensure it extends to midpalmar crease on volar palm, and to metacarpal heads on dorsal hand to allow unrestricted hand range of motion.
- Wrap splint in 4″ compressive bandage, beginning at the hand. Cut small hole in bandage to allow passage over thumb. Wrap proximally to above elbow (Fig. B.10).

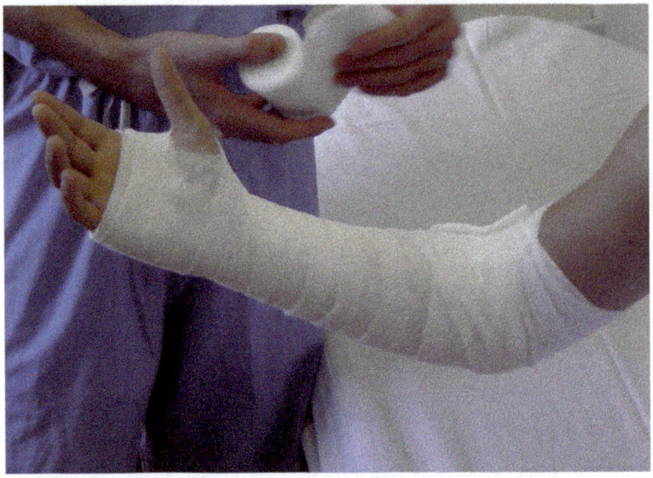

Fig. B.8 Well-padded forearm and elbow

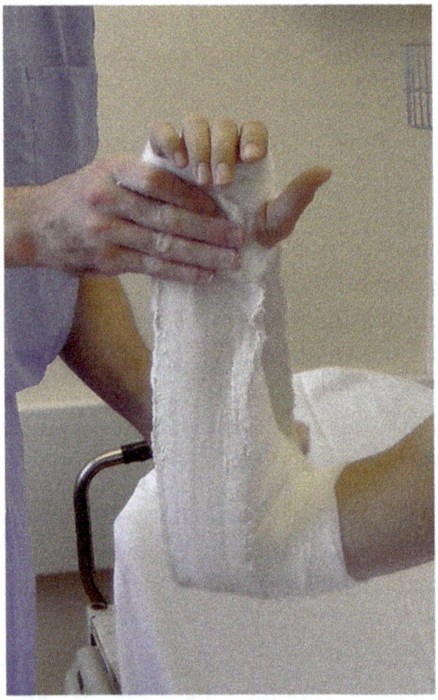

Fig. B.9 Applying plaster slab. Note the slab has been cut out for thenar eminence and stops at mid-palmar crease

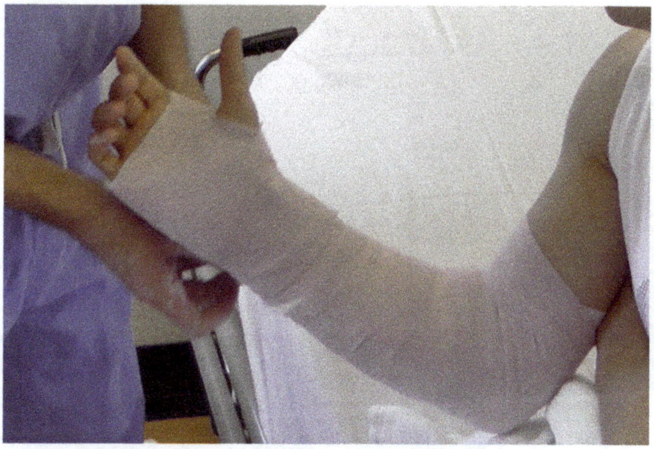

Fig. B.10 Wrapping sugar tong splint in compressive bandage

- Secure with tape and apply mold with elbow flexed to 90°.
  - The reduction of a wrist is held by a long, curved mold applied to the splint, maintaining radial height and restoring volar tilt (Fig. B.11).
- Place arm in sling.

Alternatives:

- Some prefer to create a long slab of soft roll and plaster, or using a prefabricated slab, and applying it in one step along forearm.

Pearls:

- If reduction involves axial traction and hanging arm from IV pole, the sugar tong splint may be applied while hanging, then taken down for molding (Fig. B.12).
- To achieve a well-fitting splint, over-roll the plaster with a 6″ compressive bandage under tension. After finishing the mold and plaster has hardened, remove 6″ compressive bandage and replace with untensioned 4″ compressive dressing.

5. **Ulnar gutter splint**—Forearm splint used to immobilize wrist and 4th/5th digits.

Materials:

- One roll of 3″ soft roll, one roll of 4″ soft roll, two rolls of 4″ plaster, one roll of 3″ compressive bandage, 2″ tape.

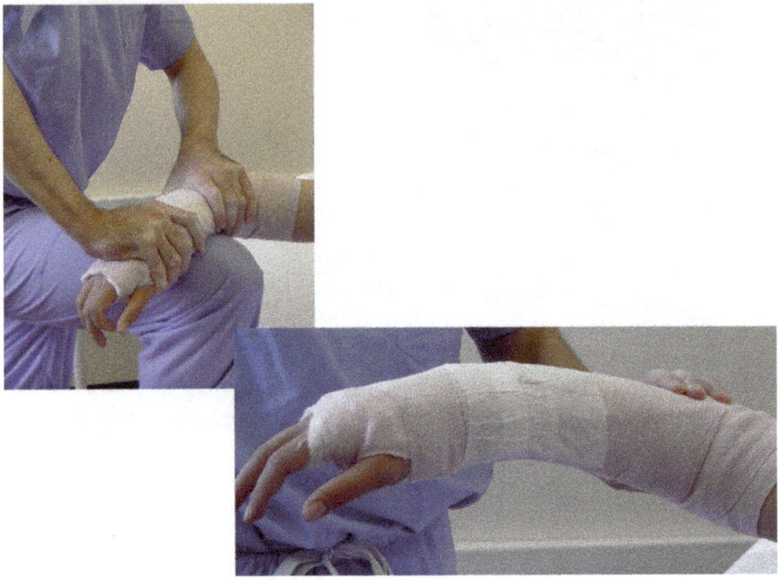

Fig. B.11 (**a**) Using three points of contact to create curved forearm mold. Note ulnar deviation of the wrist. (**b**) Long curved forearm mold in a sugar tong splint for a Colles' fracture

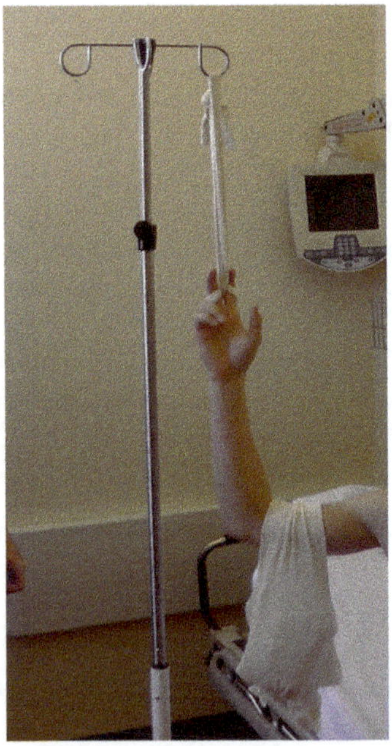

Fig. B.12 Hanging arm from IV pole with weight on upper arm

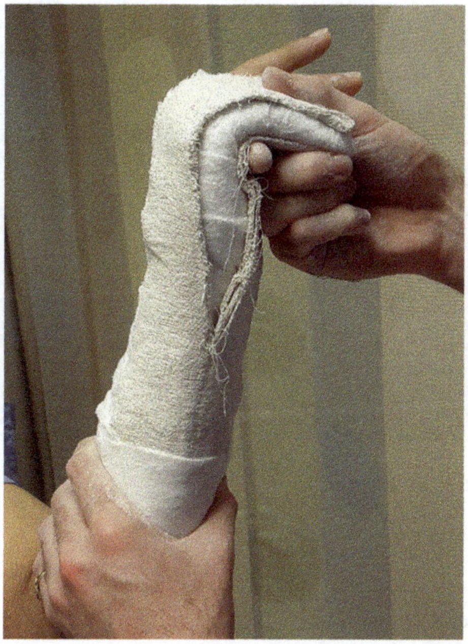

Fig. B.13 Ulnar gutter splint with plaster slab in place and digits flexed to intrinsic-plus position

Steps:

- Measure length of plaster from distal tips of 4th/5th digits along medial aspect of forearm to two fingerbreadths distal of level of antecubital fossa.
- Cut plaster longitudinally from distal end stopping at level of metacarpal bases to create two 2″ arms.
- Place piece of soft roll between 4th and 5th digits, then roll around both, keeping distal tips exposed.
- Wrap proximally with soft roll, about palm and wrist, to two fingerbreadths proximal to antecubital fossa.
- Wet plaster and lay along length of forearm, placing 2″ distal slabs over volar and dorsal 4th/5th digits. Stay medial to keep from impinging on 3rd digit.
- Flex 4th/5th digits to 90° at MCP joint, adjusting plaster so it does not wrinkle on volar aspect. Volar slab will now be longer than flexed digit and can be trimmed back with shears (Fig. B.13).
- Wrap splint from distal to proximal with 3″ compressive dressing.
- Apply mold and hold until dry.

Alternatives:

- Some practitioners prefer to splint digits in full extension.

Pearls:

- Always flex digits more than you think. Achieving intrinsic plus position with 4th/5th digits requires flexion at MCP joints of greater than 70°. This

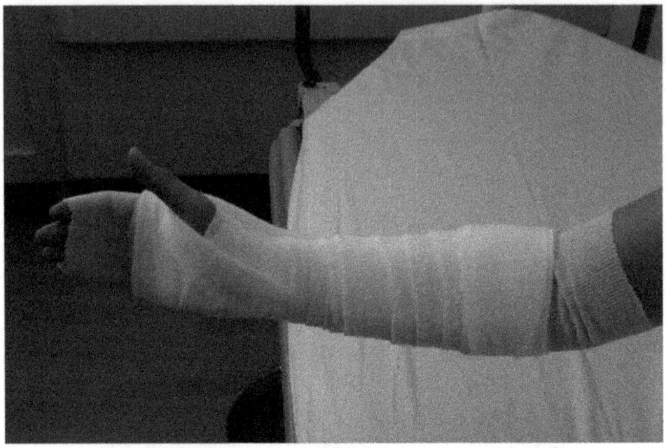

Fig. B.14 Soft roll for a short arm cast

requires more flexion than expected when viewing splint and can only be assessed on X-ray.

6. **Short arm cast:** Durable immobilization of forearm and wrist.

Materials:

- Forearm-length 4″ stockinette, one roll of 3″ soft roll, one roll of 3″ fiberglass.

Steps:

- For wrist fracture reduction technique, see Sugar Tong Splint section above.
- Roll 4″ stockinette onto affected arm from level of PIP joints to several inches above the elbow. Cut a small hole for thumb.
- Roll on soft roll from midpalmar crease to two fingerbreadths distal to antecubital fossa. Tear a hole in the soft roll to allow for passage over thumb. Tear an extra piece of soft roll to cover first web space if necessary (Fig. B.14).
- Wet 3″ fiberglass and wrap once around the wrist and move distally, up to midpalmar crease. When passing through first webspace, use shears to cut transversely through 90 % of material so only several strands of material remain, avoiding impingement in webspace. Stay clear of thenar eminence and MCP joints to allow full hand ROM (see Fig. B.14).
- Extend cast from wrist to two fingerbreadths distal to antecubital fossa (the goal is to allow full elbow flexion without impingement). Advance 50 % with each wrap (Fig. B.15).
- Cut thumb-hole in distal stockinette and pull back over thumb and hand to create padded cuff at midpalmar crease. Fold proximal stockinette over to create padded cuff distal to elbow.

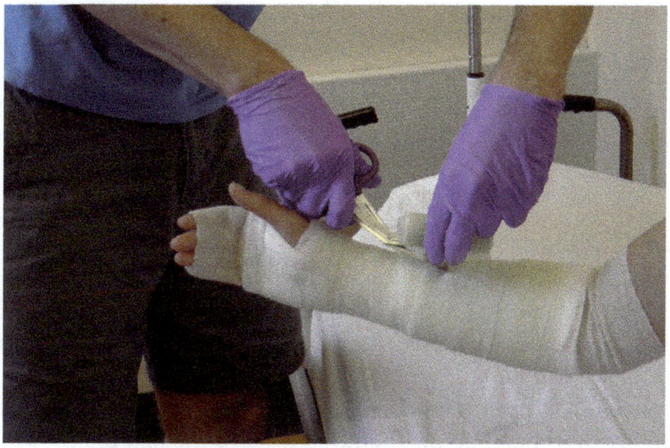

Fig. B.15 First layer of fiberglass for short arm cast

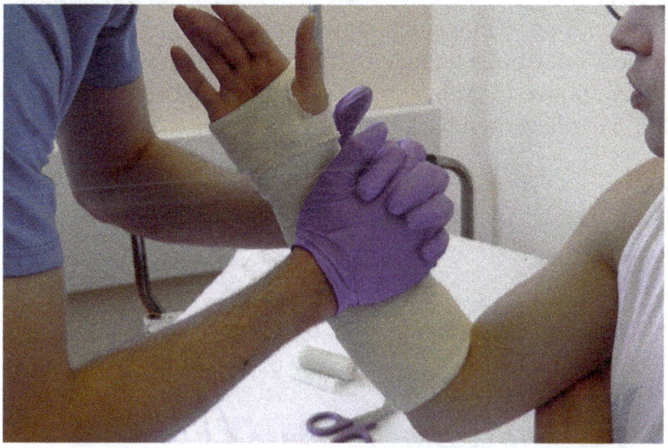

Fig. B.16 Applying interosseous forearm mold

- Use fiberglass to apply final cast layer. Stay 1 cm from edge of cuff to protect soft tissues.
- In addition to reduction mold, apply mold to forearm, ensuring ovalization about forearm with cast index 0.8. Also consider palmar mold for well-fitting cast (Fig. B.16).

Alternatives:

- If swelling prohibits circumferential casting, or casting is not indicated, a volar slab splint can be used:
  - Wrap wrist and forearm with soft roll as described and apply wet plaster slab over volar hand and forearm, from midpalmar crease to proximal forearm.
  - Fold plaster off of thenar eminence and wrap splint in compressive bandage.

7. **Thumb spica cast:** Immobilizes first MCP and wrist joints.

Materials:

- Six inches of 1″ stockinette, forearm-length 4″ stockinette, one roll of 3″ soft roll, two rolls of 2″ fiberglass, one roll of 3″ fiberglass.

Steps:

- Roll 4″ stockinette onto affected arm from level of PIP joints to several inches above the elbow. Cut a small hole for thumb.
- Cut a longitudinal slit halfway along 1″ stockinette and pull it over thumb so that slit is oriented towards first webspace, causing material to flare over lateral base of thumb.
- Roll on soft roll from midpalmar crease to two fingerbreadths distal to antecubital fossa. Extend up the thumb to level of the nail plate.
- Wet 2″ fiberglass and wrap once around the wrist and move distally, up to midpalmar crease. When passing through first webspace, use shears to cut transversely through 90% of material so only several strands of material remain, avoiding impingement in webspace.
- Continue around palm and approach base of thumb. Using shears, cut fiberglass and remove 1″ of material, turning roll into 1″ strip. Wrap distally to level of nail plate, then back to the palm, and just distal to wrist (Fig. B.17).

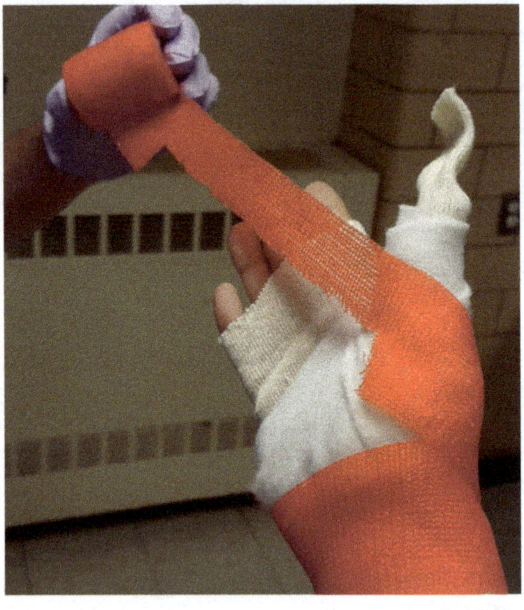

Fig. B.17 Trimming fiberglass to create 1" strip to wrap thumb for thumb spica cast

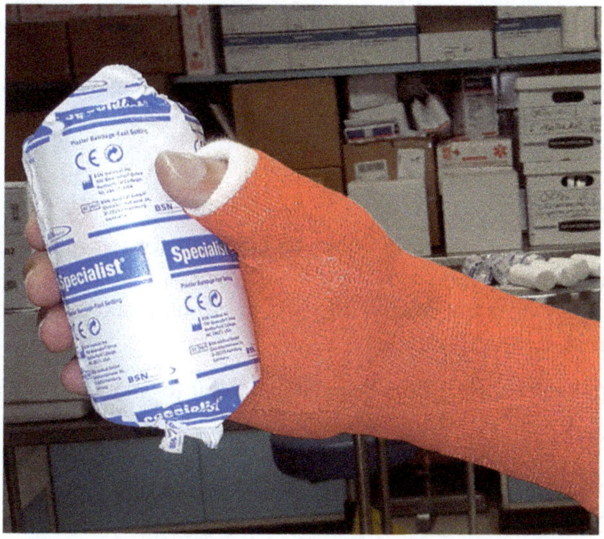

Fig. B.18 Holding a roll of plaster to achieve desired "soda can position" for thumb spica cast

- To achieve desired positioning, give patient a wrapped roll of fiberglass or plaster to gently squeeze, putting thumb in "soda can position." (abduction, extension, and pronation).
- Use 3″ fiberglass to extend cast from wrist to two fingerbreadths distal to antecubital fossa. (goal is to allow full elbow flexion without impingement) Advance 50 % with each wrap.
- Cut 3″ fiberglass roll off once proximal edge is reached and fold stockinette down to create a padded cuff. Using 3″ fiberglass, wrap two times around, 1 cm distal to cuff, and proceed distally to wrist, advancing 100 % with each wrap.
- Pull stockinette down thumb to create cuff at level of the nail, and then cut a hole in the hand stockinette and pull it proximally over hand and thumb to create cuff at the midpalmar crease.
- Use roll of 2″ fiberglass to apply final layer about hand and thumb.
- Have patient continue holding roll to achieve desired thumb positioning (Fig. B.18). Apply any further mold to forearm, ensuring ovalization about forearm with cast index 0.8.

Alternatives:

- If not planning on cast immobilization for definitive treatment, it can be easier and faster to immobilize the patient in a thumb spica splint.
- To create splint, positioning and padding are the same, with placement of 3″ or 4″ plaster slab along radial aspect of forearm, from distal to antecubital fossa, to distal thumb.
  - Cut distal 6″ of 8-layer plaster slab with two longitudinal cuts creating three equal plaster pieces. Apply wet plaster along proximal forearm and

then place one arm of plaster over dorsum of thumb, and other two arms on radial/ulnar aspects of thumb.
  - Wrap thumb to proximal forearm with compressive bandage, and have patient hold extra roll of plaster as described above to achieve appropriate thumb position.

Pearls:

- If 1″ fiberglass is available, it can be used just for the thumb, avoiding cutting the 2″ roll.
- If the injury does not involve the first proximal phalanx, it is not necessary to immobilize the IP joint.

8. **Metacarpal mitt splint:** Functional hand splint for metacarpal fractures.

Materials:

- One roll of 4″ soft roll, one roll of 4″ plaster, one roll of 4″ compressive bandage, 2″ tape.

Steps:

- Measure plaster slab from base of thumb, running over dorsum of the hand, around ulnar aspect and back along volar surface to base of thumb. Use shears to cut out space for thenar eminence on volar side.
- Wrap hand from wrist to PIP joints using soft roll, tear hole to allow passage over thumb.
- Wet plaster and apply to hand, positioning cutout to allow thumb ROM. Slab may be angled to immobilize desired MCP joint. For fifth metacarpal shaft or neck fractures, the slab can be angled to immobilize fifth MCP joint, while allowing ROM at second and third MCP joints.
- Wrap splint using compressive bandage. Apply desired mold.

Alternatives:

- Some practitioners prefer ulnar or radial gutter splints to the metacarpal mitt.

Pearls:

- Due to short length of plaster slab, overestimate length required due to shortening when plaster is wetted.

Lower extremity immobilization

9. **Long leg splint:** A long, well-padded splint for immobilization of both the knee and ankle (Fig. B.19).

Materials:

- Two rolls of 4″ soft roll, three rolls of 6″ soft roll, four rolls of 4″ plaster, four rolls of 6″ plaster, four rolls of 6″ compressive bandage, 2″ tape.

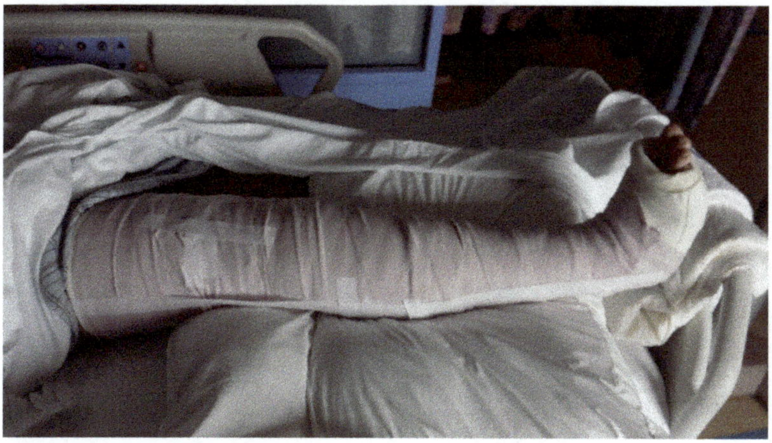

Fig. B.19 Example of long leg splint

Steps:

- Measure long 6″ plaster slab from 2–3 fingerbreadths distal to buttock crease, along posterior leg with knee flexed 10–15°, to toes. Measure two long 4″ plaster slabs from proximal thigh to plantar heel.
- Have assistant hold foot elevated with ankle in neutral position, and knee flexed 10–15°.
- Wrap foot and ankle using 4″ soft roll. Extend proximally using 6″ soft roll, ending at proximal thigh.
- Create plantar foot pad extending from toes to above ankle using five layers of 6″ soft roll.
- Wet posterior 6″ plaster slab and apply from level of toes to proximal thigh. Assistant can help hold slab in place, and several wraps of 4″ soft roll can help keep slab in place.
- Apply wet 4″ plaster slabs along medial and lateral aspects of leg, from proximal thigh to plantar hindfoot. Ensure that side and posterior slabs overlap to create rigid immobilization.
- Wrap leg from distal to proximal using 6″ compressive bandage, securing with tape.
- Apply mold and hold until plaster has set.

Alternatives:

- It is possible to first place a short leg splint, then extend proximally to create long leg splint, though without significant overlap of plaster slabs, knee immobilization will be less rigid.

Pearls:

- Extend splint as proximal as possible without impinging on inner groin or buttock to maximize immobilization.

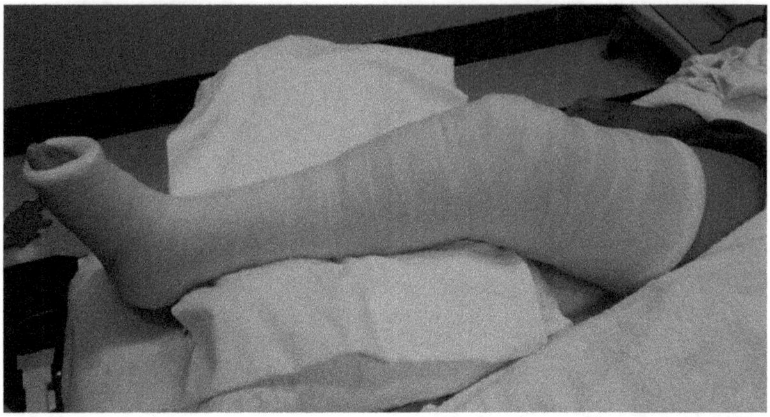

Fig. B.20 Example of long leg cast

- Knee should be flexed 10–15° to allow leg to swing through while non-weight bearing with axillary crutches, and to take tension off gastrocnemius for fracture reduction.
- This technique usually requires an assistant, though refer Honda et al. for single-provider technique. (J Orthop Trauma. 2011 Jun;25(6):385–90).

10. **Long leg cast:** Principles similar to long leg splint above (Fig. B.20).

Materials:

- Length of 4″ and 5″ stockinette, two rolls of 4″ soft roll, three rolls of 6″ soft roll, two rolls of 4″ fiberglass, three rolls of 6″ fiberglass.

Steps:

- Place 5″ stockinette about proximal thigh, with at least 4″ of material proximal and distal to intended level of cast. Place 4″ stockinette about midfoot with 4″ of material extending distal to MTP joint.
- Have assistant hold foot elevated with ankle in neutral position, and knee flexed 10–15°.
- Wrap foot and ankle using 4″ soft roll, starting just distal to MTP joint. Extend proximally using 6″ soft roll, ending at proximal thigh. Proximal and distal extent of soft roll should be four layers thick for padded cuff.
- Create plantar foot pad extending from base of toes to above ankle using five layers of 6″ soft roll. Ensure adequate padding over anterior knee, while debulking popliteal fossa of excess soft roll to avoid compression of neurovascular structures.
- Wrap foot and ankle using 4″ fiberglass, beginning at level of MTP joint, then extend proximally using 6″ fiberglass. Advance 50 % with each wrap. Ensure ankle and knee position remains constant to avoid wrinkles and soft tissue impingement.

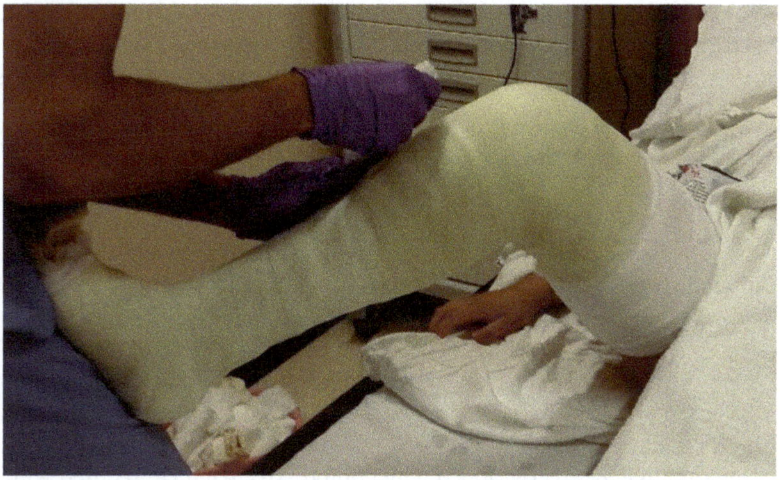

Fig. B.21 A short leg cast has been applied, then the soft roll is extended proximally and wrapped with fiberglass. The knee will be extended slightly to draw the cast out of the popliteal fossa

- Fold proximal and distal exposed stockinette back over cast to create padded cuff.
- Wrap leg again using 4″ and 6″ fiberglass, leaving 1 cm of exposed cuff proximally and distally to protect soft tissues.
- In addition to a reduction mold, the following molds should be considered for a well-fitting cast: distal femoral supracondylar mold, popliteal fossa mold, triangular anterior tibial mold and midfoot arch mold.

Alternatives:

- It is possible to first place a short leg cast, then extend proximally to create long leg cast, though any motion or change in knee flexion can weaken junction (Fig. B.21).
  - With this technique, the patient initially sits on edge of bed with leg hanging and knee flexed to 90°. Gravity aids in fracture alignment.
  - A short leg cast is applied, then with repositioning to supine position with leg elevated by assistant, knee flexed to 10–15°, and cast padding and fiberglass is extended proximally.

Pearls:

- Extend cast as proximal as possible without impinging on inner groin or buttock to maximize immobilization.
- Knee should be flexed 10–15° to allow leg to swing through while non-weight bearing with axillary crutches, and to take tension off gastrocnemius for fracture reduction.

- For patients who will be weight bearing on their cast, add reinforcement with six-layer fiberglass footplate from posterior ankle to distal extent of cast. Also ensure patient has a cast shoe to protect plantar surface from abrasion.

11. **Bulky Jones knee dressing:** Relative knee immobilization using soft roll. Can be used for any joint, though.

    Materials:

    - Three rolls of 6″ soft roll, two rolls of 6″ compressive bandage or knee immobilizer.

    Steps:

    - Wrap knee with soft roll beginning over proximal tibia and extending to distal femur. Continue wrapping back and forth over knee until dressing 5–6 layers thick.
    - Dressing may be overwrapped with compressive bandage secured with tape, or used in conjunction with a knee immobilizer.

12. **Short leg splint:** Boot-like immobilization of ankle and foot.

    Materials:

    - One roll of 4″ soft roll, two rolls of 6″ soft roll, two rolls of both 4″ and 6″ plaster, two rolls of 6″ compressive bandage, 2″ tape.

    Steps:

    - Measure out posterior plaster slab using 6″ roll from proximal tibia two fingerbreadths distal to popliteal fossa, to distal toes. Measure U-shaped plaster slab using 4″ roll from either side of proximal tibia and under plantar hindfoot.
    - Wrap foot and ankle with 4″ soft roll, with ankle held in neutral position, keeping distal toes exposed. Extend padding up leg using 6″ soft roll, stopping at level of tibial tubercle.
    - Create plantar foot pad extending from toes to above ankle using five layers of 6″ soft roll.
    - Wet 6″ plaster slab and apply to posterior leg, starting at level of tibial tubercle and wrapping under plantar foot. Fold any excess over to create foot plate ending under distal toes.
    - Apply 4″ U-shaped slab from lateral proximal calf, under plantar hind/midfoot, and back up medial calf. Overlap side and posterior slabs to ensure rigid splint (Fig. B.22).
    - Wrap splint using 6″ compressive bandage, and secure with tape.
    - Apply reduction mold while maintaining ankle dorsiflexion to neutral (unless contraindicated) (Fig. B.23).

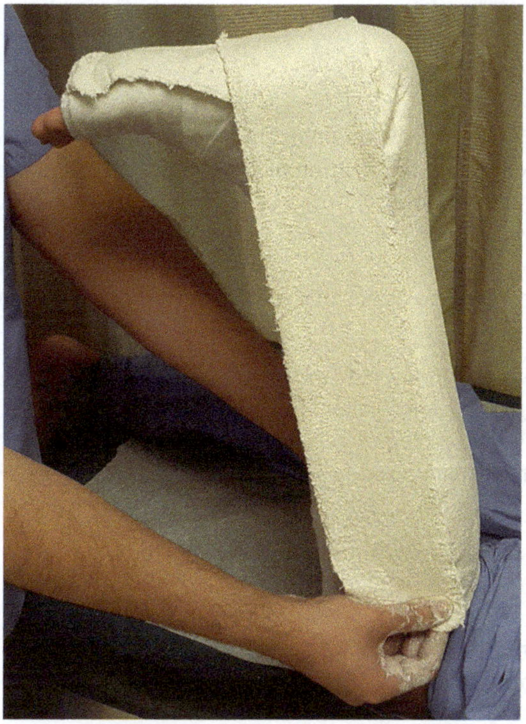

Fig. B.22 With patient positioned prone, the short leg splint can be applied by one person. Notice the u-shaped slab overlapping the posterior slab

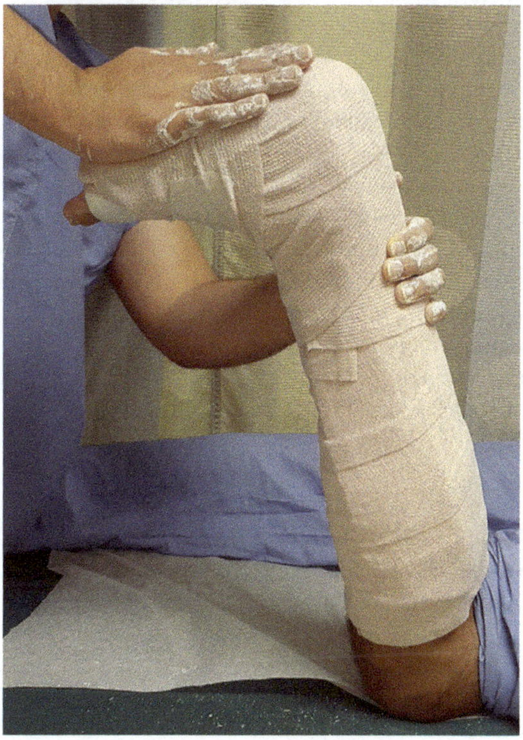

Fig. B.23 The ankle is internally rotated with dorsiflexion of the foot in this short leg splint

Alternatives:

- While less cumbersome and potentially better tolerated, short leg splints do not provide true immobilization of distal tibia and fibula. This would require a long leg cast or splint.

Pearls:

- There are various positions that aid in application of the short leg splint and cast.
  - When working alone, have the patient either sit on the edge of the bed with leg dangling, or have the patient flip prone and flex knee to 90°. The prone position allows for materials to hang from foot, making it easier for one person.
  - With an assistant, position supine and have them stand at level of knee, bend hip and knee to 90°, and have them hold patient's toes with extended arm.

13. **Short leg cast:** Principles similar to short leg splint above.

Materials:

- Two lengths of 4″ stockinette, one roll of 4″ soft roll, two rolls of 6″ soft roll, two rolls of 4″ fiberglass, two rolls of 6″ fiberglass.

Steps:

- Place 4″ stockinette about proximal calf and knee, with at least 4″ of material proximal and distal to intended level of cast. Place 4″ stockinette about midfoot with 4″ of material extending distal to MTP joint.
- Wrap foot and ankle using 4″ soft roll, starting distal to MTP joint. Extend proximally using 6″ soft roll to level of tibial tubercle.
- Create plantar footpad extending from toes to above ankle using five layers of 6″ soft roll.
- Wrap foot and ankle using 4″ fiberglass, beginning at level of MTP joint and maintaining ankle in neutral position. Extend proximally using 6″ fiberglass, ending at level of tibial tubercle. Advance 50 % with each wrap.
- Fold over stockinette at toes and proximal tibia to create padded cuff.
- Wrap leg again using 4″ and 6″ fiberglass, leaving 1 cm of exposed cuff proximally and distally to protect soft tissues.
- In addition to a reduction mold, a triangular anterior tibial mold, and midfoot arch mold, should be considered for a well-fitting cast.

Pearls:

- See positioning under Short Leg Splint above.
- For patients who will be weight bearing on their cast, add reinforcement with six layer fiberglass foot plate from posterior ankle to distal extent of cast. Also ensure patient has a cast shoe to protect plantar surface from abrasion.

Reduction Techniques:

1. **Shoulder dislocations:**
   Anterior: Most common form with over a dozen of anterior shoulder relocation techniques in the literature, here are some most commonly utilized. It is possible to try with analgesics and intra-articular blocks, though some reductions will require sedation.

   - FARES: Stands for fast, easy, reliable, and safe.
     - Lay patient supine with affected arm adducted to side with elbow extended.
     - Stand on affected side and grip hand, pulling axial traction and making small, short vertical oscillations, as though shaking their hand.
     - Gradually abducted arm with continued oscillations.
     - At 90° of abduction, externally rotate shoulder, and continue abduction and oscillations.
     - Reduction should occur by 120° of abduction.
   - Traction–countertraction (Fig. B.24).
     - Place a sheet around patient's torso, into affected axilla.
     - Lay patient supine and give sheet to assistant or tie to far bed rail.
     - Abduct affected arm 45° and pull axial and inferior traction.
     - Continue to hold traction as musculature about shoulder tires.
     - Attempts of gentle external rotation and lateral traction with maintained axial traction can aid humeral head in clearing glenoid.
   - Stimson: Gradual relocation using hanging weights (Fig. B.25).
     - Raise patient's bed and have then lie prone with affected arm hanging from bed.
     - Using 4″ stockinette, hang 5 lb weight from patient's wrist. Alternatively, using broad pieces of tape to secure weight, being careful of possible skin damage. Do not consider in patients with fragile skin.
     - Allow gentle downward traction for 15–20 min.
     - May increase weights to 10 lbs.
   - After reduction, place patient in sling and make non-weight bearing.
     - For unstable shoulders, or noncompliant patients, consider using sling with attached swath to keep arm adducted at all times.
       - If only a simple sling is available, a 6″ compressive bandage can be used to swath the affected arm.

   Posterior: Much less common; classic mechanisms include seizure and electric shock. Difficult without proper sedation.

- Forward flex the affected arm to 90°, adduct across midline and internally rotate.
- Assistant on contralateral side of body can pull axial traction while humeral head is milked anteriorly.
- External rotation can sometimes help with final reduction.

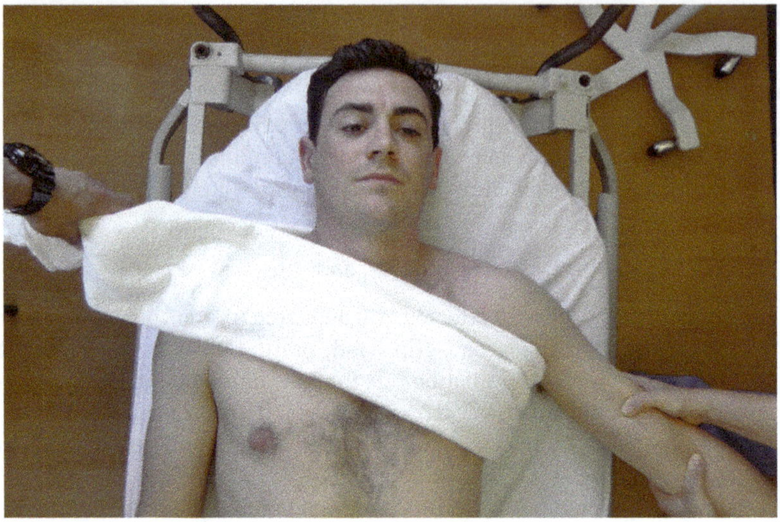

Fig. B.24 Traction–countertraction shoulder reduction technique

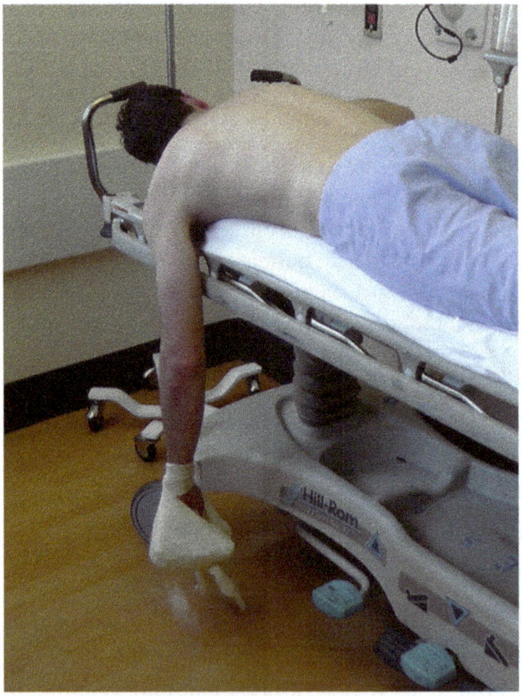

Fig. B.25 Stimson shoulder reduction technique

Inferior: Also referred to as luxatio erecta humeri, this presents as arm fixed in abduction.

- Traction–countertraction.

With setup as described above, pull axial and superior traction.
Gradually decrease abduction to reduce the humeral head.

- Two-step technique
  - Basis is to convert an inferior dislocation to an anterior dislocation, before reduction using an anterior dislocation technique.
  - Standing at patient's head, push downward directed force on lateral mid-shaft humerus, while pulling upwards on medial elbow, levering humeral head out from below glenoid, into an anterior position.

2. **Elbow dislocations:**
   - Most dislocations are posterolateral and can be either simple or complex (with associated fractures).
   - To reduce dislocation, the patient can be positioned either prone or supine on the bed (Fig. B.26).

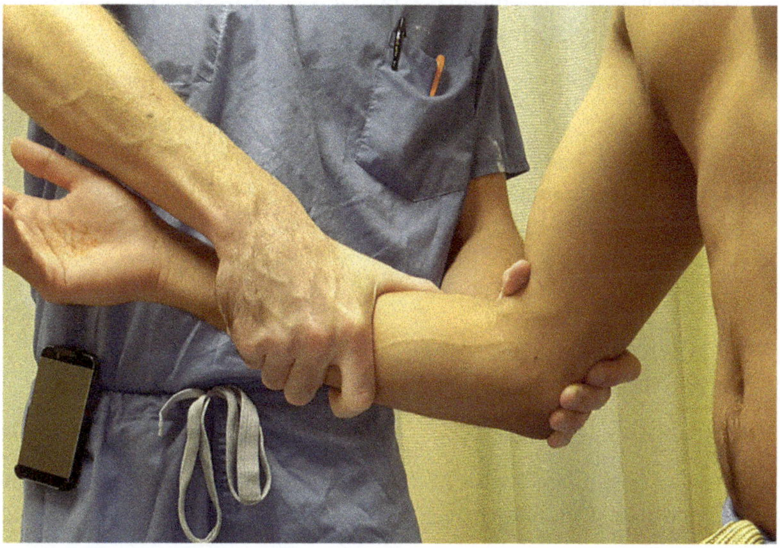

Fig. B.26 Elbow reduction technique with one hand pulling traction while the other reduces the olecranon around the distal humerus

- ◦ Flex elbow to 90° and have an assistant supinate forearm and pull axial traction in line with the deformity.
- ◦ Grip elbow with both hands, placing thumbs on posterior olecranon, pushing anteriorly while pulling countertraction, milking olecranon back around distal humerus.
- ◦ After reduction achieved, assess elbow stability. Focus on varus/valgus instability with elbow extension, supinating and pronating forearm.
- ◦ Splint elbow using long arm splint with elbow flexed to 90°.

3. **Metacarpophalangeal dislocations:**
   - Similar to interphalangeal joint dislocations, most MCP dislocations are dorsal.
   - Reduction should avoid axial traction or hyperextension, and can be achieved with joint flexion.
     - ◦ Wrist flexion also helps by relieving tension on flexor tendons.
4. **Interphalangeal dislocations:**
   - PIP dorsal dislocations
     - ◦ Simple—middle phalanx in contact with condyle of proximal phalanx.
     - ◦ Complex— shortening with bayonetting of middle phalanx over proximal phalanx.
     - ◦ Reduction should not involve axial traction, especially in complex dislocations, or volar plate may become interposed in joint.
       - ▪ Reduce with hyperextension of middle phalanx with palmar-directed force.
     - ◦ Once reduced, buddy tape to bordering digit.
     - ◦ May require open reduction if closed attempts fail.
     - ◦ Associated intra-articular middle phalanx fracture requires dorsal extension-blocking splint.
   - PIP volar dislocations.
     - ◦ Reduce with dorsal-directed force and axial traction.
     - ◦ Immobilize in extension due to central slip injury.
   - Rotatory PIP dislocations.
     - ◦ To relax lateral bands, flex MCP and PIP to 90° and pull axial traction.
     - ◦ May require open reduction.
   - Dorsal DIP dislocations.
     - ◦ Similar to PIP dorsal dislocations, there is risk of volar plate interposition with axial traction.
       - ▪ Attempt reduction with hyperextension and palmar-directed force.

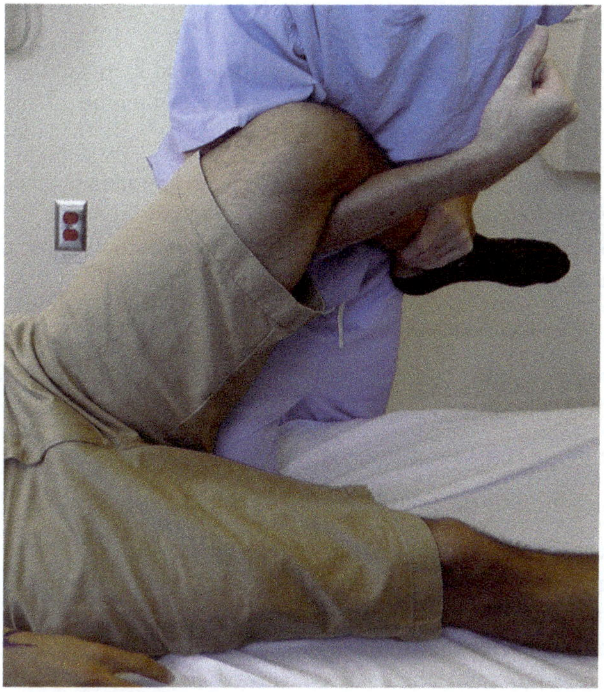

Fig. B.27 Allis hip reduction maneuver

5. **Hip dislocations**

- Hip dislocations require adequate sedation to allow for reduction without further injury to the articular surface. Reduction under anesthesia in OR should be considered if sedation is not possible in the ER.
- Hip dislocations can be either anterior or posterior, with posterior being most common.
- Reduction maneuvers, regardless of direction of dislocation, involve axial traction in line with the deformity.
  - An assistant can help placing their hands on pelvis and providing countertraction.
  - Allis maneuver involves axial traction with gradual hip flexion combined with alternating internal and external rotation (Fig. B.27).
  - Hip adduction may help complete reduction.
- Once reduced, the hip can be brought through its range of motion to assess stability and an AP pelvis X-ray should be obtained to confirm reduction.
- The ipsilateral knee should be placed in a knee immobilizer and CT should be obtained to assess for any intra-articular fracture.

6. **Knee dislocations**

- Anterior dislocations are most common, followed by posterior.
- Neurovascular injuries are common, and an evaluation of distal pulses on presentation will dictate treatment.
    - Any concern for ischemia should result in immediate reduction attempt using traction–countertraction prior to any imaging.
    - Obtain ankle-brachial index even in cases where pulses are present before and after reduction.
- Patients without concern for acute ischemia should have X-ray prior to reduction.
    - Reduction attempts should avoid unnecessary force due to risk of further neurovascular injury.
        - Sedation helps limit force required.
    - Reduction involves axial traction to distract the joint.
        - An assistant for countertraction is helpful.
        - Anterior knee dislocations require axial traction with anterior translation of distal femur.
        - Posterior knee dislocations require axial traction with anterior translation of proximal tibia.
    - Any medial/lateral translation or rotation of tibia should be corrected as axial traction is applied.
    - Splint knee at 20–30° after reduction and obtain X-ray.

7. **Ankle fracture–dislocations**

- Ankle fractures and subsequent dislocations are the result of rotational injuries. Reduction requires identifying the forces of injury, and performing the reverse.
    - Classifying the injury using the Lauge-Hansen classification helps conceptualize the injury.
- Closed injuries that present to the ED can be impending importunate fractures and should be promptly evaluated with neurovascular exam.
    - Any concern for the soft tissues requires urgent reduction prior to imaging.
- Fractures often result in lateral displacement of talus under tibial plafond due to external rotation through ankle at the time of injury.
    - Reduction requires internal rotation of the foot (Fig. B.28).
    - One hand should be placed over distal medial tibia, while the other hand is placed on lateral midfoot, firmly rotating foot internally (see Fig. B.23).
- While a provider can manually internally rotate the foot, Quigley's maneuver allows for a hands-free reduction to facilitate immobilization (Fig. B.29).

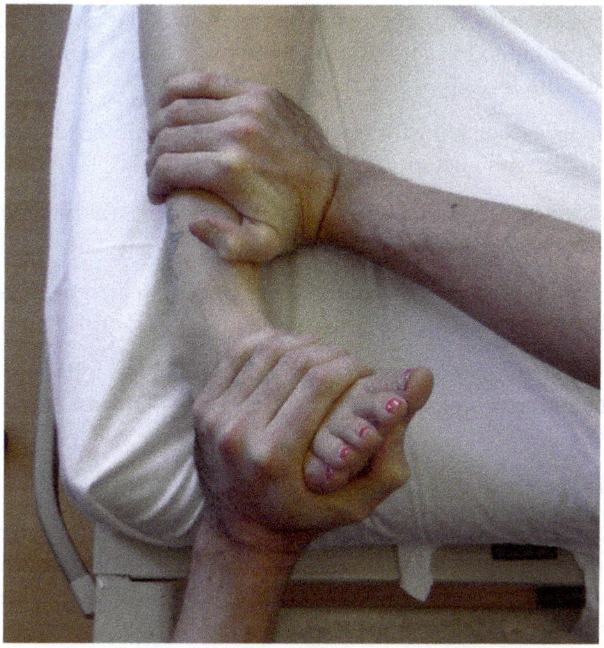

Fig. B.28 Internal rotation for reduction of ankle fracture–dislocation

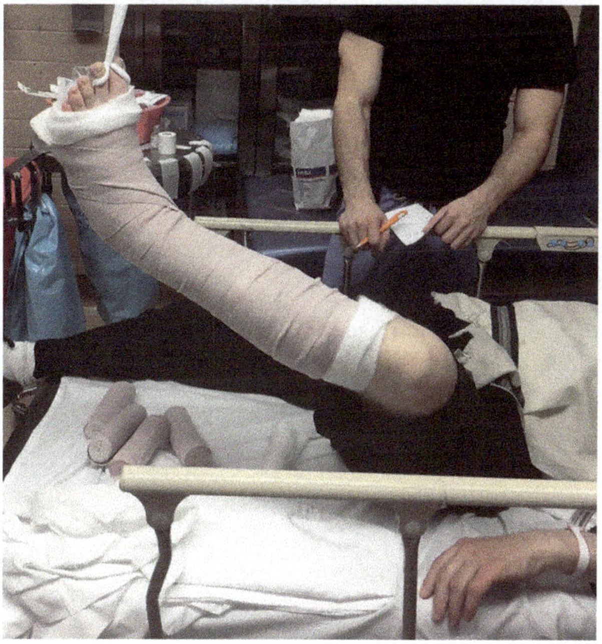

Fig. B.29 Quigley's ankle reduction maneuver

  - Suspend the affected foot by the hallux from an IV pole using stockinette.
  - Allow the hip to fall into external rotation, while will internally rotate and supinate the foot.

- Dislocations associated with fractures of the tibial posterior malleolus can be very unstable with posterior displacement of the talus.

  - Reduction requires plantar flexion of the foot, axial traction and anterior translation the hindfoot.

- Unstable ankle fracture–dislocations can be best treated by reduction, immediately followed by X-ray to confirm reduction, prior to splinting.

  - True immobilization of the ankle requires long leg splinting, though many providers elect for short leg splints in operative cases for ease of mobilization.

8. **Subtalar dislocations**

- The talus often remains in place with medial or lateral displacement of the calcaneus, dislocating both the talonavicular and talocalcaneal joints.
- Early reduction of closed dislocations is important to relieve pressure on skin and soft tissues.
- Reducing medial and lateral dislocations requires adequate sedation with knee flexion and ankle plantar flexion.

  - An assistant can hold countertraction at the knee, or the knee can be flexed over the end of the bed.

- Medial dislocations are fixed in supination.

  - To reduce, pull traction on plantar-flexed foot, hypersupinate and then pronate the foot.

- Lateral dislocations are fixed in pronation.

  - To reduce, pull traction on plantar-flexed foot, hyperpronate and then supinate the foot.

- Reduction should be confirmed via X-ray, with CT for any concern of intra-articular fracture.

  - Obtain CT in all cases of high-energy trauma.

Local Anesthesia and Blocks

1. **Local anesthesia:**

- Fast-acting local anesthesia in the ER is most commonly lidocaine, either 1 % or 2 % solutions.

  - No more than 4 mg/kg lidocaine can be safely used.
    - Up to 7 mg/kg for solutions containing epinephrine.
  - Maximum effect is reached in 5 min, and will last for 30–60 min.
- Functional anesthesia can be provided using intradermal/intramuscular lidocaine about the periphery of lacerations or infected sites.
  - Using a 22 G needle, infiltrate lidocaine by injecting through damaged tissue, first aspirating to ensure the needle is not intravascular.
    - Work in systematic fashion to infiltrate lidocaine around the entire periphery of wound.
  - Lidocaine is only moderately effective for incision and drainage of abscesses due to the low pH of infected tissues.

2. **Hematoma block:**
   - For extra-articular fractures, analgesia can be provided by infiltrating lidocaine directly into the fracture hematoma, allowing lidocaine to diffuse about injury.
     - Fractures presenting greater than one day after injury are less amenable to hematoma blocks due to clotting of hematoma.
   - Review imaging of fracture, palpate bony defect and consider local neurovascular structures to determine a safe path for injection.
     - Prepare site sterilely and use 22 G needle to inject fracture site.
     - Prior to infiltrating, attempt to aspirate hematoma. Successful access should produce small amount of sanguinous aspirate.
   - If bone is encountered when needle advanced, infiltrate small amount of lidocaine below periosteum. Walk needle along bone until it falls into fracture defect and hematoma.
3. **Intra-articular blocks:**
   - Infiltration of local anesthetic into a joint is an effective method to provide analgesia for a reduction of a dislocation or intra-articular fracture.
   - See section below for approach to performing intra-articular injections.
4. **Median nerve block:**
   - Identify the palmaris longus and flexor carpi radialis tendons by having the patient oppose the thumb and fifth digits while flexing the wrist.
     - The injection site will be between these two tendons at the level of the proximal wrist crease.
     - If the patient lacks the palmaris longus tendon, the site will be ulnar to the flexor carpi radialis tendon.

- Insert 25 G needle at the insertion site and advance approximately 1 cm, at which depth the needle will pop through the flexor retinaculum.
- Infiltrate 5 cc 1 % lidocaine into the carpal tunnel.
- Inject a further 1 cc 1 % lidocaine as the needle is withdrawn to anesthetize the superficial palmar branch.

5. **Radial nerve block:**

   - The superficial sensory branch of the radial nerve divides at the level of the radial styloid to provide sensation over the dorsum of the hand.
   - This block involves infiltrating up to 10 cc of 1 % lidocaine about the wrist to anesthetize all the sensory branches
   - Begin with subcutaneous injection of 2 cc of 1 % lidocaine over the lateral aspect of the radial styloid, lateral to the palpable radial artery.
   - Redirect the needle towards the Lister's tubercle to continue infiltrating lidocaine subcutaneously, creating a large wheal that extends to the middle of the dorsum of the wrist.
     - It may be necessary to inject several times to achieve this block.

6. **Ulnar nerve block:**

   - The injection site is located at the level of the distal ulna, proximal to the wrist, dorsal to the flexor carpi ulnaris tendon.
   - Advance needle below the flexor carpi ulnaris tendon and inject 5 cc of 1 % lidocaine to anesthetize the ulnar nerve.

7. **Digital block:**

   - Each digit is innervated by a pair of volar and dorsal digital nerves. By infiltrating local anesthetic proximal to the digit, these four nerves may be blocked, providing anesthesia of the entire digit.
   - Subcutaneous technique
     - Using a 25 G needle, create a subcutaneous wheal of 1 % lidocaine just proximal to webspace on radial side of digit. This will the block dorsal digital nerve.
     - Advance needle volarly and infiltrate 1 cc 1 % lidocaine just under volar skin to block volar digital nerve.
     - Aspirate to ensure needle is not in digital vessel.
     - Repeat on ulnar aspect of digit.
   - Transmetacarpal technique.
     - This technique targets the common volar digital nerve between the metacarpal heads prior to its division.
     - Insert 25 G needle through volar skin at the distal palmar crease on the radial side of the metacarpal neck of the digit to be anesthetized.
     - Infiltrate 2 cc of 1 % lidocaine.
     - Repeat on ulnar aspect of metacarpal.

- Circumferential ring blocks should not be used as increase in pressure can result in necrosis.

Intra-articular Injections and Aspirations

- Each intra-articular injection should be performed in a sterile fashion to minimize the risk of introducing infectious pathogens.
  - The site can be prepped with Betadine, chlorhexidine, or isopropyl alcohol as per institutional protocol.
  - Sterile gloves should be used by the practitioner and all instruments should be opened sterilely.
  - After each procedure, the site should be dressed using clean gauze.
- Aspirations should be performed using at least a 20 ga needle to allow aspiration of thick substances.
- Patients with larger body habitus may require use of a longer spinal needle in order to get intra-articular access.
- For large joints (e.g., knee), 10 cc of 1 % lidocaine is sufficient for intra-articular blocks. Smaller joints require proportionally less lidocaine. (e.g., 5 cc of 1 % lidocaine for an elbow).

1. **Shoulder:**
   - Anterior approach: (Fig. B.30).
     - Palpate the coracoid process on anterior aspect of shoulder.
     - Place needle 1 cm lateral to coracoid process and just medial to head to humerus. Advance posteriorly, angled slightly superolaterally.
   - Posterior approach: (Fig. B.31).
     - Palpate the posterolateral corner of the acromion, then mark a point two fingerbreadths inferior and one fingerbreadth medial.
     - The needle should be oriented obliquely from this point towards the coracoid process, which can be palpated with other hand on anterior aspect of the shoulder.
2. **Elbow:**
   - Lateral approach: (Fig. B.32).
     - On the lateral aspect of elbow, palpate the soft spot in the center of a triangle made by three bony landmarks:
       - Lateral epicondyle of distal humerus, radial head, and olecranon.
     - Enter the elbow joint from this point by staying parallel to the articular surface of the radial head.

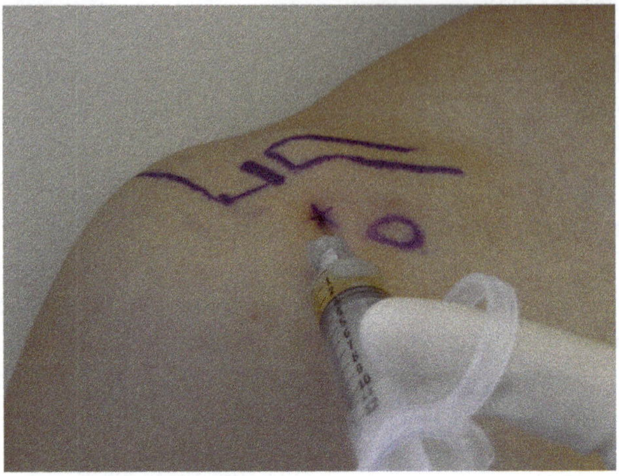

Fig. B.30 Anterior approach shoulder aspiration

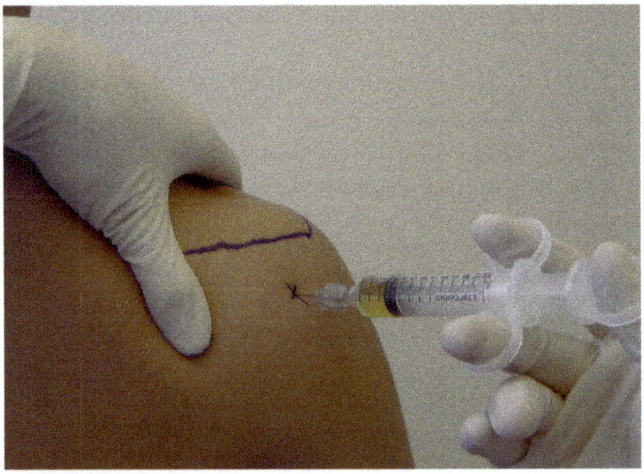

Fig. B.31 Posterior approach shoulder aspiration

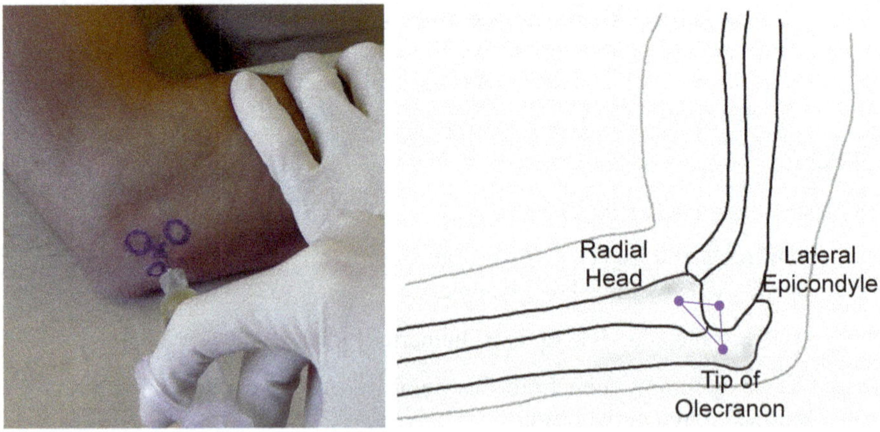

Fig. B.32 Lateral approach elbow aspiration

- Posterior approach:

With elbow flexed to 90°, palpate the soft spot approximately 5 mm proximal to olecranon process on posterior aspect of elbow.

Staying perpendicular to humerus, it is possible to pass directly through triceps and into the olecranon fossa.

3. **Wrist:**

- Dorsal approach:
  - This approach utilizes the interval between the 3rd and 4th extensor compartments of the wrist, which is the position for the 3–4 portal for wrist arthroscopy.
  - Palpate Lister's tubercle on dorsum of wrist.
  - Insert the needle distal to the tubercle, at the level of the joint, between the extensor pollicis longus and extensor digitorum communis tendons (Fig. B.33).
  - Angle the needle distally to account for the volar tilt of the articular surface.
- Medial approach:
  - Palpate the soft spot between the extensor carpi ulnaris and flexor carpi ulnaris tendons of the medial aspect of the wrist.
  - Pass the needle between the tendons distal to the ulnar styloid (Fig. B.34).

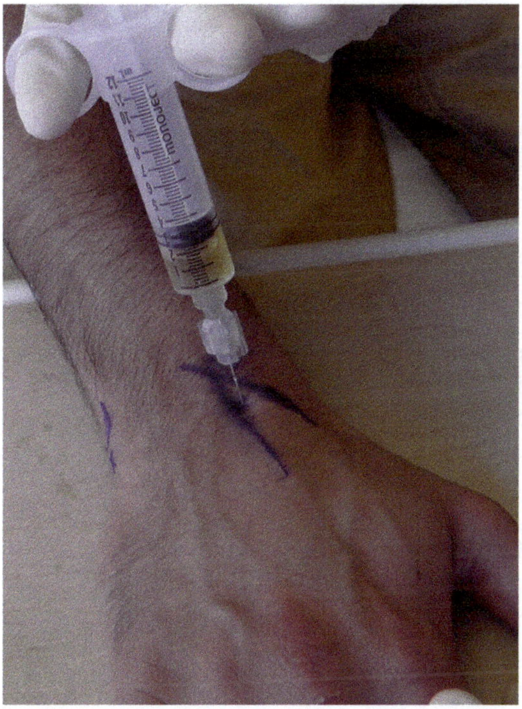

Fig. B.33 Dorsal approach wrist aspiration

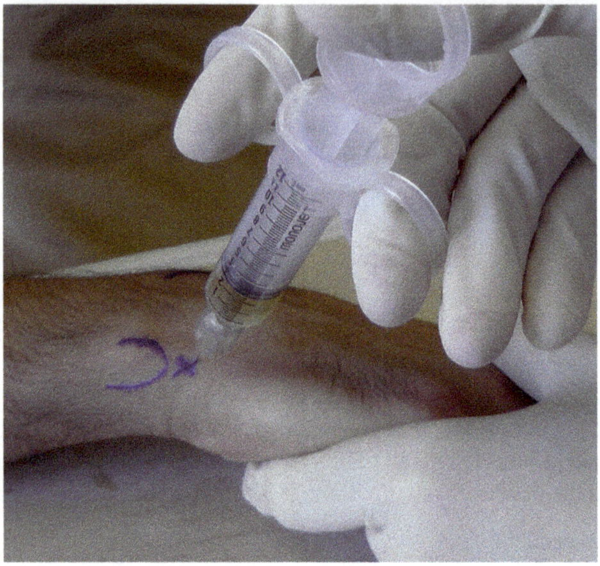

Fig. B.34 Medial approach wrist aspiration

4. **Knee:**

- Anterolateral approach: (Fig. B.35).
  - Same site as lateral portal for knee arthroscopy.
  - With knee flexed to 90°, palpate the lateral joint line and borders of the patellar tendon.
  - Mark the soft spot lateral to the patellar tendon, and above the joint line.
  - Orient needle superomedially, into femoral notch.
- Superolateral approach: (Fig. B.36).
  - Mark superolateral corner of the patella with patient supine and knee fully extended.
  - With one hand, sublux the patella laterally as the needle is passed deep into it, towards the femoral notch.

5. **Ankle:**

- Whether aspirating synovial fluid or injecting local anesthetic for an ankle fracture, an anteromedial approach to the ankle is most common.
  - Patient should be positioned supine and anterior ankle prepped in a sterile fashion.

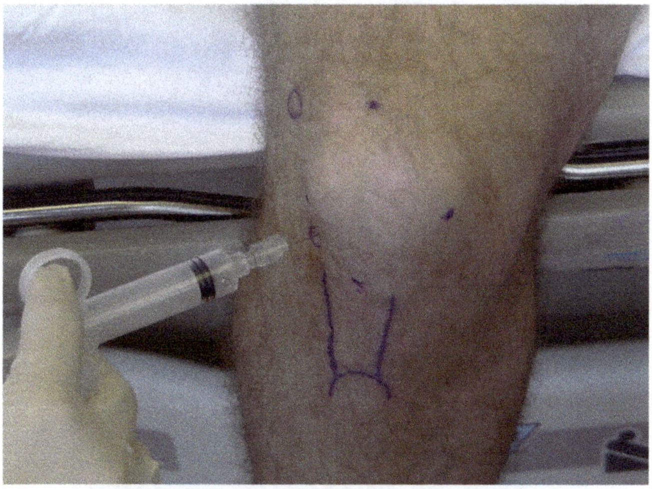

Fig. B.35 Anterolateral approach knee aspiration

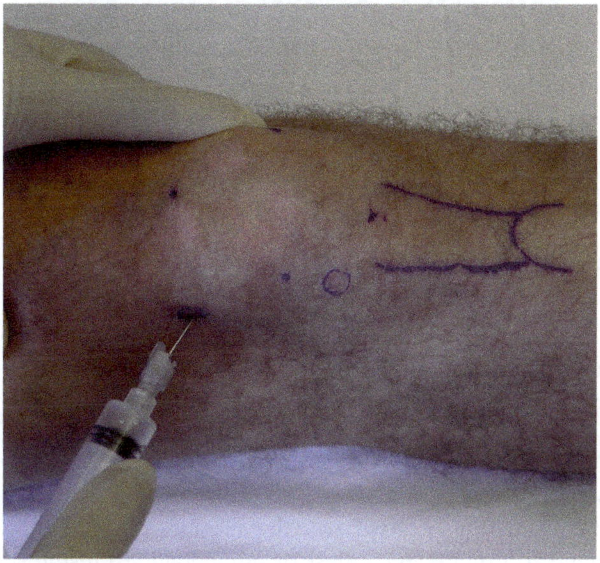

Fig. B.36 Superolateral approach knee aspiration

- Identify the tibialis anterior tendon at the level of the joint and introduce a 20 ga needle just medial to the tendon (Fig. B.37).
  - Angle needle caudal to account for slope of the dome of the talus.
  - Aspirate to confirm intra-articular placement.
- For an intra-articular block, 10 cc of 1 % lidocaine is sufficient.

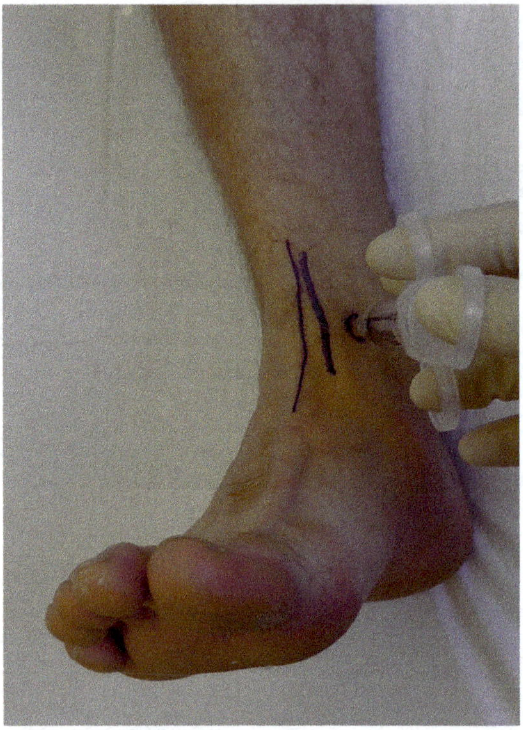

Fig. B.37 Anterior approach ankle aspiration

Saline Load Testing

- Saline load tests can help determine whether a traumatic arthrotomy is present in a periarticular laceration (Fig. B.38).
  - The sensitivity of saline load tests has been repeatedly called into question in the literature, especially when evaluating for small arthrotomies <1 cm.
    - Saline load tests still remain common practice for many practitioner during the evaluation of a periarticular laceration, though any concern for traumatic arthrotomy, regardless of saline load test result, should be taken for irrigation and debridement.
  - CT scans are a viable alternative to detect intra-articular air after traumatic arthrotomy, as described by Konda et al. (J Orthop Trauma. 2013).
- Traumatic arthrotomies require IV antibiotics and irrigation and debridement in the OR.
- This test must be performed in a sterile fashion, and involves injecting large volumes of sterile saline into the involved joint to distend the capsule.

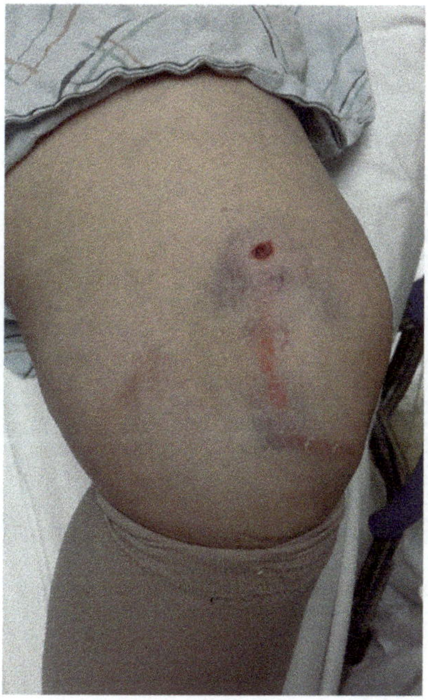

Fig. B.38 Periarticular puncture wound with concern for traumatic arthrotomy

  - A positive test is confirmed by visualization of saline in the injury site.
  - Some practitioners tint the saline using methylene blue dye to make it easier to visualize.

- Choose an approach that keeps the injection site away from the laceration, to avoid any false-positive test results (Fig. B.39).
- Capsule distension is very uncomfortable and patients should receive PO or IV analgesia prior.

  - It is also possible to consider an intra-articular block, though results vary.

- Joints require various amounts of saline corresponding to their relative sizes.

  - Knee: Inject >155 cc of saline for 95 % sensitivity.
  - Elbow: Inject >40 cc of saline for 95 % sensitivity.
  - Wrist: Inject >3 cc of saline for 95 % sensitivity.
  - Ankle: Inject >30 cc of saline for 95 % sensitivity.

- After completing the saline load test, attempt to remove as much of the injected saline as possible from the joint.

  - This can be facilitated by an assistant compressing the joint space.
  - It is very challenging to remove the full volume.

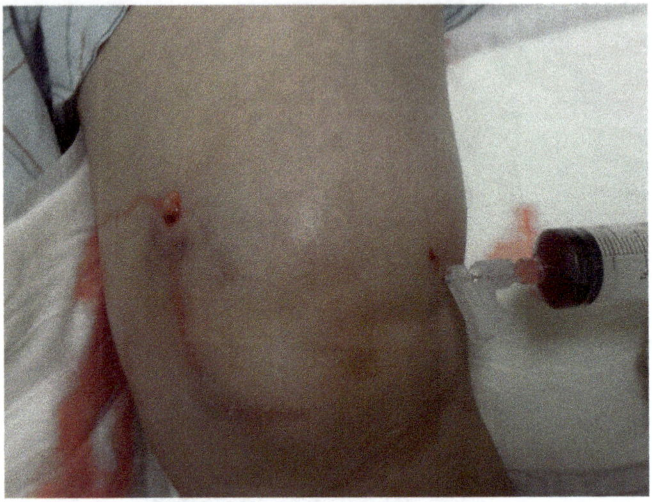

Fig. B.39 Positive saline load test with injected saline draining from puncture wound

Skeletal Traction

- Skeletal traction can be used prior to definitive surgical treatment to improve pain and prevent shortening from soft tissue contraction. The most common sites of insertion for traction pins are in the distal femur and proximal tibia. Typically insert pins from side that has neurovascular structures most at risk.
- Apply local analgesia at the proposed site of pin entry subcutaneously and also deeper until reaching tibia.
- ***Distal femur pin***
  - With patient supine, place a large bump under the knee and flex it to 90°
  - Locate a starting point two finger breadths above the adductor tubercle medially onto the anterior 1/3 of the femur.
  - Make 1 cm longitudinal stab incision and then turn knife 90° to make a small 1 cm stab transverse incision through IT band, then spread with clamp bluntly down to bone.
  - Drill traction pin bicortically through soft tissue on the contralateral side and exit through the skin, keeping the tract parallel to the knee joint.
- ***Proximal tibia pin***
  - With patient supine, rotate knee into neutral or slight internal rotation to facilitate access.
  - Make a 1 cm stab incision 2 cm posterior and 2 cm distal to tibial tuberosity on lateral aspect of leg. Avoid the common peroneal nerve which wraps behind the fibular head.

  - Spread with clamp bluntly down to bone.
  - Place a traction pin (or large K-wire) on the bone at above site.
  - Drill pin across the bone, maintaining a trajectory parallel to the joint . Avoid starting on the dense anterior cortex and then be mindful not to stray too anteriorly through the anterior tibial cortex.

- Once traction pin is in place, connect pin weight over pulley at end of bed and onto the traction pin.

Nail Bed Laceration Repair

- Nail bed lacerations are commonly associated with distal phalanx tip, or "tuft," fractures. Because of the subcutaneous location of the distal phalanx in this region, these nail bed lacerations with associated fractures are considered open fractures (Fig. B.40).
- Unlike most open fractures, these can do quite well with thorough bedside irrigation and debridement and primary closure in the emergency room.
- Before starting, explain to the patient the risk that once removed, the nail may or may not regrow, and even if it does it may be deformed.

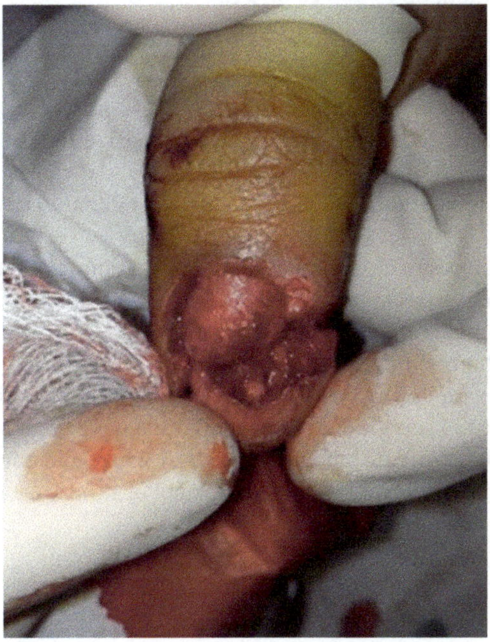

Fig. B.40 Nailbed laceration

- Begin by cleaning the digit proximally with alcohol wipes and performing digital block to the finger of interest.
- You may use a digital tourniquet to control bleeding but this is usually not necessary, and hemostasis can be maintained throughout the procedure with intermittent use of sterile gauze.
  - Very important to not forget to remove at end of procedure! Patient may still be anesthetized so may not realize if tourniquet is left on under dressing, which can result in necrosis of the digit.
  - A simple potential option for a digital tourniquet includes cutting a finger section off of a glove, then cutting the end of the digit piece, and rolling this over the finger of interest from distally to proximally.
- Wash the skin with dilute Betadine and rinse with saline solution.
- With sterile gloves, remove the nail plate if still attached. Be careful not to further traumatize the nail bed; use curved clamps with the tips pointed towards the nail and away from the underlying nail bed and spread along the undersurface of the nail until able to gently life the nail out.
- Thoroughly irrigate the wound and remove and macroscopic foreign body debris noted.
  - Use digital manipulation and sterile tools to gently manipulate the tissue to ensure the entire wound is irrigated well.
  - Ideally use a small irrigation tip such as an angiocatheter to perform high volume irrigation, up to 500 cc or 1 L.
  - Irrigation can begin with dilute Betadine but must end with saline solution as to remove the Betadine from the wound.
- Repair the nail bed laceration with 5-0 or 6-0 fast-absorbing chromic or catgut with the tails cut very short. Be very gentle as these sutures can pull out and damage the nail bed further.
- Similar results seen in literature with use of Dermabond to cover nail bed laceration (Fig. B.41).
- Use 4-0 nylon sutures to close adjacent soft tissue injuries. In the pediatric population, absorbable sutures can be used instead of nylons to avoid difficulty of suture removal in the office.
- After washing the nail plate in Betadine then saline solution, replace it into the nail fold; this (or the foil from the inner sterile wrapper holding the suture) can serve as a spacer to keep the fold open to allow the new nail to emerge.
- Dress repair with petroleum gauze, followed by gauze and compressive dressing. Extend dressing above level of the wrist to anchor it in place (Fig. B.42).

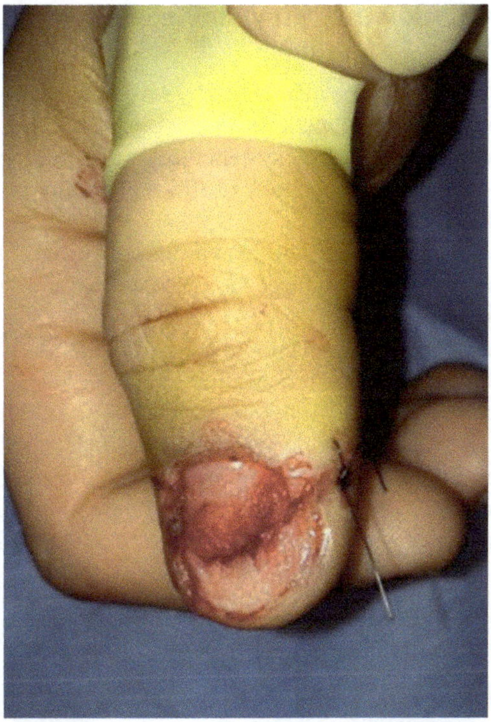

Fig. B.41 Nailbed laceration repair

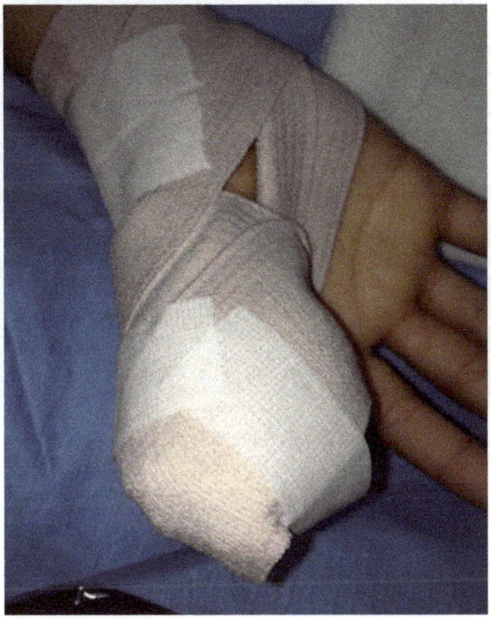

Fig. B.42 Soft dressing

Compartment Check with "Stryker Needle"

- Compartment syndrome can be manifested by several findings (see *Compartment Syndrome* section for more details).
- The conventional "Stryker Needle" system is described here; please follow package instructions for any modifications of this technology or of other compartment pressure monitoring devices.
- Superficial injection of local anesthesia at proposed site of entry.
- After turning the device on, connect the prefilled syringe with the diaphragm unit, and attach unit to needle.
- Insert the setup into the device chamber and secure closed.
- Remove air from system before proceeding.
- "Zero" the device to recalibrate it before using.
- Advance needle into desired compartment, inject 0.3 cc saline from prefilled syringe and determine pressure reading from screen. Needle should be inserted perpendicular to skin entry site, and should remain parallel to the floor. Adjustments in angle of entry can affect the device output. (Fig. B.43).

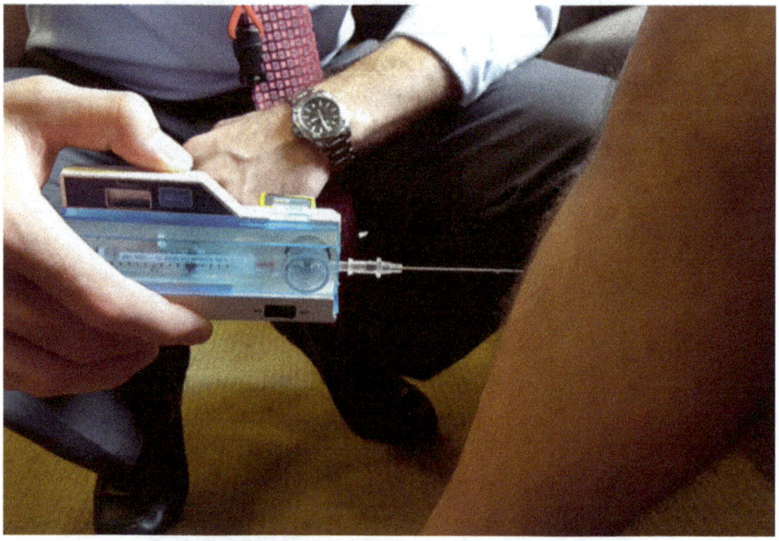

Fig. B.43 Anterior compartment measuring of leg

Gardner Wells Tongs Traction

- Gardner Wells Tongs application is a clean but not sterile procedure. They are used to apply traction force to the skull, which can enable reduction of dislocated facets.
- Assemble the tongs; make sure the pins are connected at both ends with washers and between them is a central hook which attaches to the traction weights.
- Clean the sites of interest above the ears with Betadine solution.
- Place Surgilube on the pins (or can place at the pin insertion sites).
- Place pins on skin above both ears, 1 cm above edge of the pinna and in line with the external auditory meatus. Preferably place pins slightly posterior than slightly anterior (risk of penetrating temporalis muscle, superficial temporal artery and vein) (Fig. B.44).
- Turn pins symmetrically on both sides—ensure that pin sites have remained in place on the skin.
- Pay careful attention to the indicator; stop tightening once pin is slightly palpable (about 1 mm) above the surface of the indicator base.

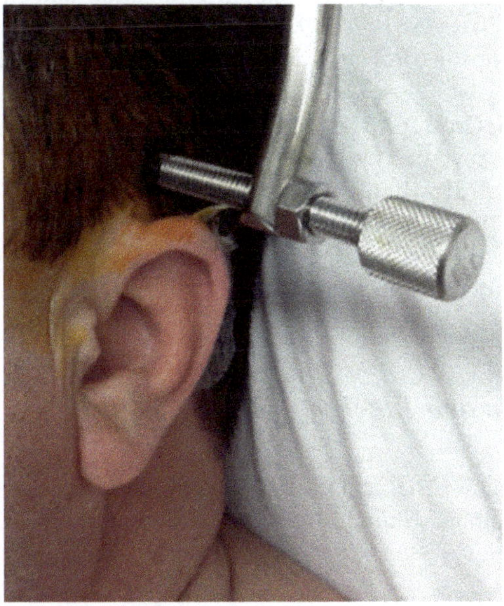

Fig. B.44 Gardner Wells Traction

References

Casting and Splinting

Bucholz RW, Court-Brown CM, Heckman JD, Tornetta P. Rockwood and Green's Fractures in adults. 7th ed. Philadelphia: Lippincott William & Wilkins; 2010.

Charnley J. The closed treatment of common fractures. London: Greenwich Medial Media Limited; 1999.

Miller MD, Thompson SR, Hart J. Review of Orthopaedics. 6th ed. Philadelphia: Elsevier; 2012.

Reductions

Bucholz RW, Court-Brown CM, Heckman JD, Tornetta P. Rockwood and Green's Fractures in Adults. 7th ed. Philadelphia: Lippincott William & Wilkins; 2010.

Cohen MA, Hastings H. Acute Elbow Dislocation: Evaluation and Management. J Am Acad Orthop Surg. 1998;6:15–23.

Foulk DM, Mullis BH. Hip Dislocation: Evaluation and Management. J Am Acad Orthop Surg. 2010;18: 199–209.

Miller MD, Thompson SR, Hart J. Review of Orthopaedics. 6th ed. Philadelphia: Elsevier; 2012.

Rihn JA, Cha PS, Groff YJ, Harner CD. The acutely dislocated knee: evaluation and management. J Am Acad Orthop Surg. 2004;12:334–46.

Saltzman C, Marsh JL. Hindfoot Dislocations: When are they not benign? J Am Acad Orthop Surg. 1997;5:192–8.

Youm T, Takemoto R, Park BK. Acute Management of shoulder dislocations. J Am Acad Orthop Surg 2014;22: 761–71.

Local Anesthesia and Blocks

Wolfe SW, Pederson WC, Hotchkiss RN, Kozin SH. Green's Operative hand surgery. 6th ed. Philadelphia: Churchill Livingstone, Elsevier, Inc.; 2011.

Injections and Aspirations

Bucholz RW, Court-Brown CM, Heckman JD, Tornetta P. Rockwood and Green's Fractures in adults. 7th ed. Philadelphia: Lippincott William & Wilkins; 2010.

Wolfe SW, Pederson WC, Hotchkiss RN, Kozin SH. Green's Operative hand surgery. 6th ed. Philadelphia: Churchill Livingstone, Elsevier, Inc.; 2011.

Saline Load Testing

Bariteau JT, Blankenhorn BD, Digiovanni CW. Evaluation of saline load test for simulated traumatic arthrotomies of the ankle. Injury. 2013; 44(11):1498–501.

Feathers T1, Stinner D, Kirk K, Kirby J, Hsu JR. Effectiveness of the saline load test in diagnosis of traumatic elbow arthrotomies. J Trauma. 2011; 71(5):E110–3.

Konda SR1, Howard D, Davidovitch RI, Egol KA. The saline load test of the knee redefined: a test to detect traumatic arthrotomies and rule out periarticular wounds not requiring surgical intervention. J Orthop Trauma. 2013; 27(9):491–7.

Konda SR, Davidovitch RI, Egol KA. Computed tomography scan to detect traumatic arthrotomies and identify periarticular wounds not requiring surgical intervention: an improvement over the saline load test. J Orthop Trauma. 2013;27(9): 498–504.

Nord RM, Quach T, Walsh M, Pereira D, Tejwani NC. Detection of traumatic arthrotomy of the knee using the saline solution load test. J Bone Joint Surg Am. 2009; 91(1):66–70.

Slikker W, Frank R, Bayne C, Al-Shihabi L, Fernandez J, Wysocki R, Cohen M. Detection of traumatic arthrotomy of the wrist using the saline load test. Poster presented at 2015 American Association of Hand Surgery Annual Meeting; 21–24 Jan 2015, Paradise Island, Bahamas.

Index

A

Abnormal gait, 469
Acetabular fractures
  acetabulum, 246
  associated types, 246
  CT, 266
  elementary types, 246
  high energy in younger patients, 245
  imaging
    AP pelvis, 245
    CT, 245
    obturator and iliac oblique, 245
  Letournel classification, 246
  low energy elderly patients, 245
  physical exam, 245
  posterior wall, 247
  transverse/posterior wall, 248
  treatment
    closed hip reduction, 249
    hip reduction technique, 249
    nonoperative, 249
    open reduction and internal fixation, 249
Achilles tendon rupture
  clinical, 332
  history, 331
  MRI, 332
  partial/complete, 333
  physical exam, 331–332
  sports injuries, 331
  Thompson test, 331
  treatment plan
    controversial, 333
    nonoperative, 333
    operative, 333
    surgical repair, 333
  ultrasound, 332
  XR ankle and foot, 332
Acromioclavicular (AC) joint injury, 123, 124, 126, 131
Acute/chronic injuries, 293, 294
Acute on chronic slip, 471
Allman classification, 118, 120
Amputation, 234–235
  eponychium, 234
  revision (*see* Revision amputation)
Angiography/embolization, 32
Ankle fracture, 336–338, 340, 342–344, 424
  anatomic/descriptive, 336
  external rotation stress, 336
  fibular shortening, 336
  history, 335
  knee exam, 335
  Lauge-Hansen classification
    PER injury, 340
    SER2 injury, 343
    SER4 fracture-dislocation, 344
    SER4 injury, 343
    supination-adduction injury, 342
  low- and high-energy injuries, 335
  pediatric (*see* Pediatric ankle fractures)
  positive stress test, 338
  rotational/axial load injury, 335
  skin exam, 335
  supination external rotation, 336
  treatment
    nonoperative, 336–337
    operative, 337–338
    reduction and immobilization, 338
  XR, 336

M.C. Makhni et al. (eds.), *Orthopedic Emergencies*,
DOI 10.1007/978-3-319-31524-9

Ankylosing spondylitis (AS). *See* Diffuse idiopathic skeletal hyperostosis (DISH)
Anterior cruciate ligament (ACL), 485
  insertion, 487
  rupture
    history, 251
    MRI, 252
    physical exam, 251
  treatment
    initial ED, 252
    nonoperative, 252
    operative, 252
  X-rays, 252
Anterior dislocations, 128
Antero-inferior shoulder dislocation, 105
Anterior posterior compression (APC), 301, 308
Apex anterior angulation, 414
Apophyseal fractures, 457
Arrhythmia, 511
Arthrocentesis, 22
ASIA Impairment Scale, 39
Asthma
  allergies, 513
  clinical manifestations, 513
  diagnosis on sideline, 513
  treatment, 513
Atlanto-axial fractures
  classification, 50–51
  history, 49
  imaging, 50
  physical exam, 49
  surgical indications, 52
  surgical options, 52
  treatment plan, 51–52
Atlanto-dens interval (ADI), 50
ATLS protocol, 32
AVOID friction massage, 515
Avulsion fractures, 75, 454, 465, 466
  injury, 194
  pelvis
    apophyseal fractures, 457
    diagnosis, 458
  treatment, 458–459
Bacteremia, 21
Balance testing, 505
Base of dens, 54
Bauman's angle, 414
Bennett's fracture, 224
Bicortical extraphyseal fractures, 479
Bilateral humerus fractures, 142
Bite wounds, 241
Body of axis, 54
Bone graft epiphysiodesis, 471
Broad-spectrum antibiotics, 29
Brown-Sequard syndrome, 38
Buck's traction, 455
Bulbocavernosus reflex, 42
Bullet/shot injury, 33
Burst fracture
  diagnosis, 79–80
  thoracolumbar region, 79
  treatment, 80–81

C
Calcaneus fracture
  axial load on heel, 347
  contralateral, 347
  CT, 348
  Essex-Lopresti injuries, 348
  non-operative treatment, 348
  operative treatment, 348
  physical exam, 347
  Sanders classification, 348
  short leg splint, 348
  tuberosity fragment, 348
  vertebral injuries, 347
  X-rays, 347
Capitate fracture, 196–197
Carpal fracture
  capitate, 196–197
  hamate, 197
  hand and neurovascular exam, 194
  lunate, 198
  pisiform, 198
  scaphoid, 193
  trapezium, 196
  trapezoid, 199
  triquetrum, 194–195
Casting and immobilization, 389
Cauda equina syndrome
  diagnostic imaging, 42
  history, 41
  non-operative treatment, 42
  physical exam, 42
  rectal examination, 42
  timing of surgery, 42
Cellulitis, 240
Central cord syndrome, 38
  imaging, 62
  management
    non-operative, 62
    operative, 62–63
  spondylosis and osteophytes, 61
  stenosis/OPLL, 61

Chance fracture
  diagnosis, 84
  flexion-distraction injury, 83
  PLC, 83
  treatment, 84–85
Child abuse-non-accidental trauma (NAT), 393–395
Chronic slip, 471
Clavicle fracture
  Allman classification, 118
  displaced midshaft fracture, 119–121
  MSK injuries, 117
  ORIF, 121
  pediatrics
    birth history, 481
    chest X-rays, 402
    classification, 402
    CT scan, 402
    difficulty breathing or swallowing, 483
    imaging, 402
    nonoperative treatment, 403
    pain, 481
    physical examination, 401
    shoulder X-rays, 402
Comminuted fracture, 487
Compartment syndrome
  diagnosis, 16
  fascial compartment pressures, 15
  fasciotomies, 15
  ischemic injury, 15
  sensory changes (paresthesias), 15
  treatment, 16
  vascular changes (decreased pulses), 15
Complete physical exam, 3
Compression fracture, 73
  classification, 73
  imaging, 72–73
  neurologic deficits, 71
  treatment
    non operative, 73
    surgery, 73
Concussion
  clinical diagnosis and evaluation, 505
  return to play (RTP) guidelines, 505
  symptoms, 505
Coracoid fracture, 124
Cord compression, 56
Coronal split fracture, 326
Coronoid fracture
  classification, 158
  diagnosis, 158
  osteology, 157
  physical exam, 157–158
  treatment, 158
Cramps, 507
CRPP, 497
Crystalline arthropathy, 22
C-spine imaging, 4, 7

D

Damage control orthopedics (DCO)
  end-organ hypoperfusion, 11
  indications, 12
  monitoring, 11
  polytrauma patients, 11
Danis-Weber classification, 336
Deep space infection, 241
Delbet classification, 474
Dens fractures, 51
  history, 53
  imaging, 53–54
  physical examination, 53
Diffuse idiopathic skeletal hyperostosis (DISH)
  anterolateral ossification, 45
  imaging, 47
  ligaments and tissues fracture, 45, 46
  treatment
    non-operative, 47
    surgery, 47–48
Digit amputations
  analgesia, 233
  fingertip amputations, 231
  hemostasis, 233
  imaging/hand X-rays, 233
  re epithelialization and wound contracture, 234
  revision amputation, 234–235
  soft tissue, 234
Digit UCL sprain, 223
Discrete fracture, 415
Displaced fractures, 115, 416
Displaced with no bony contact, 487
Distal femur fracture, 266
  associated injuries, 253
  classification
    AO classification, 254
    descriptive based, 254
    location and articular involvement, 254
    pattern, 254
    shortening and translation, 254
    skin integrity, 254
  complex intra-articular extension, 254
  full trauma examination, 253
  imaging, 253–254
  neurovascular exam, skeletal traction, 253
  saline load of knee technique, 253

Distal femur fracture (*cont.*)
simple intra-articular extension, 254
treatment plan
AO pillars, 255
articular involvement and displacement, 254
fixation of articular fragments, 255
nonoperative, 255
open reduction internal fixation, 255
typical bimodal distribution, 253
Distal humerus fractures
bimodal incidence, 145
classification, 146–148
CT, 146
diagnosis, 146–148
injury mechanism, 145
operative, 148–149
physical exam, 146
treatment plan, 148–149
Distal neurovascular exam, 454, 470
Distal radioulnar joint (DRUJ) injury
Essex-Lopresti injuries, 190
Galeazzi fracture, 190
radial shaft fracture, 189
shuck test, 189
soft tissue structures, 189
treatment, 191
Distal radius fracture
AP view, 132, 184
lateral view, 184, 185
non operative management, 131
plate fixation, 187
sugar tong splint, 131, 186
pediatrics
apex dorsal angulation, 445
apex volar angulation, 478
bicortical extraphyseal fractures, 479
buckle fracture, 478
CT, 477
history, 477
nonoperative treatment, 479
outstretched hand, 477
physical exam, 477
Salter-Harris classification, 479
surgery, 478
torus fracture, 479
wrist X-rays, 477
Distal ulna fracture, 128
Dorsal cortical fracture. *See* Avulsion injury
Dorsal PIP fracture dislocation, 227

E
Elbow capitellar fracture
arthroplasty, 175
classification, 174, 175
double bubble sign, 174
fragment excision, 175
motion and function, 173
treatment, 174–175
Elbow dislocation, 166
classification, 112
diagnosis, 112
history, 111–112
imaging, 112–115
operative treatment, 115
physical exam, 112
posterolateral, 111
treatment, 115
Encephalopathy, 509
Endocrine disorder, 472
Epiphyseal fragment, 398
Epiphysiolysis, 470
Epiphysis, 397
Epstein classification, 466
Exercise-associated hyponatremia (EAH)
clinical manifestations, 509
general diagnosis, 509
mild/moderate, 509
overdrinking hypotonic solutions, 509
severe, 509
symptoms, 509
treatment, 509
Extensor tendon zones, 215–216
Extra-articular fracture, 413

F
Fasciotomy/radical debridement, 26
Felon, 241
Femoral head fractures, 265
AP and lateral hip XRs, 257
CT, 257
full trauma examination, 257
high energy injury, 257
LE neuro exam, 257
Pipkin classification, 258
treatment
immediate treatment, 258
nonoperative, 258
operative, 258
Femoral neck fractures
diagnosis
garden classification, 285

imaging, 284
Pauwels classification, 284
osteoporotic patients, 283
treatment
non operative, 286
operative, 286
Femoral shaft fracture
balanced skeletal traction, 262
classification
AO, 261
descriptive based on, 260
skin integrity, 260
distal neurovascular exam, 259
full trauma examination, 259
history, 259
imaging
CT, neck, 260
intraoperative fluoroscopy, 260
ipsilateral femoral neck fracture, 259
ipsilateral knee films, 259
pre-operative, 260
limb shortening, 260
oblique, 261
pulmonary status, 260
transverse, 261
treatment plan
operative stabilization, 261
skeletal traction, 262
tibial traction, 262
traction technique guide, 262
Femur fracture
classification, 479
falls from climbing, 477
femoral shaft fracture, 259–262, 478
higher energy mechanisms, 477
history, 477
neurologic/pathologic bone conditions, 477
non-operative treatment, 479
osteogenesis imperfecta, 478
physical examination, 479
pre-op planning, 479
skeletal survey, 479
surgery, 480
XRs, 479
Finger fractures and dislocations
fifth MC, 224
malrotation, 222
mechanism and timing of injury, 222
metacarpal, 221
neurovascular exam, 222
open/contaminated injury, 222
phalanx, 222
pin stabilization, multiple metacarpal fractures, 225
splinting, 228
treatment plan, 222–227
visual inspection, 222
X-rays, 222
Finger, tendon lacerations, 215
Flexor tendon, zones, 215
Flexor tenosynovitis, 242
Foot injuries, 359. *See also* Metatarsal fractures
Foreign bodies, hand and wrist
history, 237
imaging, 238
physical exam, 237
surgical and nonoperative treatment, 238
Fracture, 233
classifications, 131
distal radius (*see* Distal radius fractures)
extensive soft tissue injury, 186
Galeazzi, 190
radial shaft, 189
Fracture reduction with suture/screw fixation, 487
Frostbite, 515
Frostnip, 515
Full trauma survey, 454

G

Galeazzi fracture, 190, 451, . *See also* Pediatric galeazzi fracture
Garden classification, 285
Gartland type I/II fractures, 416
Glenohumeral dislocation, 103–109
antero-inferior, 101
classification, 103–104
closed reduction
anterior, 104–109
luxatio-erecta, 107
posterior, 106
CT, 103
history, 102
inspection, 102
MRI, 103
neurovascular examination, 102
post reduction, 109
posterior, 101, 102
axillary, 107
lightbulb sign, 106
post-reduction, 102, 108
range of motion, 102
separation, glenohumeral joint, 101

Glenohumeral dislocation (*cont.*)
- and subluxation, 101
- XR imaging
  - axillary/Velpeau axillary, 103
  - grashey, 103
  - orthogonal, 103
  - scapular-Y, 103
  - stryker notch, 103
  - west point axillary, 103

Glenohumeral joint, 131
Glenoid and scapula fracture
- associated injuries, 133
- CT, 134
- floating shoulder, 135
- high-energy injury, 133
- history, 133
- non-operative treatment, 135
- physical exam, 134
- surgical treatment, 136
- X-rays, 134

Grauer classification, 54
Gunshot wound, 33, 34

H

Hamate fracture, 197
Hand infections, 131, 190, 193, 198, 215, 231, 233, 234, 237
- foreign bodies (*see* Foreign bodies, hand and wrist)
- history, 239
- *Pasteurella multocida*, 239
- physical exam, 240
- *Staphylococcus aureus*, 239
- tendon lacerations (*see* Tendon lacerations)
- treatment plan, 240–242
- XRY, 240

Hawkins classification system, 372, 373
Heat illness, 507
Heat stroke, 507
Hemiarthroplasty (HA), 115
Hemodynamically unstable pelvis fracture
- diagnosis, 32
- intra-pelvic bleeding, 31
- pelvic ring injury, 31
- treatment, 32

High-pressure injection injury
- clinical appearance, 27, 28
- diagnosis, 29
- radiographic appearance, 27, 28
- soft-tissue injury, 27
- treatment, 29

Hip aspiration, ultrasound guided, 463
Hip dislocation (native)
- anterior, 266
- classification, 266
- CT, 266
- dashboard injury, 265
- MRI, 266
- physical exam, 265
- skeletal traction technique, 266
- treatment
  - nonoperative, 266
  - operative, 267
  - planning, 266

Hip reduction technique, 258
Humeral shaft fractures, 414, 474
Humerus shaft fractures
- classification, 138
- diagnosis, 138
- history, 137
- physical exam, 137
- surgical, 141–142
- treatment plan, 139–142

I

Impending fractures
- classification, 274
- diagnosis, 273–274
- history, 273
- physical exam, 273
- treatment plan, 274

Initial cervical spine management, 4
- C-spine clearance
  - asymptomatic, 7
  - symptomatic, 8
- pathology, 7
- types, cervical collars, 8

Initial trauma assessment
- airway management, 4
- CT c-spine, 4
- neck manipulation, 4
- pelvic sheet/binder, 5
- primary survey, 3
- secondary survey, 3, 4
- sonography, 4

Interosseous membrane, 189
Intertrochanteric/subtrochanteric fracture
- classification, 279
- diagnosis, 277–279
- history, 277
- non-operative, 280
- operative treatment, 280
- treatment plan, 280

Ipsilateral injury, 185

J
Jones fracture (proximal fifth metatarsal)
  alternate classifications, 352
  athlete, 351
  CT/MRI foot, 352
  foot, 351
  injury zones, 351
  Lawrence and Botte classification, 352
  mechanism, 351
  midfoot, 351
  pain, 351
  physical exam, 351–352
  treatment
    operative treatment, 353
    zone of injury, 353
  XR foot, 352
  zone 1-3 fractures, 351, 353

K
Klein's line, 470
Knee dislocation
  high-energy injury, 289, 290
  Schenck classification, 290
  vascular surgery, 291
Kocher criteria, 22
Kyphoplasty, 73

L
Lateral compression (LC), 300
Lateral condyle fracture, 414, 497
  arthrography, 420
  elbow, 419
  history, 419
  Jakob et al. classification, 421
  Milch classification, 420
  MRI/ultrasound, 420
  nonoperative treatment, 422
  physical exam, 419
  surgery, 422
Ligamentous injury, 185
Limb length discrepancy, 469
Lisfranc injury
  boney, 357
  classification, 356
  CT scan, 356
  ED management, 357
  Fleck sign, 356
  history, 355
  hyperplantar-flexed foot, 355
  ligament complex, 355
  ligamentous, 356
  MRI, 356
  multiple TMT dislocations, 357
  non-operative, 358
  operative, 358
  physical examination, 355
  tarsometatarsal fracture-dislocation, 355
Log roll test, 461
Low/high velocity wounds, 34
Lunate, 198
Lyme disease, serologic evaluation, 462

M
Medial epicondyle fracture
  CT scan, 424
  elbow dislocation, 423
  elbow X-rays, 424
  history, 423
  minimally displaced, 424
  multiple classification systems, 425
  nonoperative treatment, 425
  physical exam, 423
  surgery, 425
  X-rays,contralateral elbow, 424
Meniscus tear
  acute/chronic injuries, 293
  ED treatment, 294
Metacarpal fractures, 221, 225
Metatarsal fractures
  classification, 360
  crush injury, 359
  fifth, 359
  history, 359
  imaging, 360
  operative and non-operative
      treatment, 360
  physical exam, 359
Midazolam, 507
Midfoot pain, 361
Milch classification, 146
Mild frostbite, 515
Monteggia fracture, pediatrics
  history, 447
  physical exam, 447
  proximal ulna fracture, 447
  radial head dislocation, 447
  treatment
    nonoperative, 448
    operative, 448
  XR elbow, 447
  XR forearm and wrist, 448
Myelopathy, 52
Myoclonic jerks, 511

N
Necrotizing fasciitis
  diagnosis, 26
  polymicrobial soft-tissue infection, 25
  rapidly progressive soft-tissue infection, 25
  treatment, 26
Neer and Horowitz classification, 466
Neurovascular exam, 462

O
Obese boys, 472
Olecranon fracture, 111–115, 157
  classification, 112, 152–153
  diagnosis, 112
  fracture pattern, 151
  history, 151
  imaging, 152
  physical exam, 151
  surgical, 154
  treatment, 153–154
Open fracture
  diagnosis, 18
  soft-tissue injuries, 17
  treatment, 19
Open wound, 437
Oral hypertonic fluids, 509
ORIF, 121, 301, 497–500
Osteochondral fracture, 303
Osteogenesis imperfecta femur fracture, 478

P
Paronychia, 240–241
Patella dislocation
  acute trauma, 303
  classification, 304
  full ligamentous knee exam, 303
  history, 303
  lateral, 303
  moving patellar apprehension test, 304
  MRI, 304
  osteochondral fracture, 303
  recurrent, 303
  subluxation with knee in extension, 304
  treatment plan
    acute injuries, 304
    non-operative, 305
    operative, 305
    pain reduction, 304
  XR knee, 304
Patella fracture
  intra-articular lidocaine injection, 299
  ORIF, 301
  transverse, 300
  vertical, 300, 301
Patellar tendon rupture, 295, 296
Pauwels classification, 284
Peak flow meter, 513
Pediatric ankle fractures, 497–500
  physeal closure, 497
  Salter-Harris I/II, distal fibula/tibia, 497
  SH2 distal tibia, 498
  tillaux (*see* Tillaux fracture)
  triplane (*see* Triplane fracture)
Pediatric distal radius fracture, 458
Pediatric forearm fracture
  clinical, 438
  Greenstick fracture, 439
  history, 431
  incomplete/Greenstick classification, 438
  nonoperative treatment, 438
  physical exam, 432
  pre- and post-reduction, 440
  radius and ulna shaft, 431
  surgery, 440–441
  X-rays, 437
Pediatric galeazzi fracture
  contralateral wrist, 452
  distal radioulnar joint, 451
  history, 451
  non-accidental trauma, 452
  nonoperative treatment, 452
  physical exam, 451
  surgery, 452
  ulna subluxation, 451, 452
  wrist X-rays, 452
Pediatric hip dislocation
  chronic, 466
  closed reduction, 466
  Epstein classification, 466
  osteoarthritis and nerve injury, 465
  osteonecrosis and coxa
    magna, 465
  post reduction, 466, 467
  Thompson classification, 466
Pediatric hip fracture
  Delbet classification, 474
  displaced fractures, 476
  hip spica cast, 475
  osteonecrosis, 474
  right hip fracture, 474
Pediatric pelvic fracture, 453
  classification, 454
  diagnosis, 454
  history, 453
  indications, 455
  physical exam, 454

surgery, 455
treatment, 455
Pelvic binder/wrapping, 32
Pelvic ring injuries
APC, 301, 308
LC, 309
VS, 309
WBAT, 310
Young–Burgess system, 300
Percutaneous pinning vs. open reduction internal fixation, 492
Perilunate dislocation
associated neurovascular complaints, 209
carpal instability complex categories, 211
CT/MRI, 210
hand X-rays, 210–211
high-energy trauma, wrist, 209
injury mechanism, 209
lunate, 210
Mayfield classification, 211
nonoperative treatment, 211
physical exam, 209
pin stabilization, 212
surgical treatment, 211–213
traction radiograph, 210
Periprosthetic hip fracture
trochanter fractures, 303
Vancouver classification, 303, 304
Periprosthetic knee femur fracture
classification systems, 316
history, 315
imaging, 315–316
operative, 316
physical exam, 315
treatment plan, 316
Phalanx fractures, 221–222, 379–381
Phalanx, tendon lacerations, 215, 218
Physeal fractures, 479
PIP fracture dislocation
dorsal, 227
simple, 226
volar, 229
Pisiform, 198
Posterior atlanto-dens interval (PADI), 50
Posterior ligamentous complex (PLC), 66, 83–85
Pre-slip, 470
Proximal humerus fracture, 405
classification, 466
CRPP vs. ORIF, 466
Velpeau bandages, 466
Proximal phalanx fractures, 221, 226
Proximal radioulnar joint (PRUJ), 189
Proximal ulnar fracture, 128

R
Radial head fracture
aspiration/injection, 158
elbow XR, 158
history, 157
intra-operative, 160
isolated/with associated injuries, 157
Mason classification, 158
minimally displaced, 159
non-operative treatment, 160
physical exam, 158
replacement, 161
surgical treatment, 160–161
XR forearm, 158
Radial head subluxation, 431, 432
Radial neck fracture
classification, 434
long arm cast, 434
percutaneous reduction *vs*. retrograde nailing, 434
pronation/supination, 433
Radius and ulna shaft fractures
description, 127
diagnosis, 128
physical exam, 127–128
treatment plan, 128–129
Rapidly progressive soft-tissue infection, 25
Reduced shoulder, 108
Return to play (RTP) guidelines, 505
Reverse total shoulder arthroplasty (RSA), 115
Revision amputation, 234–235

S
Sacral fractures
Denis classification, 92, 93
diagnosis, 92–93
pelvic ring injuries, 91
treatment, 93–94
Saline load test, 24
Salter Harris I/II fracture, 483
Salter–Harris classification
radiographs, 397
type I, 398, 399
type II, 398
type III, 398, 399
type IV, 398, 399
type V, 399
Scaphoid fracture, 193, 197, 201, 203–204
advanced imaging, 202
carpal bone, 201
classification systems, 203
CT, 202
FOOSH mechanism, 201

Scaphoid fracture (*cont.*)
missed/chronic, 201
MRI, 202
nonoperative treatment, 203
screw fixation, 204
surgical treatment, 203–204
tenderness
Snuffbox, 201
volar scaphoid tuberosity, 201
wrist X-rays, 202
Scapho-lunate advanced collapse (SLAC)
Scapho-lunate instability
acute symptoms, 205
carpal, 205
gapping, scaphoid and lunate, 206
nonoperative treatment
indications, 206
short arm vs. thumb spica cast, 206
swelling, 206
outstretched hand, 205
physical exam, 206
SLAC, 205
structures, 205
subjective, 205
surgical treatment
chronic injury, 207
indication, 207
screw stabilization, acute S-L injury, 208
Watson stages, 206
wrist X-rays, 206
Scapula fracture. *See* Glenoid and scapula fracture
SCAT-3 tool, 505
SCFE severity grading, 471
Schenck classification, 290
Sedation, pediatric patient
agent, 386, 459
bier block, 458
digital block, 457
fracture reduction, 458–459
hematoma block, 457
non-pharmacologic agents, 457
principles, 457
Seizures, 509
Septic arthritis
Kocher criteria, 462–463
shoulder, 131, 132
Septic hip vs. transient synovitis
diagnosis, 462–463
history, 461
physical exam, 461–462
treatment plan, 463
Septic joint
bacteremia, 21
bacteria and inflammatory response, 21
diagnosis, 22
synovial joint, 21
treatment, 22
Serum inflammatory markers, 22
Severe frostbite, 515
Short leg walking cast, 337
Simple PIP dorsal dislocation, 226
Single-bone fractures, 453
Skeletal maturity, 397
Sleep disturbances, 505
SLIC. *See* Subaxial injury classification (SLIC)
Slipped capital femoral epiphysis
acute slip, 470, 471
chronic slip, 471
Lorder classification, 471
MRI, 470
SCFE classification, 470–471
Southwick Angle classification, 471
history, 469
physical exam, 469–470
pre-slip, 470
SCFE severity grading, 471
treatment, 471–472
Snowboarder's fracture, 375
Soft-tissue reconstruction, 327
Spinal cord injury (SCI)
classification, 38–39
history, 37
imaging, 38
physical exam, 37–38
treatment, 39
Spinous process fracture, 76
Sports, ACL rupture, 251
Sternoclavicular (SC) joint injury, 127
diagnosis, 128
history, 127
physical exam, 127–128
treatment, 128–129
Subaxial (C3–C7) cervical spine fractures
diagnosis, 58
posterior ligamentous complex, 57
treatment, 58–59
Subaxial injury classification (SLIC), 57, 58
Sudden cardiac arrest (SCA), 511
Supracondylar humerus fracture (SCHFx)
flexion type, 414
history, 413
modified gartland classification, 415–416
physical exam, 413–414
radiographs, 414
T1, 415
T4, 416
treatment plan, 416

Surgery
  distal radius fracture, pediatrics, 480
  femur fracture, pediatrics, 480
  pediatric ankle fractures, 500
  pediatric forearm fracture, 440–441
  triplane fracture, 501
Suture/screw fixation, 487

T
Talar neck fractures, 371–373
Talus fracture, 371, 372, 375–377
Tarsal navicular fracture
  acute mechanisms, injury, 361
  chronic, 361
  CT, 362
  foot XR, 362
  nonoperative treatment, 362
  operative treatment, 362
  pain, 361
  physical exam, 361
  Sangeorzan classification, 362
Tendon lacerations
  associated neurovascular complaints, 216
  bony mallet
    after pin removal, 219
    injury, distal phalanx, 218
    pin fixation, 218
  detailed neurovascular examination, 216
  diagnosis, 216
  extensor tendon, 217
  injury mechanism, 216
  nonoperative treatment, 216
  open wound debridement, 216
  surgical treatment, 219
  tetanus and immunization record, 216
  timing/chronicity of injury, 216
Tetanus prophylaxis, 19
TFCC. *See* Triangular fibrocartilage complex (TFCC)
Thawing, 515
Thompson classification, 466
Thoracolumbar fractures
  classification, 66–67
  diagnosis, 65–68
  dislocation, 87, 88
  history, 65
  nonoperative management, 68
  physical exam, 65
  treatment plan, 69
Thumb UCL injury, 224
Thurston Holland fragment, 398
Tibial eminence fracture
  imaging, 486–487
  history, 485
  Mayers and McKeever classification, 486–487
  physical exam, 485
  treatment, 487
Tibial plafond (pilon) fracture, 365, 366
Tibial plateau fracture
  classification, 326
  diagnosis, 326
  history, 325
  physical exam, 325
  treatment plan, 327
Tibial shaft fracture
  clinical appearance, 319, 320
  complex, 321, 322
  spiral, 321
  transverse, 321, 322
  treatment, 321–323
  Tscherne classification, 321
Tibial spine, 486
Tibial tubercle fracture
  classification, 490
  history, 489
  imaging, 490–492
  overview, 489
  physical exam, 489–490
  surgery, 492
  treatment, 492
  types, 490
  Watson–Jones (with Ogden modification), 490–492
Tibial tuberosity fractures, 491
Tillaux fracture
  avulsion, AITFL, 497
  CT scan, 498, 499
  external rotation force, 497
  injury mechanism, 498
  non-operative treatment, 499
  physical exam, 498
  SHIII fracture, 498
  surgery, 500
  tender, 498
  XR, 499
Tip of dens, 54
Toddler's fracture
  diagnosis, 494–495
  history, 493
  physical exam, 493
  treatment plan, 495
Torus fracture, 479
Total hip arthroplasty (THA), 265, 266
Transphyseal plane of injury, 398
Transverse ligament injuries, 50–51

Transverse process fractures
  cervical spine, 75
  imaging, 76
  treatment, 76–77
Trapezium fracture, 196
Trapezoid fracture, 199
Trauma management, 3, 7
Traumatic arthrotomy
  diagnosis, 24
  laceration, 23
  sterile intra-articular, 23
  treatment, 24
Trendelenburg gait, 469
Triangular fibrocartilage complex (TFCC), 189
Triplane fracture
  complex pattern, 500
  CT, 501
  diagnosis, 500
  nonoperative treatment, 500
  physical exam, 500
  posterior distal tibial metaphysis, 500
  surgery, 501
  XR, 501
Triquetral body fracture, 194, 195
Triquetrum fracture
  dorsal cortical fracture (avulsion injury), 194, 195
  triquetral body fracture, 194, 195
  volar avulsion fracture, 194, 195
Trochanter fracture, 303
Type 2 dens fracture, 55
Type 3 dens fracture, 55

U
Unilateral lateral pillar fracture, 58

V
Vancouver classification, 303, 304
Varus/valgus stress test, 158
Vertebral osteomyelitis, 95, 96
Vertebroplasty, 73
Vertical shear (VS), 309
Volar avulsion fracture, 194, 195

W
Widening of joint space, 462
Wrist, 132, 190, 194, 198, 201, 215, 233
  scaphoid fracture (*see* Scaphoid fracture)
  tendon lacerations (*see* Tendon lacerations)

Y
Young–Burgess system, 299

Z
Zaricznyj modification, 486–487

Lightning Source UK Ltd.
Milton Keynes UK
UKHW02f1133261018
331253UK00002B/35/P

9 783319 315225